Second Edition

TELEPHONE TRIAGE FOR OBSTETRICS AND GYNECOLOGY

Second Edition

TELEPHONE TRIAGE FOR OBSTETRICS AND GYNECOLOGY

Vicki E. Long, MSN, CNM, RN

Certified Nurse-Midwife and Women's Health Provider
Annapolis OB/GYN Associates, PA
Annapolis, Maryland

Patricia C. McMullen, PhD, JD, WHNP-BC, RN

Associate Provost for Administration
The Catholic University of America
Washington, DC

Wolters Kluwer | Lippincott Williams & Wilkins
Health
Philadelphia · Baltimore · New York · London
Buenos Aires · Hong Kong · Sydney · Tokyo

Acquisitions Editor: Jean Rodenberger
Managing Editor: Helen Kogut
Director of Nursing Production: Helen Ewan
Senior Managing Editor / Production: Erika Kors
Senior Project Manager: Rosanne Hallowell
Design Coordinator: Holly Reid McLaughlin
Manufacturing Coordinator: Karin Duffield
Production Services: ASI Maryland Composition

Second Edition

9 8 7 6 5 4 3 2

Printed in China

Library of Congress Cataloging-in-Publication Data

Telephone triage for obstetrics and gynecology / [edited by] Vicki Long, Patricia McMullen.—2nd ed.
    p. ; cm.
  Includes bibliographical references and index.
  ISBN 978-0-7817-9099-4
 1. Maternity nursing. 2. Gynecology. 3. Triage (Medicine) 4. Telephone in medicine.
5. Nursing assessment. 6. Emergency nursing. I. Long, Vicki E. II. McMullen, Patricia C.
  [DNLM: 1. Gynecology—methods—Nurses' Instruction. 2. Obstetrical Nursing—methods.
3. Nursing Assessment--methods. 4. Telephone—Nurses' Instruction. 5. Triage—methods—Nurses'
Instruction. WY 157 T268 2010]
  RG951.T43 2010
  618.2'0231--dc22

                                                                              2008052434

Dedication

This book is dedicated to the many wonderful nurses and other providers we have worked with over the years. As we have taught them, so do they continue to teach us. Most especially, we would like to note all of the assistance that the late Dr. Felicia Stewart gave to not only us, but to literally thousands of nurses like us. She was truly an unfaltering advocate for excellence in women's health.

"Sometimes even a butterfly must miss being a caterpillar."
—Felecia H. Stewart, MD (1943–2006)

Preface: How to Use This Book

The second edition of *Telephone Triage for Obstetrics and Gynecology* builds on the purpose of the original: it is designed specifically for use by health care personnel advising patients via the telephone on topics related to obstetrics and gynecology. No book, however complete, can be a substitute for experience. However, as you become familiar with the format, you should find that it is an effective educational tool and a focal point for verifying and documenting that the advice being given has been accepted by experts in the respective fields that are covered.

The book is introduced by chapters which outline, in a didactic form, some of the medical/ legal, counseling, and practical aspects of telephone triage. A new addition is a chapter on how to incorporate the internet into this advice. Specific protocols follow on selected ob/gyn topics. Expanded and new protocols include:

- Updated infertility management and medications
- Inclusion of additional contraceptive methods such as NuvaRing and Implanon
- Current abnormal Pap smear management
- Hormone therapy advice
- Emergency contraception options

Protocol sections are arranged alphabetically for quick reference. Areas appropriate for individual practice or clinic situations are noted, taking into account differences of opinion on proper management. Hopefully you will tailor the advice contained in these protocols to your needs.

The protocol format, as with any protocol format, will take practice to be able to use quickly. We encourage you to hold "mock call" scenarios to learn the flow of questions and information presented. Due to the varying educational levels of providers who work in triage situations, some questions may seem more basic than you feel you need to assess the situation. Again, we encourage you to adapt the information to your particular educational level and experience.

Above all, this book is meant to be a "living document." Write in it, alter it, and change it as necessary for your situation. Use it as a springboard to write your own protocols. Heed the warnings and follow the advice. Telephone Triage is a growing field, one that despite the knowledge you carry in your head, demands documentation. The consequences of poor advice can be costly, and at times deadly. Use this book wisely!

Contributors and Reviewers:
First Edition

The second edition of this book exists only because of the excellent efforts of our original contributors and reviewers. They deserve credit for the book's continuance.

CONTRIBUTORS

Vicki Long, MS, CNM, RN

Patricia McMullen, PhD, JD, WHNP-BC, RN

Cynthia Grandjean, PhD, MGA, ANP/GNP-BC, RN

Felicia J. Guest, MPH, CHES

Diane Padden, PhD, FNP-BC, RN

Diane Seibert, PhD, CRNP

Col. Richard Ricciardi AN, USA, PhD, PNP/ANP-BC, FAANP, RN

REVIEWERS

Penelope Morrison Bosarge, MSN,CRNP

Diane B. Boyer, CNM, PhD, FACNM

Karen R, Hammond, MSN, CRNP

Robert A. Hatcher, MD, MPH

Teresa Marchese, CNM, PhD

James Trussell, PhD

Contributors and Reviewers:
Second Edition

CONTRIBUTORS

Cynthia Grandjean, PhD, MGA, CANP/ GNP-BC, RN
Assistant Professor
The Catholic University of America
Washington, DC

Marjorie Graziano, MSN, MPA, FNP-BC, RN
Clinical Assistant Professor
The Catholic University of America
Washington, DC

Felicia J. Guest, MPH, CHES
Director of Training
Southeast AIDS Training and Education
  Center
Emory University School of Medicine
  (SEATEC)
Atlanta, Georgia

Elizabeth Hawkins-Walsh, PhD, PNP-BC, RN
Clinical Associate Professor
The Catholic University of America
Washington, DC

M. Laurie Lemieux, MS, RN, WHNP-BC, RN
Clinical Assistant Professor
The Catholic University of America
Washington, DC

Barbara Moran, PhD, MS, MPH, CNM, FACCE
Assistant Professor
The Catholic University of America
Washington, DC

Alice Myers, MA
Director, Donley Technology Center
School of Nursing
The Catholic University of America
Washington, DC

REVIEWERS

Selected portions of the book have been reviewed by the following experts in their respective fields.

Robert A. Hatcher, MD, MPH
Professor of Gynecology and Obstetrics
Emory University School of Medicine
Atlanta, Georgia
(Selected Systemic Hormonal Contraceptive Protocols)

Gilbert Mottla, MD
Reproductive Endocrinology & Infertility
Shady Grove Fertility Center
Rockville, Maryland
(Infertility Protocol and Infertility Medication List)

James Trussell, PhD
John Foster Dulles Professor in
  International Affairs
Director, Office of Population Research
Professor of Economics and Public Affairs
Princeton University
Princeton, New Jersey
(Emergency Contraception with Plan B and Oral Contraceptives)

Susan Wysocki, RNC, NP
President and CEO of the National
  Association of Nurse Practitioners in
  Women's Health
Washington, DC
(Hormonal Therapy Overview)

Acknowledgments

We would like to thank Chris, Bill, Erin, and Ben for their patience and support. They have given up much family time as we have pursued our dreams.

Contents

Chapter 20: Natural Family Planning Overview

Chapter 21: Pelvic Complaints Overview

Chapter 22: Systemic Hormonal Contraception Overview–Combined Oral Contraceptive Pills, NuvaRing, Ortho Evra, and Progesterone-Only Pills

Guide to Abbreviations Used in This Book

Abbreviation	Term
AFP	Alphafetoprotein
AIDS	Acquired immunodeficiency syndrome
AGUS	Atypical glandular cells of undetermined significance
ASAP	As soon as possible
ASCUS	Atypical squamous cells of undetermined significance
BBT	Break through bleeding
B-HCG	Beta-human chorionic gonadotropin
b.i.d.	Twice daily
BTB	Break through bleeding
BV	Bacterial vaginosis
CF	Cystic fibrosis
COCP	Continuous oral contraceptive pills
CT	Chlamydia trachomatis
Depo	Depo-Provera injectable contraceptive
DMPA	Depot-medroxyprogesterone acetate (Depo-Provera)
DUB	Dysfunctional uterine bleeding
EC	Emergency contraception or endocerivical curratage
ECPs	Emergency contraceptive pills
EMB	Endometrial biopsy
ER	Emergency room
GC	Gonorrhea
HA	Headache
HCG	Human chorionic gonadotropin
HGSIL	High grade intraepithelial lesion
HIV	Human immunodeficiency virus
HMO	Health maintenance organization
HPV	Human papillomavirus
HSV	Herpes simplex virus
IC	Intercourse
IUD	Intrauterine device
IUS	Intrauterine system

Abbreviation	Term
LGSIL	Low grade squamous intraepithelial lesion
LGV	Lymphogranuloma venereum
LMP	Last menstrual period
Mcg	Micrograms
Mg	Milligrams
NFP	Natural family planning
NSAID	Nonsteroidal anti-inflammatory
NST	Non-stress test
OB/GYN	Obstetrics & gynecology
OC	Oral contraceptive
OCPs	Oral contraceptive pills
OTC	Over the counter
PCP	Primary care provider
PIH	Pregnancy induced hypertension
POPs	Progestin-only pill (mini-pill)
PP	Post partum
PPO	Preferred provider option
q.d.	Once daily
R/O	Rule out
ROM	Rupture of membranes
STD	Sexually transmitted disease
STI	Sexually transmitted infection
t.i.d.	Three times daily
URI	Upper respiratory infection
UTI	Urinary tract infection
VAIN	Vulvar intraepithelial lesion
VIN	Vulvar intraepithelial lesion

PART I

TELEPHONE TRIAGE BASICS

CHAPTER I

Telephone Triage in Women's Health Care: Logistical and Legal Considerations

Patricia C. McMullen

The telephone, once used merely as an appointment-scheduling device, now serves a more important role. It has become an integral part of provider–patient interactions throughout the world. Indeed, research indicates that approximately 20%–28% of all primary health care is handled over the telephone. The process of managing health complaints over a telephone line, known as telephone triage, is a double-edged sword. It is an extremely cost-effective tool that is being used increasingly to provide detailed health care advice and treat simple problems, particularly in the current cost-conscious managed care environment. However, practitioners who use telephone triage are disadvantaged because they must rely on the verbal information provided by the patient or other caller, rather than being able to use a number of physical assessment skills.

Contemporary research indicates that without proper protocols and training, telephone triage can result in improper diagnosis and management. Janssen and colleagues (2006) demonstrated that telephone triage can be a valuable tool for evaluating when women who are in labor at term and have had uncomplicated pregnancies should be counseled to come to the hospital. In this study, 731 women were managed by a telephone triage nurse and 728 women received a home visit. Rates of cesarean delivery, use of narcotic or epidural analgesia, and augmentation of labor were comparable between the two groups. However, an earlier study by Rupp et al. (1994) highlighted the importance of adequate triage in women's health settings. These investigators had a

Sample Telephone Triage Form

Patient Name: _____

Date and time of call: _____

Call handled by: _____

Current phone #: _____

Phone # to call if not at above #: _____

Caller: (If not the patient, has patient indicated you may share information with this person?) _____

_____ Patient

_____ Other

Name: _____

Relationship to patient: (Has patient indicated you may share information with this person?) _____

When will patient/caller available for return call: _____

Alternate contact approved by the patient (name and telephone number):

_____

Parity: _____

LMP: _____

Prior LNMP: _____

If pregnant, number of weeks: _____

Any problems during this pregnancy or prior pregnancies?

_____

Disposition:

_____ Teaching re: _____

_____ Office visit: _____

_____ Referred to: _____

_____ Referred to ER: _____

_____ Other: _____

Chief complaint (in caller's own words):

History of present illness:

Date of onset: _____

Symptoms: _____

Treatments used: _____

_____

Aggravating or alleviating factors: _____

_____

Any other medical problems? _____

_____

Past surgeries: _____

Current medications: _____

_____

Allergies/reactions: _____

_____

Physician/CNM/CRNP comments: _____

_____

_____

_____

Prescription called into:

Pharmacy: _____

Pharmacy Telephone No: _____

Called in by: _____

Date/Time: _____

Figure 1-1 Sample Telephone Triage Form

college student pose as a 16-year-old girl and call adolescent clinics nationwide complaining of acute-onset "belly pain." The telephone triage responses of 35 clinics were evaluated. Telephone triage was performed by nurses, receptionists, and a teenage peer advisor. An amazingly high 37% of the 35 clinics gave inadequate telephone advice by failing to rule out a possible ectopic pregnancy.

This chapter provides a brief overview of the history of telephone triage and important factors to consider when providing telephone advice to female patients. A sample triage form for triage personnel and providers is also included (see Fig. 1-1).

THE ORIGIN AND EVOLUTION OF TRIAGE

The word "triage" is of French origin and means to sort, classify, or choose. Triage was first used in medicine to set priorities for mass casualties experienced during World War I. However, it was not until the 1960s that triage techniques became widely used to set priorities for the care of patients presenting to emergency rooms for treatment.

Today, telephone triage is used in virtually every clinical setting. For example, Marklund and co-investigators (2007) assessed a telephone nurse triage system in terms of the appropriateness of referrals to the correct level of care as well as the patients' compliance with the advice that was given. Cost was also considered. A total of 362 calls were evaluated. These investigators found that the nurses provided appropriate advice 97.6% of the time. Further, study findings indicated that the telephone triage system was cost effective. Research by Giesen (2007) also considered the safety of telephone triage advice given by nurses. Triage nurses were presented with 352 triage scenarios. The nurses assigned the adequate level of urgency 69% of the time and underestimated the level of urgency in 19% of the contacts. Not surprisingly, there was a significant relationship between the nurse's training on the use of telephone triage guidelines and the correct estimation of urgency. Other research studies (Kempe et al., 2006; Marklund et al., 2007; McNeil, 2007; Van Charante et al., 2006) on the safety and effectiveness of telephone triage have produced varying results. Adequate education of those providing the telephone triage appears to be a critical factor.

Smulian and colleagues (2000) studied after-hours telephone calls received by 12 residents and nine private physicians. Calls were classified as women's health or primary care and according to whether the women were pregnant, not pregnant, or in the postpartum period. One hundred ninety-two of the 276 (69.6%) calls that were analyzed were from pregnant women. Twenty (7.2%) calls were related to postpartum concerns, and 45 (24.1%) calls were associated with a primary care complaint. Three triage dispositions were available: evaluate now, office follow-up, or home care. Callers also were asked what they would have done if they had been unable to contact their physician by telephone. Slightly more than one third of the 139 women who were triaged to the office stated they would have presented to the emergency room had they been unable to reach a provider. Of the callers who were pregnant, between 35.1% and 41.9% were told by the residents or private physicians to seek immediate evaluation. Between 10% and 11% of women in the postpartum period were triaged to immediate evaluation.

Common reasons for calling included nausea and vomiting, vaginal bleeding, leg edema, backache, pelvic pain, headache, and questions regarding oral contraceptives or hormone replacement. Symptoms of urinary tract infection, viral illness, and diarrhea also were regularly reported. There were no significant differences in disposition based on whether the provider was a resident or a private physician. The remainder of this chapter will address some of the issues relevant to the establishment of a telephone triage system. The issue of confidentiality as federally mandated by the Health Insurance Portability and Accountability Act (HIPAA) will also be discussed.

BASIC CONSIDERATIONS IN ESTABLISHING A TELEPHONE TRIAGE SYSTEM

There are some important practical and legal issues that need to be addressed before starting a telephone triage system. Any facility desiring to initiate such a system must find suitable answers to questions regarding format, personnel, documentation, and necessary information pertinent to its program.

Are "Protocols" or "Guidelines" an Appropriate Format?

The legal community often makes a distinction between a protocol and a guideline.

Protocols are rules or procedures one must follow when performing a clinical function or service authorized by a policy. Generally, the legal community views them as mandatory. That is, if protocols exist, people assume that the health care team will be instituting care according to the protocol. Thus, if the protocol states that the provider will call all patients within 24 hours of a call to determine the patient's status, failure to make the call is a violation of the protocol and implies that the provider did not comply with reasonable standards of care. For this reason, if the office or clinic elects to have protocols, they need to be realistic. If there is one triage provider fielding 300 calls per day, it may not be practical to mandate that all telephone calls receive a follow-up call from the triage provider.

In addition, protocols need to be reviewed at least once a year and revised as necessary. Unfortunately, in many instances, they are updated shortly before a Joint Commission on Accreditation of Health Care Organizations (JCAHO) visit or a managed care audit. Health care standards are ever changing. If an office protocol still advocates "leaching" and "bleeding" for an infection, it is time to do an update!

The dating and signing of all protocols by the providers and administrative personnel involved in their development helps to establish that all relevant parties concurred with the protocols and gives legal counsel an idea of when the protocol was put into effect. Outdated protocols should be kept on file in the event a question arises regarding the protocol that was in place during a certain period of time.

There are some positive aspects to having protocols as opposed to guidelines. The use of protocols means that everyone handling the telephones will give consistent information. This helps avoid conflicting advice, which often leads to patient confusion or patients playing one provider against another. Protocols also help inexperienced providers get an indication of important history information and devise appropriate management strategies. They help triage providers defend against charges that they are practicing medicine without a license. They also can serve as a foundation for later testimony in a lawsuit concerning what patient information was elicited and what advice was given.

On the other hand, guidelines are more permissive. They establish what information is important to collect and suggest appropriate management strategies. This allows more independent decision making on the part of the provider. The provider can be more creative and flexible in his or her approach to patient care. Guidelines also give the provider some legal leeway. Strict adherence to a guideline is not perceived to be legally necessary. If a lawsuit is filed concerning telephone advice given by a provider and the current literature supports the correctness of the information given, it is more likely that the provider will be assumed to have met reasonable standards of care regardless of whether the information was consistent with guidelines.

What's the First Step in Drafting Protocols or Guidelines?

After deciding whether their system will be based on protocols or guidelines, providers should begin recording the number and types of calls received each day. This allows the health care team to either employ existing protocols or draft protocols or guidelines that deal with the various types of calls received. These guidelines or protocols should be (a) symptom based, (b) offer relevant subjective and objective data associated with the problem, (c) give possible differential diagnoses, and (d) outline appropriate management strategies. Each problem should be limited to approximately one typed page.

In this book all of the pertinent elements of a sound protocol are addressed. Each symptom-based complaint is listed in alphabetical order, and protocols generally are one page in length. Both referral and home treatment strategies are suggested.

Who Should Handle the Calls?

Deciding who will handle the calls involves several issues. The clinical setting must balance cost effectiveness, accessibility, acceptability, and quality of care. For instance, it might be ideal to have a physician field all patient calls concerning treatment issues. However, is it realistic? If the physician spends much of the week doing rounds and in surgery, it is unlikely that he or she will be able to answer the calls in a timely manner. In addition, how cost effective is it to have a physician discuss routine screening measures or minor patient complaints?

Unfortunately, some clinical settings have gone too far in the other direction. They have inadequately trained or educated personnel handling complex patient calls. This can be a huge problem in the event of a lawsuit. If the provider is undereducated, inexperienced, and ill trained, you have the recipe for a legal nightmare. It will be difficult for a jury or a judge to find it acceptable to have someone with minimal education and training screening the call of a prenatal patient who is experiencing heavy vaginal bleeding.

Savvy providers make sure that all triage personnel pass a competency examination in which the triage personnel receive a mock patient call. The personnel are then required to document the call using the appropriate protocols or guidelines. Results are kept by the facility as evidence of triage personnel competency. In many cases, these "mock scenarios" are tested on an annual basis to demonstrate continued quality telephone triage care.

Some health care agencies also require that those giving telephone advice be licensed. They believe that courts and juries look more favorably on the advice given by providers who are licensed by a state to perform nursing or medical care. The National Certification Corporation now offers certification in telephone nursing practice. The examination is organized into three primary areas: principles of telephone nursing, clinical aspects of telephone nursing, and professional issues. Information about this examination is located in Box 1-1.

How Should Calls Be Documented?

All telephone calls require written documentation, and where that information is stored depends on the clinical setting. In most private practices and managed care facilities, information from the telephone call is placed in the patient's record. Some of these providers also maintain a telephone log or computerized data bank as a backup and may compile data on the types and numbers of calls received.

Lack of written documentation concerning patient telephone calls may lead to questions as to whether the patient actually called, what symptoms the patient reported, what information the provider gathered, and what management strategies were ordered. If the call is documented in a written record, these issues are relatively straightforward. If there is no written record, all of these factors will be called into question.

Box 1-1	Telephone Triage: Helpful Web Sites

Center for Telemedicine Law: This center is a nonprofit consortium of organizations dedicated to providing high-quality patient services by means of telemedicine systems throughout the United States and the world. Articles, membership information, and legislation and hearings that are concerned with telemedicine can be found at http://www.ctl.org.

National Certification Corporation (NCC): This corporation offers specialty certification in several areas of women's health. This year the group also started to offer a certification in telephone nursing practice. Information on the content of the examination and registration for it can be found at http://www.nccnet.org.

National Council of State Boards of Nursing: The Web site of this organization provides the latest information on licensure in the various states. The site can be found at http://www.ncsbn.org/files/mutual/billstatus.asp.

Privacy Rights Clearinghouse: This Web site provides important information on HIPAA Basics. The site can be accessed at http://www.privacyrights.org/fs/fs8a-hipaa.htm.

Specialty Law: This Web site contains information on health care laws in both federal and state courts, and also contains a browser for other related sites. Access this site at http://www.specialtylaw.com.

Versuslaw: This Internet site provides access to both federal and state cases and legislation. It can be found at http://www.versuslaw.com.

What Information Is Pertinent for Each Patient Who Calls?

There are some critical elements that should be gathered for every patient call. Figure 1-1 shows one example of a telephone triage data-collection tool. The dating and timing of calls is important in the event that there is a question concerning when the patient called and when the health care team returned the call. It also is important to note who made the call. Patients occasionally have a family member or significant other call for them, which can make collection of accurate data difficult. Callers other than the patient need to be questioned to establish whether the patient's acuity level is such that she is unable to make the call. In addition, providers need to be cautious about revealing potentially confidential patient information to anyone other than the patient.

Thorough providers also include when the caller will be available for a return call and an alternate telephone number where the patient can be reached. It is frustrating and costly to attempt to call a patient to no avail. These situations often lead to complaints by the patient that their telephone calls were not returned.

Other vital information to be included for all telephone calls are the chief complaint (written in the caller's own words), history of current illness, medical and surgical history, current medications, and allergies. In a women's health care practice, it is important to include the last menstrual period (LMP) to rule out such serious complaints as ectopic pregnancy, threatened abortion, septic abortion, and pregnancy-induced hypertension. In cases in which the chief complaint points to a serious problem, the patient should be seen soon in the emergency room or office.

Whether the disposition is to provide patient teaching, prescribe medications, schedule an office visit, or make the more unusual hospital referral, there must be some resolution. In all cases, it is a good idea to instruct the patient to feel free to call back if she has any questions or if the problem persists or worsens.

HANDLING OUT-OF-STATE CALLS

In 1997, the National Council Delegate Assembly of the National Council of State Boards of Nursing adopted a mutual recognition nursing compact, a legal contract between states, that applies to LPN/VNs and RNs. This compact is concerned with four areas related to the practice of nursing across state lines: jurisdiction, discipline, information sharing, and administration of the compact (National Council of State Boards of Nursing, 1998).

The compact is designed to protect the public's health and safety while allowing a nurse to have one license (in his or her residency state or "home state") and practice in other states ("remote state"), provided that the nurse acknowledges that he or she is responsible for adhering to the remote state's practice and discipline laws. States that are members of the compact allow nurses to practice in their home state and all remote states and to exchange information in the event of any administrative, civil, or criminal action. Only the home state can take action against a nurse's license, and the home state is obligated to investigate any incidents that occur in a remote state.

At this time, 22 states have passed compact legislation. These states include Arizona, Arkansas, Colorado, Delaware, Idaho, Iowa, Kentucky, Maine, Maryland, Mississippi,

Nebraska, New Hampshire, New Mexico, North Carolina, South Carolina, South Dakota, Tennessee, Texas, Utah, Virginia, and Wisconsin. It is anticipated that Rhode Island will become a compact state in 2008. Updates on compact states and information concerning the compact can be found on the Web page of the National Council of State Boards of Nursing, which is noted in Box 1-1.

A WORD ON THE HEALTH INSURANCE PORTABILITY AND ACCOUNTABILITY ACT (HIPAA)

Frequently, someone other than the patient calls the office or clinic requesting information, particular treatment advice or follow-up. As many providers know, in 1996 the federal government enacted the Health Insurance Portability and Accountability Act (HIPAA). HIPAA was designed, in part, to help ensure the privacy and security of patients' health care information. The U.S. Department of Health and Human Services was charged with writing the HIPAA Privacy Rule, which outlines what health information is protected, who can access the patient's medical records and other protected health information, who is responsible for keeping protected information private, how to file a complaint, and penalties that are available if HIPAA rights are violated. Important HIPAA resources are also noted in the reference list of this chapter.

An extensive discussion of HIPAA is beyond the scope of this chapter. However, since telephone triage sheets are typically a part of a patient's medical record, they fall under HIPAA provisions. Consequently, health care offices and triage providers will want to give them the same security they would give to any other medical records. More specifically, the triage provider will typically want to speak only with the patient regarding health care matters. In the event that the patient is not available, the triage provider should access the patient's medical record to see if the patient has given written authorization for the provider to speak to the caller, be it spouse, parent, or legal guardian. Absent written authorization, the triage provider should request that the patient herself call back to discuss any health care matter.

REDUCING LEGAL RISKS/IMPROVING PATIENT CARE

There are several relatively simple measures that can be taken to diminish the risk of liability while improving the quality of care that patients receive. Some helpful suggestions are given below:

- Make sure that personnel handling telephone triage are adequately educated and trained. Regular updates and testing should be built into the triage system.
- Licensed triage providers need to ensure that they are licensed in the state in which they are giving advice or that they are working in a compact state where their license will be recognized.
- Protocols must be in writing.
- If protocols are in place, make sure that personnel handling telephone triage adhere to them or that the patient has been triaged to an appropriate provider who can vary the protocol.

- All protocols should be dated, signed by appropriate personnel, updated regularly, and kept on file.
- Document all telephone calls and the provider's response. If the patient is told to call back to report her status, make sure her return call is also noted.
- Repeated calls, calls that are not made by the patient, calls after a recent hospitalization, and after-hours calls should be of particular concern.
- Emphasize to the caller the need to follow the care provider's advice.
- Triage providers should be open to alternative diagnoses. What may seem like a simple problem should also be analyzed in terms of potentially more serious diagnoses.
- Triage providers should avoid giving a diagnosis over the telephone but should suggest advice that may be helpful for the patient's particular complaint.
- Always invite the caller to call back if the problem persists or worsens or the caller has any additional questions.

Although this is not an exhaustive review of telephone triage in women's health, this chapter should be a good basis for developing a comprehensive telephone triage system. The protocols in the following portions of the book will give personnel handling telephone triage systems detailed instructions on handling specific complaints typically seen in women's health practices.

References

Bolcic-Jankovic, D., Clarridge, B. R., Fowler, Jr., F. J., & Weissman, J. S. (2007). Do characteristics of HIPAA consent forms affect the response rate? *Medical Care, 45*(1), 100–103.

Centers for Medicare & Medicaid Services, Health & Human Services. Exemption of certain systems of Systems of records under the Privacy Act. Proposed rule. *Federal Register, 72*(101), 289–292.

Damschroder, L. J., Pritts, J. L., Neblo, M. A., Kalarickal, R. J., Creswell, J. W., & Hayward, R. A. (2007). Patients, privacy and trust: Patients' willingness to allow researchers to access their medical records. *Social Science & Medicine, 64*(1), 223–235.

Fesko, H. L., & McGuigan, P. (2007). Prevention of HIPAA security breaches. *Health Care Law Monthly,* May 2007, 3–9.

Giesen, P., Ferwerda, R., Tijssen, R., Mokkink, H., Drijver, R., van den Bosch, W., & Grol, R. (2007). Safety of telephone triage in general practitioner cooperatives: Do triage nurses correctly estimate urgency? *Quality & Safety in Health Care, 16*, 181–184.

Houser, S. H., Howard, V. J., Hovater, M. K., & Safford, M. M. (2007). Obtaining medical records from Healthcare facilities under the HIPAA Privacy Rule: The experience of a national longitudinal cohort study. *Neuorepidemiology, 28*(3), 162–168.

Janssen, P. A., Still, D. K., Klein, M. C., Singer, J., Carty, E. A., Liston, R. M., & Zupancic, J. A. (2006). Early labor assessment and support at home versus telephone triage: A randomized controlled trial. *Obstetrics & Gynecology, 108*(6), 1463–1469.

Kempe, A., Bunik, M., Ellis, J., Magid, D., Hegarty, T., Dickinson, L. M., & Steiner, J. F. (2006). How safe is triage by an after-hours telephone call center? *Pediatrics, 118*(2), 457–463.

Knox, C., & Smith, A. (2007). Handhelds & HIPAA. *Nursing Management, 38*(6), 38–40.

Marklund, B., Strom, M., Mansson, J., Borgquist., L., Baigi, A., & Fridlund, B. (2007). Computer-Supported telephone triage nurse: An evaluation of medical quality and costs. *Journal of Nursing Management, 15*(2), 180–187.

McNeil, C. (2007). Skilled telephone triage programs streamline symptom management. *Oncology, 21* (2 Suppl. Nurse Ed), 42–44.

National Council of State Boards of Nursing. (1998; 2007). *Multi-state nursing compact.* Retrieved October 10, 2008, from http://www.ncsbn.org.

Peel, D. C. (2007). Strengthen health information privacy. *Healthcare Financial Management, 61*(11), 32–37.

Privacy Rights Clearing House. (2007). HIPAA basics: Medical privacy in the electronic age. Retrieved December 26, 2007, from http://www.privacyrights.org/fs/fs8a-hipaa.htm.

Rupp, R. E., Ramsey, K. P., & Foley, J. D. (1994). Telephone triage: Results of adolescent clinic responses to a mock patient with pelvic pain. *Journal of Adolescent Health, 15*, 249–253.

Smulian, J. C., Reeve, A. D., Donoghue, E. A., Knuppel, R. A., McCann, T. O., & Ananth, C. V. (2000). After-hours telephone calls to obstetrician-gynecologists. *Obstetrics & Gynecology, 96*, 459–464.

United States Congress. (1996). PL 104–191 Health Insurance Portability and Accountability Act of 1996. Retrieved December 26, 2007, from http://aspe.hhs.gov/admnsimp/pl104191.htm.

Uzuner, O., Luo, Y., & Szolovits, P. (2007). Evaluating state of the art in automatic de-identification. *Journal of the American Medical Informatics Association, 14*(5), 550–563.

Van Charante, E. P. M., ter Reit, G., Drost, S., Linden, L., Klazinga, N. S., & Bindels, P. J. E. (2006). Nurse telephone triage in out-of-hours GP practice: Independent advice and return consultation. *Biomed Central (BMC) Family Practice, 7*, 74–84.

Assessing the Obstetric/Gynecologic Patient by Telephone

Vicki E. Long

Assessment is a cornerstone of nursing practice. The ability to gather data in order to form an opinion about a patient's situation and ultimately participate in formulating a plan of care is integral to all that nurses are taught to do. However, assessing a patient by telephone presents some hurdles to the nursing process. The telephone, for all its convenience and immediacy, robs us of the opportunity to use many of our senses. It takes additional nursing skill to overcome the innate deficit of the medium.

Imagine a poem you may be familiar with from childhood, *The Blind Men and the Elephant* by John Godfrey Saxe (1816–1887). The poem relates the tale of six blind men who approach an elephant from different angles. The one who feels only the side of the bulky beast thinks the elephant is like a wall. The fellow who feels only the trunk equates the elephant to a snake, and the man who touches the tail is certain the elephant must be like a rope. In all, there are six different men with six different ideas of the essence of an elephant. Each is partially correct, but all of the men are wrong in their total view of the magnificent animal. That simple poem conveys the message that limited sensory input minimizes our perceptions and leads to misunderstanding. In the medical world, such limited perception can be very dangerous.

This chapter discusses some of the basics of telephone assessment. Experienced triage nurses in obstetrics/gynecology will find much of this redundant because these skills have become integrated into their daily practice. One of the difficulties of telephone triage nursing is that we do not have a large body of research or a tradition of educational processes for these skills. Nurses in triage roles tend to be experienced nurses who have gained much knowledge over time but have worked with relatively little documentation. However, we must begin to assemble our knowledge into a communicable form for the purposes of educating other nurses in triage skills and validating what we already do on a day-to-day basis.

THE BASIC DATA

The first chapter provided a sample form for collecting identifying information for each telephone encounter. No one form is perfect, and you may already be using one you think is meeting your needs satisfactorily. However, you should ensure that you routinely collect certain information for each call.

The date, time, and patient's correct name obviously are important, but sometimes the most basic data are collected in a haphazard fashion. It is hard to imagine how difficult it can be to do something as simple as obtain a "correct name." Keep in mind that many patients use hyphenated names. Some patients use one name at work and another one socially. Occasionally a patient has a different name on her health insurance card. For example, "Lucinda Doe-Smith" on your medical records may be "Cindy Smith" to her coworkers. Adequate data collection at the time the call is initiated by the patient will aid in locating her if her call needs to be returned at another time.

There is another important piece of information to be noted when recording the patient's name. Many names are similar, and particularly in practices with large patient volumes, other identifying information may be necessary. Middle initials or birth dates may be needed to adequately identify the patient at hand. Politely ask, "May I have your middle initial? We have more than one Cindy Smith in our practice." This does not offend most patients with common names. However, almost any patient could be expected to be irate if her problem is confused with another's.

Another absolutely necessary piece of information is the telephone number where the patient can be reached now and where she can be reached at a later time. If the nature of the call is such that another provider will have to return the call after routine office or clinic hours, it is imperative that alternate telephone numbers and times be obtained. In this day of multiple area codes, cell phones, and pagers, it is important to adequately identify what type of a number the patient has left. Pager numbers are particularly inappropriate for return calls because many providers may be calling from a telephone system that does not allow them to key a number for the call to be returned. For this reason, many practices will refuse to accept a pager number for return calls. You should discuss this with the providers with whom you work.

There are other telephone system pitfalls. If a patient asks to have her call returned at a place of employment after routine hours, make certain you know how to bypass her switchboard or computerized telephone system. The inclusion of the patient's personal extension or a private number may be necessary. These details may seem too simple to be mentioned. However, anyone who has worked in telephone triage is familiar with the frustration of being unable to reach a patient because of something as small as a poorly recorded contact number. The patient's location at 3:30 PM, when she calls in with her problem, could be entirely different from her location at 5:05 PM, when a provider is returning her call.

One other sensitive issue in terms of securing a return telephone number is whether the patient will be in a situation where a return call would be appropriate. The intimate nature of most OB/GYN topics necessitates sensitivity to this issue. The next chapter, "Counseling Basics and Challenges in Telephone Triage," will address this issue in more detail. For our purposes, it is enough to point out that if the patient seems uncomfortable with a return call or stipulates conditions under which a call can be received, we must take these issues into account. For example, let's say our fictitious patient, Cindy Smith, is uneasy about being called at home, which is why she called from work. If we cannot address her problem fully during the initial contact, particularly if another provider will be involved in returning the call, we may need to negotiate a time when she can call back for more instructions.

THE NATURE OF THE PROBLEM

Once we have established who the patient is and how to reach her should a return call be necessary, it is important to get to the nature of the problem that precipitated the call. For the purposes of this book, we have included a Basic Triage Assessment Form at the beginning of major sections containing protocols for specific problems. These forms are designed to prompt you on the information needed to adequately triage certain problems. Again, experienced triage nurses may find these forms less relevant than will nurses new to triage, but it is important to realize that these basic bits of information should always be in the back of your mind when speaking with patients.

The required information does not always need to be directly asked of the patient. For example, our patient "Cindy Smith" calls in with complaints of spotting while she is taking birth control pills. If her record is in front of you, you may know which product she takes. You may know from having briefly reviewed her record how long she's been taking this oral contraceptive and whether or not she has had other complaints while taking it. Instead of going through each question on the Basic Triage Assessment Form for Oral Contraceptives, you may confirm the information you have at hand by asking, "Cindy, has there been a change in your prescription since you were in the office for your last Pap smear?"

Sometimes, particularly if the patient has made multiple calls, it may be best to verify the information directly with the patient. It is important in this phase of basic data gathering to not frustrate the patient. If a patient has experienced numerous problems recently, she may feel as if she has described the problem already, even though this is the first time you have talked with her. In our mock situation with Cindy, a simple point of clarification may ease the way for you to ask more detailed questions. For example, you can broach the subject of which birth control pill she is currently taking by saying, "Cindy, it looks like we have changed your birth control pills a couple of times recently. My notes say you are currently taking Ortho Tri-Cyclen. Is that correct?" Convey to the patient that you are trying to get the correct information so you can help her address her problem adequately.

In many instances, you may not have access to the patient's record or previous calls. In these situations, it is important that you know which questions you need to create a basic structure for evaluating the problem. Box 2-1 and Box 2-2 outline the most basic of questions for a call related to obstetrics and a call related to gynecology. You will use the Basic Triage Assessment Forms organized throughout the book to fill in the gaps for each individual type of problem. Remember that these questions are not all-inclusive. If you find there are other points you deem important or that are required by the providers with whom you work, please add them to the Basic Triage Assessment Forms included in the book.

THE REAL NATURE OF THE PROBLEM

We are all familiar with the type of patient call in which it seems we can't get to the core of the problem. Sometimes it is because the patient isn't quite sure what is wrong. Sometimes it is because she is reluctant to admit what is bothering her. Sometimes it is because we have asked the wrong questions. Often, it isn't what we have asked; it is how we have asked it. Part of the skill of assessing over the telephone is the ability to listen and speak with empathy, compassion, and true interest in the person on the other end of the line, despite the problem. In their classic book *Telephone Triage: Theory, Practice and Protocol Development*, Wheeler and Windt (1993) called this "telephone charisma." Let's return to Cindy Smith and her breakthrough bleeding for an illustration.

Cindy has called her OB/GYN provider's office with a complaint of spotting while taking her birth control pills. What she doesn't initially share is that she has missed two pills and is fearful of pregnancy. Cindy has missed pills before. She knows what to do when she misses a pill, but because she underwent a termination of pregnancy 6 months ago for a similar situation, she is worried, despite having followed what she thinks is the correct procedure. She is hoping beyond hope that history will not repeat itself. She may be embarrassed to be in a similar situation. She may be angry with herself and her boyfriend for not routinely using condoms. However, she simply says she has been spotting while taking her oral contraceptives. She's hoping the voice on the other end will hear what she's not saying.

It is Monday morning when Cindy calls. Nora, the nurse who receives her call, has a stack of prescriptions in front of her that must be called into various pharmacies. Nora has just hung up after talking to Mrs. Jones, who is upset about her abnormal Pap smear result and upcoming colposcopy. It is only 10:00 AM, and already Nora is behind.

Nora asks Cindy most of the questions on the office protocol used to evaluate patients who are bleeding while taking oral contraceptives. She queries as to when in

Cindy's cycle she missed pills, how she made them up, and whether or not she used a backup method for 7 days after missing the pills. She advises Cindy to wait for two missed cycles and take a pregnancy test if her period doesn't come. What she doesn't do is pick up on the anxiety in Cindy's voice. She notices that Cindy had called before about bleeding while taking birth control pills, but she doesn't research to see what happened in those circumstances. She doesn't stop to think that perhaps Cindy isn't able to manage taking oral contraceptive pills correctly in a consistent fashion. She dismisses the lack of use of a backup method,

Box 2-2	The Most Basic Gynecologic Data to Be Obtained

1. Date and time of call
2. Caller identification
   Complete name
   Relationship to patient, if someone else is calling
   Accurate telephone number and times it is valid
   Alternate telephone number and times it is valid
3. Gynecologic-related data
   Patient's age
   Last menstrual period
   Last normal menstrual period
   Nature of problem
   Duration of problem
   Recurrence rate of problem
   Associated symptoms
   Method of contraception or hormone replacement
      therapy (if applicable)
   Other medical problems
   Current medications
   Known allergies to medications
Add any information your practice deems necessary.

admonishing her to do better next time. She doesn't notice that Cindy grows quieter as she talks. Cindy hasn't been forthcoming in her real concern, but Nora hasn't given her an opportunity to work through to that point. Nora is still thinking about the other calls she needs to make. Nora has heard the nature of the problem, but she hasn't really listened to Cindy's larger concerns. Just as one of the six blind men with the elephant, Nora is partially correct but doesn't see the whole picture.

Let's see what could have happened to make the response to Cindy's call more satisfactory. Penny, an experienced triage nurse, receives Cindy's call. Penny has her chart in front of her and glances through the last few calls. She notices that Cindy's pills have been changed frequently because of her problems with spotting. She notices the referral for the termination. She quickly picks up on the fact that, although Cindy has admitted to missing pills when questioned, she's never called in with that specific complaint.

Penny begins her call by greeting Cindy and identifying herself. As she goes through the questions on her office's protocol, she begins to interject some statements that may hint at the nature of Cindy's concerns without putting Cindy on "the witness stand." She says, "Many women have trouble remembering to take their pills. We can suggest some ways to remember, but some women decide to try another method. Would you like to talk about other options?" If she senses Cindy is interested, she uses that opportunity to make suggestions. As Cindy relaxes in the conversation, Penny adds, " I know some package inserts recommend to wait until a second missed period to take a pregnancy test. But peace of mind is worth a lot. It probably is too early to do one now, but if your next period isn't normal, you'll feel better if you go ahead and do a urine pregnancy test anyway." She takes the issue further and asks Cindy if she knows about emergency contraception. She gently talks about more consistent backup method use. By the time they are finished, Cindy feels less anxious, even though she knows it is too early to have absolute confirmation that pregnancy hasn't occurred.

Getting to the real nature of the problem is not an accident. It involves a disciplined approach to data gathering combined with the time-honored nursing skills of compassion and caring. In his book on the fundamentals of relationships between patients and healers, *The Lost Art of Healing* (1999), Nobel Peace Prize winner Dr. Bernard Lown writes of the power of sympathetic listening and touch. Skilled telephone triage nurses learn to touch with their voice. Although the long-distance physical separation imposed by the medium of the telephone minimizes some of a nurse's senses, she can heighten others to facilitate communication.

EXPLORING SYMPTOMS

The example we've used to illustrate the fundamentals of assessing by telephone is fairly straightforward, but the patient often isn't that certain what is wrong. Bleeding while taking birth control pills is a specific problem. However, abdominal pain is a vague complaint that requires additional investigation before a nurse can even begin to decide which line of questioning to pursue. This process is much like peeling an orange. The patient's complaint is dissected section by section in an attempt to understand what she is experiencing.

In traditional assessment of patients, history taking provides as much as 75% of the information that leads to a correct diagnosis—much more than physical examination and laboratory testing (Lown, 1999). A thorough history takes time, however, and brief telephone encounters may not afford the luxury of taking a complete history. One technique of formal history taking that is easily adapted to the telephone is the list of questions often referred to as "the anatomy or attributes of a symptom" (see Box 2-3). This series of questions should be memorized by every nurse working in telephone triage.

It is helpful for nurses employed in a telephone triage setting to regularly review Chapter 2, "An Approach to Symptoms," in *A Guide to Physical Examination and History Taking* (Bates et al., 1995). Although the book is intended for practitioners doing classic history taking and physical examination, this chapter presents detailed questions for every body system, many of which are adaptable to history taking via the telephone. Knowing which questions the patient may be asked if she is brought in for an examination may expedite the initial assessment phase that is so important in triaging patient concerns.

Box 2-3	Anatomy of a Symptom

Its location
Its quality
Its severity
Its timing
Its setting
Its triggers
Its accompanying manifestations

TIME MANAGEMENT IN TELEPHONE TRIAGE

We have alluded to the time constraints imposed on telephone triage nurses. The volume of calls in many busy practices is reason enough to be concerned about time. However, there are other practical reasons for being sensitive to the time limitations faced by most nurses in these positions. It may seem as if the need to be realistic in approaching this issue is a direct affront to our emphasis on compassion and empathy for patient concerns.

One way we can help patients get the most from their health care encounters is to be respectful of their time. Patients are subjected to being "on hold" to make appointments and speak to nursing personnel. Even when the patient is seen in person, there is a reason reception areas are called "waiting rooms." The terms alone arouse frustration. Although telephone triage nurses enjoy the one-on-one interaction with patients (or they would not be in their positions), it is easy for inexperienced nurses to err on the side of being too talkative.

Being overly personal in one's conversation is not the same as being sensitive to a patient's personal needs. It takes professional discipline to delve into touchy subjects with authentic concern. The ability to listen, delineate problems, offer suggestions, and suggest resources in a timely fashion demands intense focus and concentration. Patients appreciate adequate time being allotted to their needs, but most understand that other patients are waiting to have similar calls returned and problems solved.

There is no way to learn time management in telephone triage without practice. In our mock patient situation, our experienced nurse was able to quickly glance through the patient's chart and glean several bits of information. She wove information she wanted to deliver to the patient among her pertinent questions. Deciding how to balance the personal touch with professional requirements takes an active understanding of how to ask questions.

Reviewing the basics of questioning techniques can be helpful. Open-ended questions probably are best described as "the gold standard" when it comes to giving patients the freedom and time to describe their problems. As mentioned, telephone triage nurses do not always have time. Direct questions with "yes" or "no" answers, multiple-choice answers, or rating scales ("Where would you rate your pain on a scale of 1 to 10?") can be a means of controlling the pace of the conversation during the detailed data-gathering section. Using the communication techniques of clarification ("What do you mean by heavy bleeding?") or interpretation ("You have asked a lot of questions about depression. Are you worried you are depressed?") may help patients to focus on issues you are assessing. When time is precious, reserve your open-ended questions for the topics you have identified as important by your more directed questions.

Time and trust go hand in hand in developing telephone triage skills. Regular mock calls help nurses decide what sounds right and what time allotment is realistic for certain problems. Reviewing traditional history and physical components will help hone nursing skills. Triage nurses need to be focused, organized, and professional while being attentive to the individuals whose problems they are assessing. For a nurse's advice to be deemed legitimate, she must exude confidence in her knowledge. This comes only with time and practice.

References

Bickley, L. S. & Hoekelman, R. A. (1999). *An approach to symptoms. In: A guide to physical examination and history taking* (7th ed.). (pp. 1–42). Philadelphia: Lippincott Williams & Wilkins.

Lown, B. (1999). *The lost art of healing.* New York: Ballantine Books.

Wheeler, S. Q., & Windt, J. H. (1993). *Telephone triage: Theory, practice and protocol development.* Albany, NY: Delmar Publishing.

CHAPTER 3

Counseling Basics and Challenges in Telephone Triage

Felicia Guest

This is a postliterate age. Unless you work in a college health service, it is likely that some portion of your patient population cannot read educational materials, at least not in the language(s) you have them available. For some health care providers, functional literacy rates among their patients are so low that print materials don't feel like an educational option.

This also is a do-it-by-telephone age. Round-the-clock toll-free numbers for banks and stores are ubiquitous, and most of us are now quite comfortable, if impatient, doing business via telephone, punching our way through verbal menus ("For your account balance, press one . . .").

Health care services cannot afford to ignore these paradigmatic shifts in the national culture, and so you accommodate, translating the intimate, personal skills of patient counseling and education to the telephone.

TELEPHONE COUNSELING FUNDAMENTALS

Telephone counseling is a form of instrument flying. You make your way as best you can without being able to give and receive body language cues, making do with reading a voice when you need also to read a face, hands, and shifts in position. You make do with comforting words when you might wish also to grasp a hand or touch a shoulder. Literally, you can't see where you are going.

Using the telephone to deliver bad health news or to cope with other demanding situations sometimes is unavoidable and often is the only practical access route for linking nurse and patient. You can be separated from your patients by too many miles, by too many competing priorities such as work or child care, by too few evening or weekend clinic or office hours, or by too little trust. So you make do.

Because you can't see your patient, you must always begin by ascertaining whether she has enough privacy to talk and whether she has time to talk (you can estimate for her whether you need 5 minutes, 15, or more). And because she can't see you, either, tell her who you are, where you are, whether anyone else can hear the conversation, and whether you are recording the conversation or taking notes.

This chapter explores counseling concepts that can be helpful for breaking bad news to patients by telephone. It then explores telephone techniques for being helpful when patients express strong feelings.

BREAKING BAD NEWS

Your ultrasound (or x-ray or MRI or CT scan) shows something abnormal.
Your HIV test result is positive.
Your Pap smear result is abnormal.

Each and every patient brings the potential for breaking bad health news, a time when you will tell her some unwelcome fact about her own health or the health of someone close. The news may be disappointing: a negative pregnancy test after months and months of trying. It may be temporarily dismaying: an abnormal Pap smear result that has detected cell changes early enough for definitive treatment and cure. Or it may be devastating, marking life with a milestone for "before I knew" and "after I knew": a diagnosis of cancer or HIV, for example. This conversation deserves your highest level of skill as counselor, teacher, and advocate.

GETTING STARTED

Begin by giving your patient a clear statement of why you have called and then ascertaining whether this is a time and place that will work for such a conversation.

- "Ms. Green, your lab tests are back, and I need to tell you what we found. Can you talk now? Or would you prefer to come in, or to set up another time to talk by telephone later today?"
- "Hi, Brenda, I have your test results. Is this a good time to talk? Do you need to close your office door or anything?"
- "Good morning, Ms. Powell, this is Betty Connor from the clinic. I need to go over your test results with you. Are you okay to talk privately now?"
- "Hello, Ms. Miranda, it's Donna in Dr. Weinman's office. Can you talk for a few minutes?"

Once you have established that the conversation can go forward, use a preparatory remark such as, "We've found something we need to check out," or "I'm afraid I have bad news." Then state the bad news simply and plainly. As one woman said, "It just made it worse when they kept stalling around!" Use two or three straightforward sentences to explain the situation. Then say, "I'm so sorry," or something similar in your own speaking style, and then stop talking. Even on the telephone, the patient needs time to absorb your words. You might add, "I'm going to be quiet for a minute so you can think, okay?"

Once she seems ready to talk, you might suggest that she get pencil and paper to jot down notes, especially if you will be giving telephone numbers, appointment times, addresses, or other details that are hard to remember under the best of circumstances.

In addition, she will have a bit of time to take a deep breath, move around a bit, and continue to absorb your news. If you hear a television or radio, ask, "I hear your TV or radio. Would you like a moment to turn it down?" If you hear live conversation, ask her again if she can talk freely.

EMOTIONAL RESPONSE TO BAD HEALTH NEWS

Ten patients will respond to bad news 10 different ways, so remember that reactions are varied and unpredictable. Be careful not to assume you know in advance how your patient will feel. When nurses and other care providers in workshops were asked to recall their own experiences of hearing bad health news, their emotional responses included the following, in roughly this order of frequency:

- numb or dazed; short-circuited;
- frightened or scared;
- angry at self, others, or God;
- "it's not fair";
- "there must be some mistake";
- helpless; and
- guilty ("if only . . .").

It may be easy or difficult to read your patient's emotional response on the telephone. If her emotional state isn't apparent to you, ask, "Can you tell me how you're feeling right now?" Offer comfort and quiet presence, such as "I'm here, take your time," if she needs to regain composure.

NURSING GOALS AND PATIENT GOALS

Nurses and other health care providers usually are in agreement about their goals for this difficult counseling conversation:

- to help the patient (and any other people the patient wants to include on an extension or speakerphone) understand the health situation as clearly as possible;
- to be as comforting as possible on a telephone;
- to be as reassuring as possible, without false reassurance;
- to reach mutual agreement on the next step for appropriate health care; and
- to assess whether the patient is distraught enough that some immediate intervention is warranted.

These are straightforward and noncontroversial goals, from the health care provider perspective. It is important to remember that patient goals for this conversation may or may not be the same. When workshop participants were asked, "Right at that moment, what did you want and need from your health care provider?," they recalled an impressive variety of wishes and goals.

- Hug me and show me you empathize with how bad this is. (Patients with this goal will not get what they need from telephone counseling. If you hear this need being expressed by a patient, you might say something to her such as, "I'm sorry I can't be there right now to give you a hug!")

- Let me think for a minute and pull myself together.
- Tell me what happens next. What's the next step?
- Tell me everything will turn out all right.
- I have no idea what I want or need.
- I need to talk to my husband/mom/sister/other support person. (If a patient is eager to hang up and call someone for support, try to contract for a few more minutes of discussion first, until you feel comfortable that the patient is composed and safe, posing no danger to self or others. Schedule a time to continue the counseling session that day or as soon as possible.)
- Tell me I didn't do anything wrong.
- Tell me where to go for another opinion.
- Tell me this is just a bad dream and I'll wake up in a minute.
- Tell my family for me.
- Tell me what to read from the library/bookstore/Internet to learn more about this.
- Tell me how I'm going to pay for this.
- Give me the worst-case scenario.
- Tell me we can get started fixing this today.

With patient goals and wishes as varied as these, it is important not to guess or assume you know what your patient will need from you! You might launch into education when comfort is needed. You might offer comfort when time to think is needed.

Some patients are able to state clearly what they want at that moment. Others don't know, or are hesitant to say aloud their wishes. Ask, "How can I be helpful right now?" "Do you want to know more?" When we don't ask what patients want, we tend to assume they want what we would want in similar circumstances. For example, clinically trained nurses might tend to be comforted by facts, by a fuller understanding of the science of the situation. Science might be lost on a patient who needs reassurance. And reassurance might be lost on a patient who needs to talk to her partner. Think about your personal style for coping with crisis, by reviewing how you have reacted in the past. Be careful that you don't assume patients will need what you needed.

HELPING PATIENTS UNDERSTAND

Remember that a key goal for this telephone conversation from the nursing perspective is to help the patient (and others) understand the health issue as fully as possible. However, information doesn't comfort everyone, so let the patient cue how much you impart. Consider a question such as, "Are you the kind of person who would like to know everything about what's going on, or just an outline?" Be careful to pace your instructional messages at a speed the patient can follow, pausing frequently to allow for questions, or to ask her to repeat in her own words what you said.

We tend to go too fast with education for patients because we are so familiar with the material ourselves. One workshop participant remembered a conversation about an abnormal Pap smear result. She called the patient, spent several minutes telling her about colposcopy, biopsy, and some of the possible treatment options, then said, "Do you have any questions?" The woman replied, "Did you say this was about my Pap smear?" Slow down!

Nurses are ethically bound to educate patients about their health problems in a manner consistent with full disclosure, informed choice, and informed consent. However, this initial breaking-bad-news discussion on the telephone may not be the ideal time for teaching because a woman experiencing strong and distressing emotions may not be able to absorb much technical information. When you feel confident you will soon be face to face with a patient, consider deferring most of the full-disclosure education during the initial telephone call and return to it at the later in-person encounter.

COMFORT AND REASSURANCE

From the nursing perspective, another key goal for this telephone conversation is to comfort and reassure the patient as much as possible. Attending is comforting for most people, so stay with her on the telephone as long as she wishes, if you can. If what is worrying the patient is not apparent, ask, "What worries you most right now? What concerns do you have?" Most (but not all) patients want to know what to expect. Spoken or silent questions can include:

- What will it be like?
- Will it hurt?
- Is it curable?
- If not, will it shorten my life? How much?

Avoid false reassurance, and follow your patient's lead about looking into the future. If your patient asks, share any available science-based outcome data about her condition, cautioning that you cannot predict with certainty the outcome of her particular case. Some patients want to discuss the future right away, whereas others look no further ahead than telling other people the news and preparing for next-step medical procedures.

Some patients face a health crisis with hope and optimism, and others do not. Workshop participants often have credited a healthy and intact personal support system, a strong faith community, and an optimistic personality with enabling them to face a health crisis with a positive outlook.

THE NEXT STEP, COMPOSURE, AND CLOSURE

Another key nursing goal for this telephone conversation is to reach a joint commitment with the patient on the next step, whether it will be a counseling visit, a biopsy, a referral, a second opinion, a medication regimen, or another option.

Time pressures can become critical at this juncture. For example, if you call a pregnant woman with bad news about an abnormal CVS, AFP, or amniocentesis result, you will want to give her as much time as possible to consider her options, even before she returns to the office or clinic. You and your patient do not have the luxury of time for her to absorb the news because the passage of time can become a limiting factor in her range of choices. Unfortunately, this reality means that the patient will need to consider complex medical choices at a time of emotional distress. You can empathize with the pressure on your patient: "I'm sorry we have to push ahead and talk about your choices right now. It's the only way I know to give you time to think about what you want to do."

Seeking agreement on the next step also functions as a natural way to bring closure to the telephone discussion, a stopping point that usually makes sense to both the nurse and the patient. Once you have broken the bad news, responded to immediate emotional needs, provided comfort and reassurance, and offered appropriate education, begin to close down the discussion by assessing her understanding of the medical issues.

Remember to begin this assessment by saying, "Let me be sure I'm doing my job to teach you, by hearing how you would tell your best friend what we've talked about," rather than, "Let me see what you have learned." Put the burden of educational success or failure on yourself, not your patient, who has enough to cope with at this stressful time. If you are making an immediate referral to another care provider, be sure the patient can tell you in her own words where to go, when, what to take along, and how to prepare for her appointment. Referred patients sometimes feel "handed off" and abandoned, so be sure that you close the referral loop and track your patient's care as closely as you can. Invite her to keep you informed.

The next step toward closure is to evaluate her composure. One way that nurses can assess a patient's emotional equilibrium on the telephone is to ask, "What will you do after we hang up?" Not surprisingly, responses to this question can vary widely. Workshop participants reported these activities, in roughly this order, as their first action after receiving bad news:

- connecting with husband or partner, family, other supporting people;
- returning to work or home, "going through the motions";
- crying;
- going to a library or bookstore or computer to read about the medical issue;
- praying;
- walking, exercising, "anything to keep moving";
- eating, drinking, or taking drugs ("I went straight to the ice cream store for a huge sundae!"); and
- getting affairs in order.

It can be very difficult to assess composure during telephone conversations, when no body language cues are provided. Your patient may hang up in distress, or distraction, before you feel confident about her status. Three possible red flags that a patient could need immediate support or intervention are:

- suicidal ideation ("I might as well go ahead and kill myself and get it over with!");
- magical thinking ("Maybe I'll just get run over by a bus or something and not have to deal with this pregnancy!");
- and, most common of all, the inability to formulate a plan ("What am I going to do when I hang up? I have no idea . . .").

If you are worried about your patient's possible danger to self or others, consider an immediate referral to a mental-health crisis line. You also might offer to call her husband or partner, parent, or other support person, if she is alone. And you might elicit a promise that she will call you back (or await your call) within a few hours or the next day.

Once you have assured yourself that the patient is composed and safe and has a plan for what to do when she hangs up, ask, "What else would you like us to talk about? Can I help with anything? Is there anything else you want to say?" Then pause long enough for her to gather her thoughts. You can finish up the conversation by repeating that you are sorry to bring bad news, and by reminding her to call your office whenever she needs more information and support.

SPECIAL COUNSELING SITUATIONS

If you are breaking bad news to an adolescent, even a young woman from a big family, remember that she may feel very isolated and alone, so assess her perception of a personal support system carefully. Some teens are unable to tolerate waiting for test results and other outcomes and thus may struggle with your suggested care plan: "Why can't I have it taken care of today?" Young people can be impulsive, so be diligent about assessing what she plans to do after hanging up the telephone.

Power is an important issue in these stressful telephone conversations, and patients sometimes want to delegate responsibility for decision making to the health care provider. Be careful not to usurp autonomy from a patient who has just heard bad health news, even if she invites you to make all her decisions about whom to tell and what to do next.

In some cultures, patients are told the truth about ominous health conditions, and in other cultures, they are not. Learn the practices of the cultural groups represented in your patient population, so you will have an idea of what to expect. Nevertheless, always assess each patient as an individual with personal and particular wishes and needs.

Health care providers are sometimes patients themselves. Remember that these women need the same emotional support, the same careful education as any other patient, and their professional knowledge and skill can desert them in times of personal crisis.

CARE FOR THE CARE GIVER

Breaking bad news is hard, demanding work. You will need to take care of yourself. Prepare for occasional "blame the messenger" experiences and for patients who have unrealistic expectations that medicine or surgery can solve any problem. Expect the frustration of not knowing what has happened to patients whom you refer for care.

Some health care offices and clinics use simple, formal grief rituals to comfort nurses and other staff members when a patient dies. One common practice is to place a small table in a staff area with a blank book and a candle. When a patient dies, write her name in the book, and light the candle for a day in her memory.

WHAT MATTERS ABOUT BREAKING BAD NEWS

An educator in an HIV clinic asked all new patients what they recalled about finding out they had HIV. Very often, the answer was, "Well, they were real nice, but I don't really remember much about what they said." This does not mean the discussion was a counseling failure. The important part of the answer, what the patient values enough to remember about the breaking of bad news, is "they were real nice."

COPING WITH STRONG FEELINGS ON THE TELEPHONE

Angry patients can be counseling challenges on the telephone because you wish you could hang up, and sometimes they do hang up! When you hear, "I had this Pap test almost 3 weeks ago, and you are just now calling to tell me there may be a problem," or a similar, angry statement, try this three-step response (Beresford, 1988):

- let her know you heard her anger, and name it: "I know you are angry, Ms. Lee."
- let her know it is okay for her to feel it and talk about it: "I certainly understand how frustrating it is to wait so long. Thank you for telling me."
- help her return to feeling in control of her situation by offering her an option: "Would you like to talk about what the test means, and where we might want to go from here?"

   Patients who are fearful in response to your telephone counseling may have generalized a longstanding medical fear, expressing such ideas as, "Hospitals give me the creeps," or "I always hate going to the doctor!" They may fear and anticipate pain, especially if they already have been experiencing pain from an injury or illness. They may be afraid of dying, whether or not that is a rational fear in the present counseling situation. If you detect a fearful response from your telephone patient, the following techniques may be helpful.

- Give the patient permission to be afraid, and to express the fear, even when you want to break in with "don't worry" statements. She may need to vent first. If you can live calmly with her fearful thoughts, it will help her to live calmly with them herself.
- Clarify the fear, if she does not express it in specific terms herself. "What worries you about this?" "What part sounds worst?" Sometimes patient fear is grounded in a genuine understanding of what lies ahead. Sometimes it can grow out of myth, rumor, or even guilt.
- Help relieve fear then and there on the telephone. You might practice deep breathing with the patient, giving her comfort in the moment, your compassionate collaboration, and a skill to use for herself later.
- Reassure her as much as you can without giving false reassurance. Use statements such as, "Some women say it feels like . . ." or, "The nurse will be there to tell you what to do if . . ." Avoid making promises you might not be able to keep, such as, "You won't have any trouble with this," or "It's not very painful."

THINKING POSITIVELY ABOUT TELEPHONE COUNSELING

Telephone counseling isn't ideal. However, this task is more likely to be a satisfying part of your work experience if you are able to cast it in a positive light. Remember that telephone counseling:

- saves precious time for the patient and the nurse;
- may save the patient money she did not have to spend on transportation costs or child care costs;
- may save her wages or leave time;
- may sometimes provide distance and privacy so that patients can more freely discuss risky or intimate issues; and
- usually allows counseling in a more private, confidential manner than office visits can offer.

Best wishes for enjoying the rewards of this very 21st century form of nursing. Can Internet counseling be far behind?

References

Beresford, T. (1988). *Short term relationship counseling* (2nd ed.). Baltimore, MD: Planned Parenthood of Maryland.

Bibliography

Buckman, R., & Kason, Y. (1992). *How to break bad news: A guide for health care professionals.* Baltimore: Johns Hopkins University Press. [This 223-page book includes a six-step protocol for the counseling discussion, and a sample interview using the protocol.]

Girgis, A., & Sanson-Fisher, R.W. (1995). Breaking bad news: Consensus guidelines for medical practitioners. *Journal of Clinical Oncology, 13,* 2449–2456. [Contains national consensus guidelines.]

Ptacek, J.T., & Eberhardt, T.L. (1996). Breaking bad news: A review of the literature. *Journal of the American Medical Association, 276,* 496–502. [Contains an excellent overview of works on breaking bad news.]

CHAPTER 4

The Use of Online Information Retrieval in Telephone Triage

Alice Myers

We literally are experiencing an information explosion. Frequently, patients call and ask providers about some piece of information they found on the Internet and seek the advice of the triage nurse. For example, over the past year, patients have seen a great deal of conflicting information on such women's health matters as hormone replacement therapy, the use of CA-125 testing as a screening tool for ovarian cancer, and whether or not they should discontinue the contraceptive patch because of concerns over blood clots.

As a triage provider, you will need to decide whether Internet information is credible. You may also have to do some independent "Internet hunting" to help patients and your practice determine whether the newest information is valid and how your practice should formulate a response to patients' questions. Finding valid clinical information on the Internet can be daunting. By understanding how Internet search engines work and performing efficient Internet research, you'll be much better prepared to help both your patients and your practice interpret current clinical evidence.

This chapter is designed to give you a basic overview of important terms and features of the Internet, and will also help you decide whether information available on the Internet is credible. It is important to remember that the Internet can be a valuable tool as you work to develop sound patient care standards in your practice.

IMPORTANT TERMS

Let's begin by defining some important terms you will need to understand to navigate Internet information.

A browser is software on your computer that enables you to access and browse the Internet. There are several different types of browsers that may be found on any given computer. These include Microsoft Internet Explorer, Mozilla Firefox, and Apple Safari.

The Uniform Resource Locator (URL) is a unique address for a specific Web site or page of information on the Internet. URLs often end with .com, .gov, .org., or .edu, depending on the Web site (http://www.iana.org/gtld/gtld.htm).

.com–denotes a for-profit company Web site
.gov–denotes a government Web site
.org–denotes a nonprofit organization or association Web site
.edu–denotes an educational Web site

Example URLs are www.abc.com and www.nih.gov.

Once the browser is open, the user can enter a URL or Web address. After several seconds, the browser displays the requested Web site. Each Web site is made up of several Web pages that concern topics relevant to that particular organization.

WEB PAGE ORGANIZATION AND NAVIGATION

A Web site is a series of Web pages that are connected on the computer by means of something called "hyperlinks," or "links" for short. A Web site's home page is the first page displayed when a Web site address is entered. The home page provides an overview of the Web site you have accessed, as well as links and a directory to other pages within the Web site or to other Web sites. Hyperlinks are often underlined, bold, highlighted, or colored. A hyperlink is available when your computer cursor changes from an arrow to a hand as your computer mouse pointer moves across the link. To access the new Web page, click on the hyperlink. To return to the previous Web page, click on the back button. The back button is located in the upper left-hand corner of the browser window.

INTERNET SEARCH ENGINES

Finding information is simple when the Web site address is known, but what about when the Web address is unknown (McKeown, 1997)? In such cases, you can use Internet search engines, which are Web sites that accept the keywords you enter to locate other Web sites matching specific terms or criteria. Once a keyword or words are entered, the search engine displays a list of Web page titles with hyperlinks and a brief description of each Web site that matches the keyword(s). Search engines are used frequently for Internet research, and they are designed with easy-to-remember names (Franklin, 2007). Here are some of the popular Internet search engines that are often used:

www.google.com
www.ask.com
www.yahoo.com
www.msn.com
www.yahoo.com
www.live.com
www.pubmed.org

How do Internet search engines know about all these different Web sites? Search engines have programs called spiders that traverse the Internet looking for new Web pages. The search engine maintains a catalog of Web pages and then matches user-entered keyword(s) to that catalog. The matches are displayed on the results page(s). Different search engines have different ways of operating spiders and indexing and retrieving results. The way the catalog of Web sites is generated may produce different results for different search engines.

CHOOSING KEYWORDS

Selecting keywords for Internet research is as much an art as it is a science. A good approach is to imagine the title or text for the perfect article. What words or phrases might appear in that article? Once a few keywords are identified, you can list possible synonyms for those keywords. It is helpful to include singular and plural versions of keywords. This sometimes produces different results (Haase et al., 2007). Different keywords, even small variations, can produce different types of results.

For example, imagine that you are a nurse looking for information to help a patient quit smoking. You first enter "quitting smoking" into the search engine, and the number of Web site results is over 6 million. You then enter "quit smoking" into the search engine. The number of results is lowered to 4 million. This is still a large number of sites to review, and you realize that most of the Web sites are targeted to people who are trying to quit smoking. Finally, you change the keywords to "smoking cessation clinical" and the number of results drops 1.8 million. The number of results is now more manageable and more focused on what you are actually looking for. As a triage example, imagine you are a nurse who receives a call from a patient who needs current information on abnormally heavy periods. You may want to begin your search with the keywords "abnormally heavy periods." Possible synonyms that you will want to include in your search are "heavy menstrual flow," "heavy menstrual bleeding," and "menorrhagia."

It is important to track the keywords and search engines you use when you are conducting extensive research. It is very easy to become so involved in Internet searches, listing keywords and search engines, that you wind up reviewing the same information over and over again. Table 4.1 is an example of an Internet Search Tracking Form. The column on the far left is used to list keywords and phrases. Across the top, search engines are listed. The use of a tracking form helps you avoid confusion and duplication of effort while conducting Internet research.

Table 4.1 Internet Search Tracking Form

Keywords	Google	Yahoo	PubMed
Abnormally heavy periods			
Heavy menstrual flow			
Heavy menstrual bleeding			
Menorrhagia			

Generating keywords is somewhat of a "trial and error" process. After reading some of the Web sites, you may identify additional keywords. You can add new keywords to your form if you find them helpful.

ENTERING KEYWORDS

Operator names used in computer search engines typically use such terms as AND (+), OR, and NOT (−). Entering these operators between keywords or phrases tells the search engine what type of results you want.

- **Using AND (+):** The default operator for most search engines is AND. For instance, when you enter "weight loss programs" into a search engine, the search engine looks for pages that include weight AND loss AND programs. Whether you use the words "and," "or," or "not" makes a big difference in terms of how much information you will retrieve.
- **Using OR:** Web sites that contain either "labor" or "delivery" in the text can be located by entering the keywords "labor OR delivery" in the search engine.
- **Using NOT (−):** NOT is used to eliminate a word or phrase from your search results.
- **Using Quotation Marks (" "):** Websites that contain a phrase in a specific order can be identified by putting the phrase inside double quotation marks (" "). Web sites that contain the separate words are not listed on the results page.

Table 4.2 contains examples of the results that may be found by using specific keywords and operators.

RESULTS DISPLAY

The exact format of the results that are displayed varies with the search engine used; however, there are common elements among the different results displays. These include the keyword textbox, number of results found, sponsored sites, related searches, and results entries. The keyword textbox contains the keywords you entered on the search engine's main page. This textbox gives you the opportunity to make changes to the keywords and resubmit a search or start a new search. The number of results lets you determine how many Web pages were found that match the keywords you entered, as well as the time it took the search engine to complete the search. Table 4.3 shows the results that were generated when the words "high risk pregnancy" were searched for.

If the number of Web page results is in the millions, adding additional keywords to the search may narrow the focus of the search and generate better results. If the number of results is less than 200, you have probably done a comprehensive search, and making the search less specific may yield results that are not as helpful.

When reviewing search results, a common pitfall people make is to access the Web pages that are the first ones listed on the results page. They are easy to access, no scrolling is required, and no clicking to the next page of results is necessary. However, by understanding the order of results of the search engine, you can gain insight into the Web page's content.

Table 4.2 Examples of Keywords, Operators, and Results from Internet Searches

Information needed	Keywords used	Example of keywords entered	Results
Heavy menstrual bleeding	*Heavy menstrual bleeding*	*Heavy menstrual bleeding*	Pages containing *heavy*, *menstrual*, and *bleeding* somewhere.
Weight-loss programs excluding crash diets	*weight loss crash diet*	*weight loss* NOT *crash* *weight loss* NOT *crash diet*	The results for this search include all the pages that contain the words *weight*, *loss*, and *programs*. If the page includes *crash*, it is not displayed. If the page includes *crash diet*, it is not displayed.
Labor without inducing labor	*Pregnancy labor inducing*	*Pregnancy labor* NOT *inducing* Note: In Google the keywords would be entered *pregnancy labor-inducing*.	Pages that contain *pregnancy* and *labor*, discarding all the results that contain the word *inducing*.
Web pages or articles with the specific phrase *removing uterine fibroids*	*Removing uterine fibroids*	*removing uterine fibroids*	Pages containing the words *removing uterine fibroids* in that order. Pages that contain those words but not in that order are not displayed.

Popular Web sites are frequently listed at the top of the results page. Consequently, Web sites such as Wikipedia frequently appear as one of the first results during a search. Unfortunately, Wikipedia is fraught with problems, since information on Wikipedia is usually not peer reviewed by a group of recognized experts in the field.

Sponsored links are frequently found at the top of a search and along the right side of the results window, or at the top of the screen. These sites are prominently listed

Table 4.3 Results from Keyword Search *High Risk Pregnancy*

Search engine used	Number of web site / web page results
www.live.com	One of 742,576 results
www.google.com	Results 1–100 of 4,280,000 for *high risk pregnancy* (0.27 seconds)
www.yahoo.com	Results 1–10 of approx 12,000,000 for *high risk pregnancy* (0.53 seconds)

because a company or group has paid to have its link appear prominently on the results page when certain keywords are entered. The location on the results page does not indicate the quality of the sponsored link's content, only that the placement of the link has been purchased.

When the search results in a large number of hits, a search engine may provide related search links (or "also try" links) that focus the results. For example, in Yahoo a search for "high risk pregnancy" may produce related/also try links such as sites dealing with "high risk pregnancy symptoms" and "high risk pregnancy management." This is the search engine's attempt to assist you in narrowing the search.

While you are using a search engine, you will probably find it helpful to scan the results for the bold text that indicates the keywords and check to see if they are in the necessary order for the search you are conducting. Be sure to look at the Web site address or URL for that result. Is it for a recognized organization? For example, the address for the Mayo Clinic is www.mayoclinic.com (not hospitalinminnesota.com), and the Center for Disease Control's address is www.cdc.gov.

EVALUATING WEB PAGE CONTENT

Once you have identified important Web sites, you must evaluate the information on the site. It is good to be cautious about the information found on the Internet until you look at the background of those who created the site and determine whether they have expertise in an area or if they have an agenda they want to advertise. Here are some key elements that you'll want to consider:

A recent phenomenon on the Internet is user-generated content. User-generated content is found on Web sites, blogs, message boards, etc., where individuals can post information on the Internet without having any particular knowledge on the topic. Some Web sites are designed so that many different users can contribute to its content. Wikipedia is an example of a user-generated, collaborative Web site. Anyone in that user community can add, delete, or modify the information. This can be done without demonstrating any particular knowledge about the subject matter. Consequently, there is no way to verify the credentials of a person who enters content into the site. These sites themselves cannot be a reliable source of information. However, the references on these sites may provide reliable references for that subject.

The identity of the Web page creator sometimes provides insight into the context of the site's content. This information is frequently located at the top of the Web page.

Sometimes it is difficult to determine who wrote the content on a particular Web site. The sponsor of a Web site can often be found by clicking on the "About Us" link on a Web site's home page. Information about a Web site's author/sponsor may also be found at the bottom of the main page or in the copyright or disclaimer information. For example, a site sponsored by a drug company may have a much different view of a topic than an article that has been peer reviewed. It is important to keep this in mind while reviewing Web content.

PATIENTS AND THE INTERNET

Research by Pew Internet & American Life Project indicates that millions of patients access the Internet each year in search of health information. In addition, research by these groups confirms that these same patients believe Internet content impacted their health care decisions. Consequently, providers need to help patients decide on the credibility of information that is accessible on the Internet (Fox and Rainie, 2006; Spink et al., 2004).

SCHOLARLY SEARCH ENGINES/DATABASES

Google, Yahoo, Live, and Ask are search engines that help users find Web pages using specific keywords. There are special databases you can search to find scholarly articles. Different types of scholarly databases are accessible over the Internet. Some provide electronic versions of abstracts, while others provide electronic versions of abstracts and full-text articles.

There are two steps to the process of conducting research using scholarly databases: a) identifying relevant articles on your topic, and b) locating those articles in either electronic or paper form. You may find Box 4.1 helpful when you want to search for evidence-based information on a particular women's health subject.

Once you have searched one of these sites and printed out any pertinent abstract, you can evaluate the abstract to determine whether the article seems relevant. When the online citation displays hyperlinks labeled "full-text," "full-text html," and/or "full-text pdf" as an option on the citation display, this means that you can get the entire article text online. Whether or not an entire article is available online depends on the type of database subscriptions offered by a particular publisher or organization.

Some large organizations have subscriptions that permit database access from a particular network or building. When this is the case, clicking on the full-text hyperlink will bring up the online article. This can be printed for later use. If the database allows individual access, you will usually need a login and password that you must purchase. Some Web sites will allow you to purchase 24–hour access to their database articles at a discounted price. There are other databases that allow users to purchase a single copy of an article for a fixed fee.

When a "for fee" article is identified, it is a good idea to look for other Web sites that may have a free online version of the article. In a search engine (such as Google, Yahoo, or Live), enter the title of the article. Remember that the search engine retrieves Web pages in which all the keywords are listed on the page. Consequently, the results page may display many results, but not all of them will have the correct title.

Box 4-1	Scholarly Search Engines (Giustini)

scholar.google.com
academic.live.com
pubmed.org
scirus.com
http://www.tripdatabase.com
http://www.cochrane.org/index.htm
http://www.uptodate.com/
Medline
Cindhal

PROPER USE OF THE INTERNET

In summary, the Internet has the potential to be a powerful tool for triage nurses. At the same time, there exists a tremendous potential for misuse by providers and patients alike. Make certain you familiarize yourself with the Internet utilization techniques mentioned in this chapter before you recommend Web sites to patients or assess the credibility of information retrieved online.

Once you are comfortable with this powerful resource, be sure to build time into your schedule to review and update recommended resources. As instantaneous as the "Net" can be, sites can become outdated quickly if not properly maintained. This is perhaps more important in the health care field, where information, new research, medications, and treatments change frequently. Make certain you are not pointing patients to obsolete information.

References

Fox, S. & Rainie, L. (2006). The online health care revolution: How the Web helps Americans take better care of themselves. Pew Internet and American Life Project: Online life report. Retrieved July 12, 2008, from http://www.perInternet.org.

Franklin, C. (2007). How Internet search engines work. Retrieved July 12, 2007, from http://computer.howstuffworks.com/search-engine.htm.

Giustini, D. (2005). How Google is changing medicine. *British Medical Journal, 331*, 1487–1448.

Haase, A., M. Follmann, G. Skipka, & H. Kirchner. (2007). Developing search strategies for clinical practice guidelines in SUMSearch and Google Scholar and assessing their retrieval performance. *BMC Medical Research Methodology, 7*, 28.

Haynes, R., Wilcznski, N., Wong, S., et al. (1994). Developing optimal search strategies for detecting clinical sound studies in MEDLINE. *Journal of the American Medical Informatics Association, 1*(6), 447–458.

Internet Assigned Numbers Authority. Retrieved September 6, 2007, from http://www.iana.org/gtld/gtld.htm.

McKeown, M. (1997). Use of Internet for obstetricians and gynecologists. *American Journal of Obstetrics and Gynecology, 176*, 271–274.

Spink, A., Yang, Y., Jansen, J., Nykanen, P., Lorence, D. P., Ozmutlu, S., & Ozmutlu, H. C. (2004). A study of medical and health queries to Web search engines. *Health Information and Libraries Journal, 21*, 44–51.

PART II

OBSTETRIC PROTOCOLS

CHAPTER 5

Preconceptual and Infertility Overview

All women who are considering a pregnancy warrant a preconceptual counseling visit. A number of issues should be covered during this appointment, including:

- institution of relatively simple measures that may improve pregnancy outcomes (folic acid, altering work place hazards);
- identification of medical factors that may have an impact on a pregnancy;
- consideration of psychosocial factors that may place the woman at greater risk (poverty, abuse);
- screening and testing for certain diseases and genetic conditions; and
- adjustment of medications and treatments that may be harmful to a fetus.

Unfortunately, not all women attempting a pregnancy will be successful at conceiving. Generally, if a woman is younger than 35 years and has not conceived after 1 year without using contraception, she should be scheduled for an infertility evaluation. If the woman is 35 years or older, most practices will schedule such a visit if she is unable to conceive after 6 months. Many practices will request that the woman's partner have a semen analysis as the first step in an infertility evaluation. A semen analysis is inexpensive and provides a good assessment of potential male factor infertility problems. The initial evaluation of female-related factors is determined by the practice but often includes fertility monitoring, assessment of tubal patency, evaluation of the lining of the uterus, and hormonal testing.

Infertility testing and management can become quite involved and expensive, often requiring rather exotic procedures at specialized infertility centers. Most womens' health care providers, if unsuccessful with routine infertility measures, will refer their patients to such centers.

Despite the many advances in infertility technology, many couples fail to conceive or decide not to pursue assisted reproductive technologies. Some pursue adoption options, and others decide to remain childless. In all cases, it is important to support the choices made by the couple.

This section provides a simple 30-day infertility workup for women who have regular menstrual cycles. Common infertility tests and medications often prescribed to assist with conception are given. It is important to establish the infertility standard in your practice. Only those issues practical for telephone discussion are included here.

BASIC TRIAGE ASSESSMENT FORM FOR AN OBSTETRIC PATIENT'S EXPOSURE TO ENVIRONMENTAL AND HOUSEHOLD CHEMICALS

1. How many weeks pregnant are you? _____
2. What substance do you think you have been exposed to? _____
3. Where did this exposure occur (workplace, home, friend's house)? _____
4. What was the nature of the exposure (inhaled, poured on skin, came through air duct)? _____
5. If this exposure occurred at work, what action was taken? _____
6. If this exposure occurred at work, is this a substance with which you regularly work and for which a Material Data Safety Sheet exists? _____
7. Have you experienced any symptoms since the exposure? _____

BASIC TRIAGE ASSESSMENT FORM FOR AN OBSTETRIC PATIENT'S EXPOSURE TO COMMUNICABLE DISEASES

1. How many weeks pregnant are you? _____
2. When do you think the exposure occurred? _____
3. Have you ever been exposed to _____ before?
4. Did you have _____ as a child?
5. Did you previously receive a vaccination against _____?
6. Do you have any symptoms indicative of a communicable disease? _____

Exposure to Selected Communicable Diseases in Pregnancy

(Note: Please refer to STI chart for some additional diseases.)

Name of Disease	Presenting Symptoms	Incubation Period	Mode of Transmission	Usual Course	Important Facts in Pregnancy
Chicken pox (Varicella)	Low-grade fever, followed by rash beginning on face and scalp in 24 hours, spreading quickly to trunk	12–18 days	Droplets or aerosols from vesicle fluid; secretions of the upper respiratory tract of infected individuals. Virus is disseminated across the placenta.	After initial rash, lesions appear for approximately 5 days; intense pruritus is characteristic. Antibodies appear after 5 days. Crusted lesions are not infectious.	Symptoms are more pronounced in adults; 14% of infected pregnant women develop varicella pneumonia. Relatively low frequency of anomalies in first half of pregnancy. Most extreme manifestation is varicella embryopathy, reported in approx 1%–2%.* Preterm labor occurs in 14%. Infection 5 days before and 2 days after delivery may result in neonatal disease.
Fifth disease (Parvovirus B19)	Mild prodrome with low-grade fever, headache, malaise, often unnoticed, followed by hallmark "slapped-cheek" rash. Adults may present with symmetrical arthralgias.	4–20 days	Probably by droplets from oral or nasal secretions. Virus found in upper respiratory tract secretions and blood several days before symptoms. Placental transmission possible in primary maternal infections.	In adults, most common course is malaise and arthralgia; rash may not be evident. Rash, if present, usually resolves in about 3 weeks. Patients with underlying hemoglobinopathy may have a transient aplastic crisis.	Chance of infection of a susceptible pregnant woman from an infected household member is 50%–90%; daycare or classroom exposure 20%–30%. Fetal risk is greatest in 1st trimester maternal illness, rate of maternal-fetal transmission is 5%–15%. Fetal hydrops results, leading to an aplastic anemia and congestive heart failure. No structural anomalies seen.

Measles (rubeola)	Fever, malaise, coryza, conjunctivitis, photosensitivity; generalized maculopapular rash; Koplik's spots.[†]	10–12 days	Respiratory droplets; virus can cross the placenta.	Typical rash begins on face and neck, spreading to trunk and extremities, lasting approximately 5 days, receding in order of appearance. Disease associated with an increase in maternal mortality during pregnancy, primarily because of pulmonary complications.	Infected pregnant women need close monitoring for hepatitis, encephalitis, and pneumonia. Slight increase in preterm delivery and spontaneous abortions. Congenital anomalies not significant. Neonatal measles develop within 10 days of delivery in infants of acutely infected mothers.
Rubella (German measles)	Half of affected individuals have no symptoms. Simultaneous occurrence of low-grade fever, mild upper respiratory tract infection, and macular pruritic rash.	14–18 days	Respiratory transmission; virus shed from 1 week before to 3 weeks after acute illness.	Rash fades within 1 to 3 days of onset. Posterior cervical and occipital adenopathy may be the only presenting symptoms, peaking at the time of rash. Usual recovery is 3–4 days. Major complication is acute polyarthralgia, possibly persisting for days to weeks.	Timing of gestation is most critical in the fetal/natal course. Infection as early as 12 days after LMP may cause fetal infection. Maternal infection before 16 weeks may lead to ocular, cardiac, and CNS systems being adversely affected. Approximately 20% of exposed individuals, even as late as exposure in the 6 month of gestation, have manifestations 10–20 years later.

Continued

Exposure to Selected Communicable Diseases in Pregnancy—cont'd
(Note: Please refer to STI chart for some additional diseases.)

Name of Disease	Presenting Symptoms	Incubation Period	Mode of Transmission	Usual Course	Important Facts in Pregnancy
Toxoplasmosis (*Toxoplasma gondii*)	No real course of disease is noted in immune-intact individuals. Manifestations are seen in immune-compromised individuals and the fetus.	No real incubation period. After inoculation or ingestion, the organism invades cells directly or is affected by phagocytosis.	Ingested in under-cooked meat; oocysts in cat feces; blood transfusion; placental transmission during maternal parasitemia.	Course of infection is influenced by size of inoculation, virulence of organism, and immune status of the patient. For immunosuppressed individuals and the fetus, infection may result in massive tissue destruction in multiple organs, primarily the brain and eye in the fetus.	Acute maternal infection is necessary for fetal/neonatal manifestations; 40% of infants born to acutely infected mothers have signs of infection. Congenital infection is most likely in 3rd trimester exposure. Less than 40% of infants whose mothers are infected develop toxoplasmosis complications. Wide range of clinical presentations.

*Varicella embryopathy has multiple anomalies, including limb hypoplasia, cutaneous scarring, microcephaly, psychomotor retardation, malformed digits, and ocular abnormalities.

†Koplik's spots are blue-gray specks with a red base, developing across from the 2nd molars on the buccal mucosa.

Cleaning Agents

ASSESSMENT

1. Are you planning on using a cleaning agent during pregnancy?

ACTION

YES Go to Step A.
NO No action.

ACTIONS

STEP A: Use of Cleaning Agents

Read product labels and cautions closely before using any household cleaner.

Most cleaners are safe in pregnancy. However, to be on the safe side, always wear gloves and use in a well-ventilated room.

Avoid mixing cleaning products, especially those with chlorine bleach and those containing ammonia. Toxic fumes may develop.

Cleaners with strong fumes, such as tile cleaners and oven cleaners, should be used by someone who is not pregnant.

Pump sprays deliver fewer droplets than do aerosol sprays, decreasing the amount of cleaner that can be inhaled.

Cord Blood Banking

ASSESSMENT	ACTION
1. Do you know what cord blood banking is?	**YES** Go to Question 2.
	NO Go to Step A.
2. Are you interested in cord blood banking?	**YES** Go to Step B.
	NO Go to Patient Education.
3. Are you aware of controversies surrounding core blood banking?	**YES** Go to Patient Education.
	NO Go to Step C.

ACTIONS

STEP A: Definition of Cord Blood Banking

Cord blood is the blood that remains in the newborn's umbilical cord after the cord has been cut. This blood is rich in stem cells. Stem cells are used to treat, and sometimes cure, several life-threatening diseases. These diseases include cancers, such as various forms of leukemia and lymphoma; diseases of bone marrow failure, such as aplastic anemia; blood disorders, such as sickle cell anemia; and diseases of inborn metabolic errors and immunodeficiency origin. New uses for stem cells are under constant research because of the unique ability of these cells to heal and regenerate.

Cord blood must be harvested at the time of delivery. Arrangements must be made before labor to obtain a collection kit that the delivering physician or midwife will use to collect the blood. You will be provided with a special kit and instructions for mailing the specimen back to the company you contract with. Typical fees cover the collection kit, shipping, processing, and testing, and the first year of storage. There are yearly storage fees. The person delivering your baby may charge a collection fee, which may or may not be covered by insurance.

The harvested stem cells are a genetic match to your infant and may be used by other family members in some situations. It is common for the baby's mother or siblings to receive benefit. Cord blood has been used in medical treatment 15 years after collection with proper storage, and there is no current expiration date for properly collected, shipped, and stored stem cells derived from cord blood.

STEP B: Arranging for Cord Blood Banking

Your OB/GYN practice may have literature and/or collection kits onsite from one of the major companies involved in cord blood banking. You may sign up at any time, but signing up early guarantees that you are prepared in case of premature delivery. You should research more than one company before deciding where you will "bank" your cord blood. Two reputable sources are listed below:

CBR	1-888-932-6568	http://www.cordblood.com
ViaCord	1-866-668-4895	http://www.viacord.com

STEP C: Controversies Surrounding Cord Blood Banking?

Controversies abound regarding the value of private cord blood banking. Professional medical organizations caution against over-optimistic claims and believe patients should not see it as insurance against future illness. There is concern there is latent disease (perhaps the disease intended to be treated) in the preserved blood. No one knows for certain how long blood can be stored. Official recommendations from the American Academy of Pediatrics and the American Society for Blood and Marrow Transplantation advise against private banking except in cases where an existing close relative has already been diagnosed with a condition for which a stem cell transplant would offer a therapeutic option. Here are two sources from professional medical organizations to help you form your own opinion. Watch their Web sites for continued updates:

American College of Obstetricians and Gynecologists	http://www.acog.org
American Academy of Pediatrics	http://aappolicy.aappublications.org

Unfortunately, public banking does not exist in all states. The National Marrow Donor Program includes a list of public banks by states and is included as a reference to refer patients to who are interested in public banking:

http://www.marrow.org/index.html

PATIENT EDUCATION

Many patients are confused about stem cells because of the political and ethical controversies surrounding *embryonic* stem cells. Cord blood is a readily available source of stem cells that if not "banked" will simply be thrown away. There is no controversy in cord blood banking. This point needs to be clarified to ensure that patients make an informed decision.

Many patients wonder if there is chance they or a family member will ever need to use the banked cells. It is currently estimated that the odds of being diagnosed with a condition that may benefit from treatment with cord blood stem cells is variable with 1 in 2,700 reported most frequently. Those odds will increase as these cells are used in the treatment of more diseases, such as other cancers, multiple sclerosis, heart disease, and diabetes.

Food Safety in Pregnancy

KEY QUESTIONS

ASSESSMENT	ACTION

1. Do you know the basic rules of clean, separate, cook, and chill for food safety?

YES Go to Question 2.
NO Go to Step A.

2. Do you eat fish?

YES Go to Step B.
NO Go to Question 3.

3. Do you eat cheese and/or unpasteurized dairy products?

YES Go to Step C.
NO Go to Question 4.

4. Do you eat deli meats, paté, smoked fish, or hot dogs?

YES Go to Step D.
NO Go to Question 5.

5. Do you have cats that hunt and eat prey or are fed raw meat?

YES Go to Step E.
NO No action.

ACTIONS

STEP A: Basic Rules of Food Safety

The basic rules of food safety are: clean, separate, cook, and chill. First, "clean" means to thoroughly wash your hands with soap and water before handling food, especially after using the restroom or changing diapers. Fresh fruits and vegetables should be cleaned by rinsing them under running water. Surfaces on which raw foods are prepared should be cleaned after use. Plastic cutting boards are safer than wooden ones because they are not porous. "Separate" refers to keeping raw foods and foods to be cooked from coming in contact with each other during preparation. There should be separate surfaces for preparing meats and fresh fruits and vegetables prior to cooking. Next, all foods to be cooked should be cooked thoroughly. Undercooked meat or eggs can be dangerous. Finally, "chill" refers to proper refrigeration of perishable foods. Never leave perishable food out of the refrigerator for more than 2 hours.

STEP B: Food Safety Advice for Consuming Fish

One of the greatest controversies in food safety currently is the issue of methyl mercury in fish. Methyl mercury can harm the developing nervous system of a developing baby. The controversy is fueled by economic issues in the fish industry as well as by a lack of knowledge about how methyl mercury "invades" the fish. As a source of food, fish is a wonderful low-fat protein. Because fish generally lack fat, harmful substances can be stored in the flesh. The larger, long-lived fish are the biggest problem. Four fish should not be eaten during pregnancy: shark, swordfish, king mackerel, and tilefish.

Controversy also surrounds the other fish selections. The current FDA regulations recommend no more than 12 ounces per week of seafood. Freshwater fish should be eaten in amounts recommended by local authorities. Tuna is currently a fish in the "suspect" category. Follow the 12-ounce per week rule, noting that the average tuna sandwich contains 2 oz of fish. Smaller tuna, such as yellowfin, may be less harmful than larger tuna, such as albacore. Other canned fish are not considered suspect. Shellfish are not currently in question, but the source of the shellfish should be known. Do not purchase from unknown roadside vendors whose basic food safety rules may be in question. Do not eat uncooked sushi while pregnant. In this case the issue is not methyl mercury but rather bacteria and parasites.

STEP C: Food Safety Advice for Selected Dairy Products

Unpasteurized or "raw" dairy products, notably cheese, may be a source of the food-borne illness listeriosis, which is caused by the bacteria *Listeria*. Although the symptoms are flulike, the onset of the disease may be greatly delayed, causing the pregnant woman to pass the disease to her unborn baby without feeling sick. *Listeria* can survive in cold temperatures. It is important to keep the refrigerator clean and make sure the temperature is at or below 40°F. Fortunately, in the United States, almost all types of cheese can be found pasteurized, including soft cheeses like brie and feta. Most cases of listeriosis in the United States can be traced to a soft cheese called queso fresco, a Hispanic cheese made with raw milk.

STEP D: Food Safety Advice for Deli Meats, etc.

Listeriosis can also be cause by improperly handled deli meats, smoked fish, patés, and hot dogs. Remember, it can survive in the cold. Hot dogs should only be eaten thoroughly cooked. Canned smoked fish and patés are acceptable. Use caution or avoid processed deli meats altogether. Any purchased meats that will not be cooked prior to eating should be stored in refrigeration under 40°F and used within 5 days of purchase.

STEP E: Safety Advice for Avoiding Toxoplasmosis Exposure

The parasite *Toxoplasmagondii* causes toxoplasmosis. It is a disease often associated with cats. This is unfortunate since cats in general are not the problem. Cats that hunt and eat their prey, or are fed raw meat, can be a problem because the parasite is passed through feces. Pregnant women who have cats should have someone else clean the litter box or should wear disposable gloves when cleaning it themselves. Daily litter box cleaning will prevent the problem because the parasite is not infective in feces for 1–5 days.

In actuality, toxoplasmosis infection is more likely to be caused by ingested meat. Pigs, sheep, and deer can carry the parasite. Fruits and vegetables grown in soil infected with the parasite are also a source of transmission. Follow the rules of clean, separate, cook, and chill.

PATIENT EDUCATION

Instruct patients to pay attention to local guidelines, recommendations, and potential warnings for fish and shellfish.

Federal updates can be found on the FDA's Web site: http://vm.cfsan.fda.gov

Hair Dye and Permanent Wave Exposure

KEY QUESTIONS

ASSESSMENT

ACTION

1. Are you planning to dye your hair or treat it with
   a permanent wave?

YES Go to Step A.
NO No action.

ACTIONS

STEP A: Hair Dye or Permanent Wave

Animal studies have indicated that hair dyes and permanent waves may be toxic to a
fetus. However, these studies used concentrations that were much higher than those
used by women.

For women who decide to use hair dyes or permanent waves, some simple suggestions
may reduce the degree to which the fetus is exposed to these chemicals.

- Avoid using during the first 3 months of pregnancy, when many of the fetal organ
  systems are developing.
- Don't "scrub" or "rub" the permanent wave or dye solution into the scalp. Most of
  the chemicals in these products are absorbed through the skin, so minimizing
  skin/scalp exposure probably is helpful.
- Use semipermanent dye and wave solutions. These usually are less concentrated
  than the permanent forms of such products.
- The use of highlights, where just the tips of the hair or small sections of the hair are
  treated, may result in less exposure.

Paint Exposure

KEY QUESTIONS

ASSESSMENT	ACTION
1. Are you planning to use latex paint?	**YES** Go to Step A.
	NO Go to Question 2.
2. Are you planning to use spray paint?	**YES** Go to Step B.
	NO Go to Question 3.
3. Are you planning to use oil- or lead-based paint?	**YES** Go to Step C.
	NO Go to Question 4.
4. Are you planning to use a sealant or shellac?	**YES** Go to Step D.
	NO Go to Question 5.
5. Are you planning to use art supply types of paint?	**YES** Go to Step E.
	NO No action.

ACTIONS

STEP A: Latex Paints

Latex paints generally are safe for use during pregnancy. Avoid latex paints manufactured before 1990 because some may contain mercury, which was added to some latex paints before 1990.

As with all paints, try to use in a well-ventilated room.

Using a roller or brush results in less inhalation of the paint than does using a sprayer.

STEP B: Spray Paints

Avoid spray paints with m-butyl ketone (or MBK) because it has been associated with neurological damage in newborns who were exposed during pregnancy.

As with all paints, try to use in a well-ventilated room.

Using a roller or brush results in less inhalation of the paint than does using a sprayer.

STEP C: Oil- or Lead-Based Paints

Oil- and lead-based paints should be avoided during pregnancy. Research studies indicate that lead can be toxic to developing fetuses, and many oil-based paints may contain mercury as a preservative.

STEP D: Sealants and Shellacs

Some animal research has shown sealant and shellac fumes may be hazardous during pregnancy. If they are used, avoid using a sprayer, and keep the room well ventilated, or better yet, try to do the project outdoors.

STEP E: Artists' Paints

There are many types of art supplies available. To check the safety of a particular supply, the patient can call The Arts, Crafts, and Theater Safety Group at (212) 777-0062.

PATIENT EDUCATION

Many paint thinners and cleaners produce potentially toxic fumes. Latex paint and many art paints can be cleaned with soap and water. If turpentine or paint thinner is required, have someone who is not pregnant clean up the supplies. In all cases, use gloves and avoid the fumes.

Pesticide Use

ASSESSMENT

1. Are you planning to use a pesticide?

ACTION

YES Go to Step A.
NO No action.

ACTIONS

STEP A: Pesticide Use

Almost all pesticides have been found to be harmful when a woman has been exposed to them for long periods of time. Studies indicate pesticide use can be associated with limb deformities and neurological problems. Thus, pregnant women generally should not use pesticides or be exposed to them for long periods of time.

Because there are hundreds of different pesticides, we recommend that the patient call the Pesticide Hotline at (800) 858-7378 for questions about a specific pesticide.

Common 30-Day Female Infertility Workup for Women With 28- to 30-Day Cycles

Women experiencing irregular cycles, certain medical problems, or gynecological problems should be evaluated and treated by a health care provider.

KEY QUESTIONS

ASSESSMENT	ACTION
1. Are you on the first day of your menstrual period?	**YES** Go to Step A. **NO** Start this infertility workup on the first day of your menses.
2. Once you are on the first day of your menstrual period, count this as Day 1 of your cycle. Begin the procedure as outlined in this protocol.	**YES** Go to Question 3 on Day 2 to 3 of your cycle. **NO** Return to Question 1.
3. Are you on Day 2 to 3 of your cycle?	**YES** Have blood drawn for serum follicle stimulating hormone (FSH) and estradiol levels and begin charting basal body temperature. **NO** No action.
4. Are you on Day 6 to 10 of your cycle?	**YES** Have hysterosalpingogram (HSG) performed. **NO** Return to Question 1.
5. Are you on Day 10 of your cycle?	**YES** Begin using ovulation predictor kit daily until the color change occurs (LH surge). **NO** Return to Question 1.
6. Has the color change occurred on the ovulation predictor kit?	**YES** Begin having intercourse. **NO** Return to Question 1.

7. Are you on the day after the color change?	**YES** Perform postcoital test 2 to 24 hours after intercourse.
	NO Return to Question 1.
8. Are you on Days 7 to 9 after the color change?	**YES** Have serum progesterone level assessed.
	NO Return to Question 1.
9. Are you on Days 14 to 17 after the color change?	**YES** Are you menstruating? If so, call treating physician and go to Step A.
	NO Schedule a B-HCG test and go to Step B.
10. Are you late for your menstrual period?	**YES** Go to Step C.
	NO Return to Question 1.

ACTIONS

STEP A: Getting Started

Ensure the patient is receiving adequate folic acid supplementation.

Most women should be receiving 0.4 mg folic acid/day supplementation; this can be accomplished by taking daily prenatal vitamins.

Women who experienced a prior pregnancy that resulted in a baby or a fetus with a neural tube defect should be given 4 mg folic acid/day supplementation.

STEP B: Menses After Completion of the Infertility Workup

Schedule consultation with attending provider to discuss results of the tests that were performed and to determine a plan of care; continue basal body temperature charting unless otherwise instructed.

STEP C: No Menses After Completion of the Infertility Workup

Call office within a few days after laboratory studies are done to review results.

If results of the B-HCG test are positive and the serum progesterone level is normal, schedule a follow-up appointment for ultrasound in 2 weeks; you may also be instructed to have the B-HCG level assessed again 2 days after the initial positive result to confirm normalcy of the rising levels.

If the serum progesterone level is low and the pregnancy test result is negative, schedule a follow-up appointment with the physician for additional evaluation.

PATIENT EDUCATION

Emphasize the need to begin the workup on the first day of the menstrual cycle and that the timing of each test is critical.

Make sure the patient receives folic acid supplementation, either in the form of plain folic acid or by means of prenatal vitamins.

Be available to answer any questions or review instructions, as needed.

BASIC TRIAGE ASSESSMENT FORM FOR PREGNANCY

1. What was the first day of your last menstrual period?_____
2. What is your parity? _____
   a. Full-term pregnancies? _____
   b. Premature deliveries? _____
   c. Abortions? Spontaneous abortions? Therapeutic abortions? _____
   d. Living children? _____
   e. Ectopic pregnancies? _____
3. Have you had any pregnancy-related problems in either this pregnancy or in a past pregnancy? _____
4. Do you have any medical problems? _____

Commonly Used Infertility Medications*

Medication	Pharmacology	Typical Dosage	Nursing Considerations
Clomiphene citrate (Clomid, Serophene)	Antiestrogenic drug. Stimulates the pituitary to release FSH by effectively reducing the circulating estradiol levels. Consequently increases follicular development. Used for ovulatory disorders in patients with an intact hypothalamic-pituitary-ovarian axis. May be particularly useful in patients with infrequent or long menstrual cycles.	50 mg every day for 5 days, beginning on days 3–7 of the menstrual cycle. Increased in increments of 50 mg/day, to a maximum of 200 mg/day for 5 days.	Side effects include possible hot flushes, headaches, ovarian hyperstimulation (cysts), poor cervical mucous. Avoid more than 6 months of therapy because longer duration of therapy may not be of clinical benefit. The multiple-pregnancy rate is 5%–9%, generally twins. Symptoms of ovarian hyperstimulation (rare) may include increased pelvic pressure/pain, fluid shift, and abdominal bloating, and can be serious. If a patient is taking this medication and calls with pelvic complaints, she should be evaluated promptly for possible ovarian hyperstimulation.
Follicle stimulating hormone (recombinant) (Follistim, Gonal-F)	Used to induce ovulation in an anovulatory woman or to increase the number of mature follicles produced in a single cycle. Most commonly prescribed for patients who have no response to clomiphene citrate, have unexplained infertility, or are undergoing *in vitro* fertilization. Can be used in combination with clomiphene citrate.	Supplied in 75-IU ampules. Subcutaneous or intramuscular administration. Dosage is highly individualized. Generally, the initial dose is 150 IU/day, but it may be increased or decreased based on current or previous response.	These medications should only be prescribed by a physician who is thoroughly familiar with the risks, benefits, and potential complications that may result from gonadotropin therapy. (S)he also should be able to perform necessary monitoring with ultrasound and same-day estradiol level assessments 7 days a week. The patient may experience mild burning, stinging, or redness at the injection site.

Gonadotropin releasing hormone (GnRH) analogs (leuprolide, Lupron, nafarelin, Synarel)	Synthetic medication with pituitary-binding properties. Acts to decrease FSH and LH stores and suppress production and release of FSH and LH. Used to suppress estradiol production from the ovary for treatment of endometriosis and uterine fibroids. Also used commonly as an adjunct in in vitro fertilization treatment.	Intramuscular administration: (Depo-Lupron) 3.75 mg monthly or 11.25 mg every 3 months for treatment of endometriosis or uterine fibroids. Treatment may be continued for a total of 6 months. Subcutaneous administration: To 1 mg per day as an adjunct to in vivo fertilization with gonadotropins.	Patients should be apprised of the risks of multiple pregnancy and ovarian hyperstimulation syndrome (which can commonly occur). These medications are generally self-administered or administered by the patient's partner.
	Rapid fall in testosterone levels occurs within 1 week of administration.	Nasal spray (Synarel, nafarelin): 1 spray/day, alternating nostrils each day. Most commonly used as an adjunct to in vivo fertilization treatment with gonadotropins, but may be used for as long as 6 months for treatment of endometriosis or uterine fibroids.	Side effects include hot flushes, dyspareunia (uncomfortable intercourse) resulting from vaginal dryness, headache, insomnia, and moodiness. Decreased libido may be experienced by some patients. Use refrigeration to store an open vial.
Gonadotropin releasing hormone antagonist (Antagon, Cetrotide)	Intended for the inhibition of premature LH surges in women undergoing ovulation induction with gonadotropins. Ultra-rapid onset of action and short half-life.	Subcutaneous administration: Treatment is begun approximately 6 days after the start of gonadotropin stimulation.	Should not be given in the same syringe with gonadotropins.

Commonly Used Infertility Medications*

Medication	Pharmacology	Typical Dosage	Nursing Considerations
Human Chorionic Gonadotropin (hCG) (Ovidrel, Pregnyl, Profasi, Novarel)	Bioactivity similar to LH. Used to mimic the LH surge and signal ovulation of mature follicle(s) or to facilitate the maturation of oocytes in IVF prior to the oocyte retrieval procedure. Most commonly used to induce ovulation after gonadotropin administration.	Subcutaneous injection (Ovidrel): 250 mg. Intramuscular injection (all others): 5000–10,000 IU Generally administered after mature follicles are documented by ultrasound.	Patients should be instructed not to do a pregnancy test before 14 days because a false-positive result is likely. The risks of ovarian hyperstimulation and multiple pregnancy should be reviewed with the patient before drug administration. These risks are related to the total number of ovarian follicles, the number of mature follicles, and the estradiol level. If the risks are deemed too high by the patient or physician, hCG may be withheld, thereby minimizing the chance of ovulation.
Human menopausal gonadotropin (purified urinary gonadotropins) (Pergonal, Repronex, Humegon Menopur)	Consists of FSH and LH extracted from human menopausal urine. Used to induce ovulation in anovulatory women or increase the number of mature follicles produced in a single cycle. Most commonly prescribed for patients who have no response to clomiphene citrate, have unexplained infertility, or are undergoing IVF.	Intramuscular administration or subcutaneous administration. Dosage is highly individualized. Generally, the initial dose is 150 IU/day, but it may be increased or decreased based on patient's current or previous response.	These medications should be prescribed only by a physician who is thoroughly familiar with the risks, benefits, and potential complications that may result from gonadotropin therapy. (S)he should also be able to perform necessary monitoring with ultrasound and same-day estradiol level assessments 7 days a week. The patient may experience mild burning, stinging, or redness at at the injection site.

| Steroids (dexamethasone, Decadron) | Used to suppress adrenal secretion of male hormones (DHEA-S), which may interfere with ovulation. | Oral administration: 0.5 mg/day | Patients should be apprised of the risks (multiple pregnancy and ovarian hyperstimulation syndrome [which can commonly occur] and benefits of this medication before it is prescribed. These medications generally are self-administered or administered by the patient's partner. | Most patients do not have any side effects with low dosages. However, possible side effects include increased appetite, abdominal distension, insomnia, mood swings, and weight gain. |

*All infertility medications warrant **careful** monitoring. These medications should only be prescribed by a health care provider who is thoroughly familiar with the use, side effects, and risks, and is capable of providing the necessary monitoring and interpretation of results. In addition, other causes of infertility must be investigated, such as hyperprolactinemia, thyroid disorders, male factor infertility, and tubal revome vomiting disease, before therapy is begun. Calls from patients concerning a side effect other than mild vomiting, hot flushes, slight depression, acne, slight weight gain, or vaginal dryness should be referred to the prescribing provider **immediately.**

Shady Grove Fertility Center has an excellent Web site for both health care providers and couples who require specialized fertility services. Its Web site address is http://www.shadygrovefertility.com.

CHAPTER 6

Prenatal Screening Overview

Many women contemplating pregnancy may want to consider their chances of a normal pregnancy and risk for potential problems. For some women, it may come as a surprise that they are at greater risk for developing problems than anticipated. Some women do not know their family background or the background of their baby's father until questions are prompted of them by their obstetrical care providers. Regardless, all women should be offered prenatal screening and have the opportunity to make informed decisions. In fact, in some states it is mandatory for obstetrical care providers to offer certain tests to pregnant women and document their response. It is imperative that you know your responsibilities based on your state of employment.

The decision to undergo *any* type of prenatal screening requires that the prospective parents ask themselves, What will this information mean to us in the course of our pregnancy? There are personal moral and ethical considerations inherent in these decisions. In short, there is no one *right* answer for every prospective parent. It can be an emotional experience to face the reality of a possible poor pregnancy outcome just at the time one is excited about being pregnant.

For many prospective parents with known risks, the potential for a poor outcome and definitive tests to ascertain the degree of risk have prompted them to undergo this step as part of their preconceptual planning. This is the ideal situation. Individuals wanting a genetic assessment should be referred to a qualified genetic counselor to get the full benefit of such planning.

This section contains descriptions of the major tests available to all patients seeking prenatal screening.

Early Prenatal Genetic Screening

KEY QUESTIONS

ASSESSMENT

ACTION

1. Are you interested in any genetic screening or testing?

YES Go to Question 2.

NO No further action.

2. Is it important for you to know with 99+% certainty whether your baby has Down syndrome or other chromosomal problems?

YES Go to Step A.

NO Go to Step B.

ACTIONS

STEP A: CVS and Amniocentesis

Chorionic villus sampling (CVS) is a genetic test that detects chromosomal abnormalities such as Down syndrome, as well as other genetic disorders such as trisomy 13, trisomy 18, cystic fibrosis, sickle cell disease, Tay-Sachs disease, and sex chromosome abnormalities such as Turner syndrome and Klinefelter syndrome.

For the procedure, an ultrasound is performed to determine the position of the placenta. A small sample of cells is taken from projections on the placenta, called the chorionic villi, for genetic analysis. This is usually done between 11 and 12 weeks of pregnancy. Depending on where the placenta is lying, the tissue sample is taken through either the cervix or the abdominal wall. This test is more than 99% accurate in diagnosing these conditions. There is a slight risk of a miscarriage associated with a CVS that is estimated to be between 1 in 100 and 1 in 200.

Since the test is done early in pregnancy, CVS cannot detect neural tube defects, such as spina bifida. If you undergo CVS, you'll be offered a blood screening test, called an alpha-fetoprotein (AFP) test, in your second trimester to determine whether you're at increased risk for neural tube defects.

Amniocentesis is another genetic test that detects chromosomal abnormalities. For this test, a small amount of amniotic fluid is taken from the amniotic sac surrounding the fetus for genetic analysis. This test is used to detect the same disorders as CVS, as well as neural tube defects such as spina bifida, and is more than 99% accurate in diagnosing these conditions.

Neither CVS nor amniocentesis can detect birth defects such as heart malformations or a cleft lip or palate.

STEP B: Nuchal Translucency (NT) Screening and Quad Screening

NT screening is also called first-trimester screening.

NT screening is a test to assess your infant's risk for Down syndrome and trisomy 13 and 18. This screening is done between weeks 11 and 13 6/7 of pregnancy.

This screen involves two steps. First, a sonogram is used to confirm the gestational age and to evaluate the skin thickness of the fetus's neck (known as the NT) and the fetus's nasal bone. Second, a maternal blood test measures substances in the blood known as human chorionic gonadotropin (B-HCG) and pregnancy-associated plasma protein-A (PAPP-A). With first-trimester screening, the detection rate is 90% for Down syndrome and 97% for trisomy 18 and 13, with a false-positive rate of 5%.

In the second trimester (between 15 and 20 weeks), a second blood test, the AFP, may be taken to test for neural tube defects such as spina bifida.

Keep in mind that the results of these tests do not tell you with absolute certainty whether or not the infant has a chromosomal problem. The results of the NT screening are then combined with those of the blood tests and the mother's age to assess the risk for the fetus. The results are given in the form of a ratio that expresses the chance of the fetus having a chromosomal abnormality. The detection rate for the first-trimester combined screening is approximately 90%. There is a 5% false-positive rate. You may need other tests to confirm or rule out a diagnosis. A level II ultrasound at 18–20 weeks is often offered with this testing.

Quad screening is a blood test that is done between 15 and 22 weeks of pregnancy to screen for Down syndrome, trisomy 18, and neural tube defects. This test measures AFP, which is a substance found in amniotic fluid, fetal blood, and the mother's blood; estriol, which is a hormone made by the placenta and the liver of the fetus; human chorionic gonadotropin, which is hormone made by the placenta; and Inhibin-A, a hormone that is also produced by the placenta. An elevated screening score may indicate neural tube defects (opening in the spine), and a lower screening score may indicate Down syndrome. This screening test is not as accurate as the first-trimester screening. The quad screen detects Down syndrome in 81% of cases. The AFP test detects neural tube defects in 80% of cases. Because levels of the substances measured change during pregnancy, it is important to ensure that the gestational age is accurate.

PATIENT EDUCATION

There is a window of opportunity for many of these tests. Evaluating gestational age is important for accurate screening and testing.

Prior to January 2007, genetic screening/testing was only offered to women over the age of 35. New American College of Obstetricians and Gynecologist (ACOG) guidelines recommend that all pregnant women should be offered genetic screening or testing.

Before starting any conversation about genetic screening or testing, it is important to ask the woman and her partner how important it is to know the information, and whether the information will change the course of her/their course of action. Pregnant women and their partners fall along a continuum from not needing to know the information because it would not change the course of her pregnancy to needing to know with absolute certainty the information because she/they might terminate the pregnancy, and knowing that these tests have small risks associated with them. There is no one right decision. People have different feelings about what risks are acceptable.

Cystic Fibrosis Screening

ASSESSMENT

ACTION

1. Are you interested in cystic fibrosis screening?

YES Go to Step A.
NO No further action.

2. Have you had a positive screening test?

YES Go to Step B.
NO Go to Step A.

ACTIONS

STEP A: Cystic Fibrosis Screening

Cystic fibrosis (CF) is an inherited disease that affects many systems, including the mucous and sweat glands. Approximately 30,000 people in the United States have CF. Although it affects people from all racial and ethnic groups, it is most common among Caucasians whose ancestors are from Northern Europe or of Ashkenazi Jewish origin. In these two groups the incidence is about one in every 3,000 babies born in the United States. CF is also common in Latinos and Native Americans, but less common among African Americans (one in 17,000) and Asian Americans (one in 90,000). Approximately 12 million Americans are carriers of an abnormal CF gene. CF is caused by a defect in a gene called the cystic fibrosis transmembrane conductance regulator (CFTR) gene. This gene makes a protein that controls the movement of salt and water into and out of certain cells, including those that line the lungs and pancreas. When the gene is not working effectively, the mucus becomes thick and sticky. The mucus builds up in the lungs and blocks the airways, which causes respiratory problems and provides a breeding ground for bacteria to grow, leading to frequent lung infections and lung damage. This thick mucus can also block ducts in the pancreas, resulting in digestive enzymes being blocked from reaching the intestines, which hinders fats and proteins from being absorbed.

Symptoms of CF vary widely from milder versions that are discovered in adults to more severe versions, with serious lung and digestive problems, that are discovered shortly after birth. Symptoms include frequent coughing, shortness of breath, poor growth, frequent episodes of bronchitis and pneumonia, salty-tasting skin, dehydration, intestinal blockage, male infertility, and digestive symptoms of diarrhea or greasy stools. There is no cure for CF. The main treatments for CF include antibiotics for infections, chest physical therapy, and exercise. Respiratory failure is the most common cause of death in people with CF.

Prenatal genetic testing can help patients find out if either parent is a carrier of this defective gene. Screening is now offered routinely to all couples who are pregnant or contemplating pregnancy.

STEP B: Positive Screening Test

A positive result tells you that the patient is a carrier of one or more genetic changes in the CF gene. A positive test is over 99% accurate and detects about 90% of all CF mutations. If the mother tests positive in this screening, it is important that the father also be tested. An infant is not at risk of CF unless both parents carry the abnormal gene.

It is important to remember that not all CF mutations are detected and that this test is not 100% accurate. There are many mutations of this gene and the test screens for the most common of these. So even if the test shows that a person is not a carrier, there is a very small chance that this is a false negative.

PATIENT EDUCATION

Genes come in pairs from the mother and the father. To inherit CF, an infant must receive two CF genes, one from each parent who is a carrier of the CF gene. When both parents carry the abnormal CF gene, there is a 25% chance that the infant will have CF, a 25% chance that the infant will not have the abnormal gene, and a 50% chance that the child will be a carrier like the parents. The risk is the same with each pregnancy. If only one parent is a carrier of the gene, there is no chance that the children will have CF.

CHAPTER 7

1st Trimester Overview

The 1st trimester of pregnancy is characterized by overwhelming physical and emotional changes. Numerous physiologic issues surround patient concerns, and complaints are numerous. From a telephone triage standpoint, a few issues dominate the picture. Risk of ectopic pregnancy and miscarriage are great until a viable intrauterine pregnancy has been documented. In the case of multiple miscarriages, even early viability may not be reassurance enough.

Ectopic pregnancy accounts for 10% of maternal mortality. The failure to recognize the signs of ectopic pregnancy is an issue of great medicolegal concern. It also is a cause of much patient suffering. Patients who have experienced repeated ectopic pregnancies have greatly reduced fertility potential and higher risk for another ectopic pregnancy.

Within the 1st trimester, miscarriage occurs in 20% of documented pregnancies. The rate of repeat miscarriage is high for some patients. The emotional cost of miscarriage is of concern. Although little can be done to alter the course of pregnancy loss in most 1st trimester cases, the emotional impact can be minimized by sensitive, supportive care.

Ambivalence is common during the 1st trimester as patients adjust to the reality of assuming parenthood. Depression may surface for the first time. Domestic violence often is increased. These emotional issues, coupled with the physical complaints of nausea, vomiting, and fatigue, make the 1st trimester a telephone triage challenge.

1st Trimester Abdominal Pain

KEY QUESTIONS

ASSESSMENT

	ACTION

1. Are you having any vaginal bleeding associated with the pain?

YES Go to Step A.
NO Go to Question 2.

2. Is the pain severe in nature, and did it start during the last 24 hours?

YES Go to Step B.
NO Go to Question 3.

3. Is the pain mild/moderate in nature, and has it been present longer than 24 hours?

YES Go to Question 4.
NO Go to Question 4.

4. Is the abdominal pain accompanied by nausea, vomiting, bowel changes, fever, dysuria, lightheadedness, or dizziness?

YES Go to Step C.
NO Go to Patient Education.

ACTIONS

STEP A: Vaginal Bleeding

If the patient is experiencing vaginal bleeding, determine how much. If she is soaking one or more pads per hour or six or more in a 12-hour period, or if she is lightheaded, she meets the criteria for serious vaginal bleeding. The patient should be instructed to come to the office immediately or go to the nearest ER. The patient should not drive herself. If there is any question of loss of sensorimotor skills, the patient or her agent should call 911.

If the bleeding is not heavy, determine the history of the following ectopic risk factors: prior ectopic pregnancy, prior tubal surgery, prior pelvic infection, endometriosis, prior abdominal surgery, and prior ruptured appendix.

Determine the history of prior pregnancy loss, miscarriage, more than three spontaneous abortions, or five or more voluntary pregnancy terminations.

Continue to Question 2.

STEP B: Severe Abdominal Pain

If abdominal pain is severe regardless of the risk factors, immediate referral to an available obstetric care provider, on-call provider, or ER is warranted. The patient should not drive herself. If there is any question of loss of sensorimotor skills, the patient or her agent should call 911.

STEP C: Problems to Consider

Threatened pregnancy loss: If the pregnancy has been confirmed by a sensitive testing method, the patient may be experiencing the early symptoms of spontaneous abortion. Have her rest, drink at least 8 ounces of water/hour, and call the office again within the next 24 hours for a status report. If vaginal bleeding develops, pain worsens, fever occurs, or she experiences additional symptoms, she should call back immediately.

Urinary tract infection: If she experiences pain on urination or unusually frequent urination, she should see a provider in the next 24 hours for urine culture and sensitivity and possible treatment. In the meantime, the patient should increase her intake of water and/or cranberry juice by 1 quart during the next 24 hours. If she is experiencing low-back ache, flulike symptoms such as nausea or vomiting, or a fever, she should be given a same-day appointment to be evaluated for a kidney infection (pyelonephritis).

Appendicitis: If the patient still has her appendix, the pain is in the right lower abdominal quadrant, she has a fever, or she is experiencing bowel changes, she should be given a same-day appointment or sent to the ER or urgent care center for an acute abdominal evaluation.

Gastrointestinal problem: If the patient has any bowel changes, such as constipation or diarrhea, or associates the pain with eating, it is a good idea to have her contact her primary care provider to see if a gastrointestinal evaluation is warranted.

PATIENT EDUCATION

Some women may experience mild to moderate abdominal pain as a normal part of early pregnancy. If she does not have any other accompanying symptoms, urge her to continue to monitor her symptoms and call if they persist for more than 48 hours, additional symptoms develop, or if she has any questions or concerns.

1st Trimester Ambivalence/Depression

KEY QUESTIONS

ASSESSMENT	ACTION
1. Are you feeling ambivalent about this pregnancy or having doubts about being pregnant?	**YES** Go to Step A.
	NO Go to Question 2.
2. Are you feeling depressed or especially anxious about this pregnancy?	**YES** Go to Step B.
	NO Go to Question 3.
3. Do you have any history of depression, postpartum depression, or mental illness?	**YES** Go to Step C.
	NO Go to Question 4.
4. Are you experiencing feelings that you want to harm yourself or someone else?	**YES** Go to Step D.
	NO Return to Step B.

ACTIONS

STEP A: Ambivalence in Pregnancy

Research indicates that four of five women experience some degree of ambivalence during pregnancy. Even during a planned pregnancy, a woman may not feel totally sure about the concept of being pregnant.

Suggest that the patient make a list of the positive and negative aspects of being pregnant to aid in decision making.

Talking with a partner, significant other, close friend, or family member may be beneficial for some patients.

In the event of an unplanned pregnancy, the patient may find it helpful to talk to a counselor about whether or not to continue the pregnancy.

In our practice, we recommend the following counselors who may be of value in helping to sort out feelings of ambivalence and pregnancy continuation: _____
_____.

STEP B: Possible Underlying Depression or Anxiety

Major life events may unmask or precipitate depression or anxiety. If there is any question that the patient is experiencing uncontrolled mood swings, thoughts about harming herself or others, feeling out of control, or becoming withdrawn, do the following:

- Make a same-day appointment with a mental health provider and ensure that a friend, family member, or social services worker accompanies the patient to the appointment.
- Ensure that a high-risk patient is not left alone.
- If necessary, have another person in your office call Emergency Services and remain on the line with the patient until help arrives.
- Notify a provider in your practice of the problem and your actions.

If the patient is of no danger to herself or others, do the following:

- Refer her to a mental health counselor for an appointment within the next 3 to 5 days.
- Reassure the patient that she may call back at any time if the symptoms worsen.

Your practice should have a system for identifying patients possibly at risk for depression early in pregnancy.

In our practice, we do the following to identify patients at risk for depression during pregnancy (and thus, possibly postpartum depression). _____

STEP C: History of Depression or Mental Illness

Patients with a history of depression or mental illness may be at greater risk with a new pregnancy.

Repeat the actions in Step B.

STEP D: Desire to Harm Oneself or Others

If the patient is experiencing uncontrolled mood swings, thoughts about harming herself or others, feeling out of control, or becoming seriously withdrawn, make a same-day appointment for her with a mental health counselor and ensure that a friend, family member, or social services worker accompanies her to the appointment.

Ensure that a high-risk patient is not left alone.

If necessary, have another person in your office call Emergency Services and remain on the line with the patient until help arrives.

Notify a provider in your practice of the problem and your actions.

PATIENT EDUCATION

1. Reassuring a patient that ambivalence is common in early pregnancy may be reassurance enough that her thoughts are not abnormal.
2. Do not be judgmental if the patient sounds as if she is considering termination of pregnancy. Patients need to talk through their feelings for validation; it does not necessarily mean that you agree with her decision if you listen without passing judgment.
3. Patients with a history of depression during pregnancy or the postpartum period need education regarding the possible recurrence and to know that help is available. Avoid being judgmental. Many patients have the misconception that all feelings can be controlled by will.

1st Trimester Bleeding

KEY QUESTIONS

ASSESSMENT	ACTION
1. Has your pregnancy been confirmed?	**YES** Go to Question 2.
	NO Go to Step A.
2. Is this bleeding as heavy as a normal period?	**YES** Go to Step B.
	NO Go to Step C.
3. Are you experiencing any abdominal pain or cramps?	**YES** Go to Step D and E.
	NO No action.

ACTIONS

STEP A: Pregnancy Confirmation

If the patient has not had pregnancy confirmed by a highly sensitive pregnancy test, determine the following:

- last menstrual period (LMP);
- normalcy of LMP;
- history of abnormal menstrual cycles;
- history of previous early pregnancy risk factors (prior ectopic pregnancy, ≥3 spontaneous early pregnancy losses, ≥5 voluntary pregnancy terminations, abdominal surgery, pelvic infection).

Question the patient regarding symptoms of early pregnancy that she may be experiencing, such as:

- breast tenderness,
- fatigue,
- nausea, and
- urinary frequency

Ask the patient if she was attempting a pregnancy.

Question the patient regarding her contraceptive pattern if she was not actively attempting a pregnancy.

If the patient is taking oral contraceptives, question her regarding medication use that may have interfered with oral contraceptive effectiveness, such as certain antibiotics or antiseizure medications.

Under any circumstances, suspected pregnancy with bleeding needs immediate pregnancy confirmation. Have patient perform a self-test or follow office protocol for pregnancy confirmation. (See the Patient Education section.) Continue to Step B.

STEP B: Vaginal Bleeding, Heavy

If the patient is experiencing vaginal bleeding, determine how much. If she is soaking one or more pads per hour or six or more in a 12-hour period, or is lightheaded, she meets the criteria for serious vaginal bleeding. The patient should be instructed to come to the office immediately or go to the nearest ER. She should not drive herself. If there is any question of the loss of sensorimotor skills, she or her agent should call 911.

Irregular bleeding in early pregnancy may be associated with an ectopic pregnancy. The risk factors for ectopic pregnancy include prior ectopic pregnancy, prior tubal surgery, prior pelvic infection, and endometriosis history. In addition to irregular vaginal bleeding, women experiencing an ectopic pregnancy also may report abdominal, shoulder, or back pain. Suspected ectopic pregnancy requires immediate consultation with an obstetric care provider.

STEP C: Vaginal Spotting or Irregular Bleeding

If the bleeding does not meet the criteria for severe bleeding, question the patient as to the following:

- ectopic pregnancy risk factors, which are prior ectopic pregnancy, prior tubal surgery, prior pelvic infection, endometriosis, prior abdominal surgery, and ruptured appendix; and
- spontaneous abortion risk factors, including ≥3 spontaneous abortions or ≥5 voluntary pregnancy terminations.

Continue to Steps D and E.

STEP D: Ectopic Pregnancy Considerations

Irregular bleeding in early pregnancy may be associated with an ectopic pregnancy. The risk factors for ectopic pregnancy include prior ectopic pregnancy, prior tubal surgery, prior pelvic infection, and a history of endometriosis. In addition to irregular vaginal bleeding, women experiencing an ectopic pregnancy may report abdominal, shoulder, or back pain. Suspected ectopic pregnancy requires immediate consultation with an obstetric care provider or ER referral if such a provider is not available.

STEP E: Spontaneous Abortion Considerations

If ectopic pregnancy is not suspected, the patient needs evaluation within 24–72 hours, based on the severity of her symptoms.

Patient needs to be instructed to call back immediately if symptoms increase.

Patients with a history of frequent pregnancy losses need to be seen earlier, rather than later, for additional reassurances.

PATIENT EDUCATION

All practices should have an agreed upon standard for confirmation of pregnancy and diagnosis of possible ectopic pregnancy. These include quantitative HCG testing, transvaginal ultrasound, and serum progesterone. In our practice, we recommend that pregnancy be confirmed by: _____.

1st Trimester Constipation

KEY QUESTIONS

ASSESSMENT	ACTION
1. Is the onset of your symptoms pregnancy related?	**YES** Go to Step A.
	NO Go to Question 2.
2. Is the constipation accompanied by prolonged nausea, vomiting, abdominal distension, or failure to pass gas?	**YES** Go to Step B.
	NO Go to Question 3.
3. Do you have a pre-existing problem with constipation?	**YES** Go to Step C.
	NO Go to Question 4.
4. Is there blood in your stool?	**YES** Go to Step D.
	NO Return to Step A.

ACTIONS

STEP A: Pregnancy Related

Constipation is a common complaint throughout pregnancy. Causes in the 1st trimester are primarily hormonal in nature, with progesterone causing relaxation of smooth muscle of the bowel.

The following suggestions may be helpful:

- Increase fiber in the diet.
- Increase clear fluids by 1–2 quarts daily.
- Add stool softeners as determined by office/clinic protocols (see list of approved stool softeners).
- Increase exercise within limits of the 1st trimester. Keep pulse rate below 140 beats/minute.
- Change prenatal vitamin to one with time-released iron or avoid iron altogether until the end of the first 12 weeks of pregnancy.
- Assess calcium intake. Many patients mistakenly take more calcium supplementation than is needed.

Avoid laxatives.
Continue on to Questions 2, 3, and 4.

STEP B: Constipation With Additional Symptoms

Ileus is uncommon in early pregnancy but must not be overlooked. If patient has additional symptoms, she should call her primary care provider immediately.
Continue on to Questions 3 and 4.

STEP C: History of Constipation

Patients with a history of constipation or irritable bowel syndrome may have a worsening of symptoms.
Assess laxative and other medication use.
Encourage recommendations in Step A. If patient is a chronic abuser of laxatives or experiences no response after trying the suggestions in Step A, refer her to an obstetric care provider or gastrointestinal care provider.

STEP D: Blood in Stool

Blood in the stool may be a sign of straining or hemorrhoids but also may be a signal of a more serious medical problem. The patient should have this symptom evaluated by her obstetric care provider at her next scheduled appointment or sooner if the symptoms worsen.

PATIENT EDUCATION

1. There are many available iron preparations that may be more easily absorbed if the patient is known to be anemic but is reluctant to take iron because of constipation.

   Our practice recommends: _____.

2. Calcium (particularly calcium carbonate) can be constipating and can directly interfere with iron absorption.

   Our practice recommends: _____.

3. All minerals probably are best absorbed when obtained through foods consumed. Encourage the patient to eat foods rich in iron and calcium.

1st Trimester Dizziness/Fainting

KEY QUESTIONS

ASSESSMENT	ACTION
1. Is the dizziness accompanied by severe headache, visual changes, numbness, or tingling?	**YES** Go to Step A.
	NO Go to Question 2.
2. Have you fainted or lost consciousness?	**YES** Go to Step B.
	NO Go to Question 3.
3. Is the dizziness accompanied by inner ear pain or sinus pressure?	**YES** Go to Step C.
	NO Go to Question 4.
4. Is the dizziness associated with position changes, temperature changes, prolonged sitting, or prolonged standing?	**YES** Go to Step D.
	NO No further action.

ACTIONS

STEP A: Sudden, Severe Headache or Neurological Changes

The onset of a sudden, severe headache usually is not a problem related to obstetrics and needs immediate referral to the patient's primary care provider or the ER, as appropriate. The patient should not drive. If the headache is accompanied by loss of sensorimotor skills, the patient or her agent should call 911. Likewise, visual changes and numbness and tingling are not normal 1st trimester symptoms and require medical evaluation.

STEP B: Fainting, Loss of Consciousness

Does the patient have a history of epilepsy or fainting? If so, the provider who has been treating her for epilepsy or fainting spells should be contacted by the patient ASAP to determine the need for additional evaluation or medication changes.

Assess if the patient actually lost consciousness or merely felt as if she would "black out."

Assess if anyone was with her at the time and could provide an accurate account of the event.

A patient who has fainted or lost consciousness needs to be evaluated for possible head injury or seizure activity. Whether or not the patient or a witness is positive the patient had a seizure, the patient needs to discuss her symptoms with her primary care provider ASAP to decide if additional evaluation is warranted.

STEP C: Ear Pain or Sinus Pressure

The patient may be experiencing vestibular disturbance caused by an upper respiratory tract or sinus infection.

Recommend the patient take a decongestant in accordance with the practice/clinic protocol.

If there is no improvement in 24–72 hours, the patient should contact her primary care provider.

STEP D: Syncope

Syncope may be caused by vasomotor instability as blood pools in the lower extremities or splanchnic and pelvic areas, causing transient disruption of blood flow to the brain.

Explain causes to the patient.

Recommend she:

- avoid prolonged sitting, standing, or lying flat on back;
- alternate elevation of each foot approximately 8 inches when performing routine tasks while standing (ironing, washing dishes, standing in grocery line, standing at work);
- rise slowly;
- avoid excessively hot baths, showers, and sitting in a hot tub.

PATIENT EDUCATION

1. Hypoglycemia (low blood sugar) may be another cause of dizziness. A diet that is high in protein and frequent consumption of high-fiber snacks may prove helpful.
2. Later in pregnancy, the fetus may compress the vena cava, a major blood vessel that returns blood from the legs to the heart, causing a relative drop in blood pressure. Lying on the back or long periods of sitting may lead to this occurrence. Try changing positions.
3. Assess situations that may contribute to symptoms and be particularly careful with safety issues, such as driving, carrying small children, or potentially hazardous conditions at work.
4. Maintain adequate fluid intake. The patient should be drinking at least 1–2 quarts of fluids in addition to what she normally drinks.

1st Trimester Fatigue

KEY QUESTIONS

ASSESSMENT	**ACTION**
1. Is the onset of your symptoms pregnancy related?	**YES** Go to Step A.
	NO Go to Question 2.
2. Do you have a history of a chronic medical condition, such as anemia or thyroid or cardiac problems?	**YES** Go to Step B.
	NO Go to Question 3.
3. Do you have extenuating circumstances that could be contributing to your fatigue, such as small children or a demanding work schedule?	**YES** Go to Step C.
	NO No further action.

ACTIONS

STEP A: Pregnancy-Related Fatigue

There are several causes of onset of fatigue in early pregnancy. Physiologic and hormonal changes are the predominant causes.
The following suggestions may prove useful:

- Take more frequent naps or rest periods.
- Go to bed earlier or arise later.
- Eliminate nonessential activities.
- Decrease personal expectations.
- Enlist help from family members or friends.

STEP B: Pre-existing Illnesses

Patients who have a pre-existing medical condition that may be contributing to the fatigue should have that condition re-evaluated at their initial pregnancy appointment and at any time during the pregnancy if the condition worsens. Pregnancy may change the amounts or types of medications the patient should be taking or may cause an alteration or worsening of their condition.

STEP C: Outside Stressors

Many patients underestimate the demands in their lives that may contribute to the already-draining adaptation to pregnancy.
Refer to Step A actions.
Evaluate resources for support.

1st Trimester Headache

KEY QUESTIONS

ASSESSMENT	ACTION
1. Was the onset of this headache sudden and severe?	**YES** Go to Step A.
	NO Go to Question 2.
2. Is the headache accompanied by any numbness, tingling, loss of bowel or bladder control, or seizure behaviors?	**YES** Go to Step A.
	NO Go to Question 3.
3. Is the headache accompanied by visual changes?	**YES** Go to Step B.
	NO Go to Question 4.
4. Is the headache accompanied by debilitating neck stiffness or high fever?	**YES** Go to Step A.
	NO Go to Question 5.
5. Is the headache accompanied by upper respiratory tract infection symptoms (congestion, fever, cough, or facial or tooth discomfort)?	**YES** Go to Step C.
	NO Go to Question 6.
6. Is the headache dull and not debilitating in nature?	**YES** Go to Step D.
	NO No further action.

ACTIONS

STEP A: Sudden, Severe Headache

The onset of a sudden, severe headache usually is not a problem related to obstetric care and needs immediate referral to the patient's primary care provider or ER, as appropriate.

The patient should not drive. If the headache is accompanied by loss of sensorimotor skills, the patient or her agent should call 911.

STEP B: Neurological Symptoms

Question the patient as to history of migraine headaches. Are these headaches like the migraines that she has experienced before?

Refer the patient to an on-call provider to determine if additional neurological evaluation is warranted and to determine the safety of any medications the patient may have on hand for treatment of her migraines.

Instruct the patient to lie in a dark room and apply compresses to the area where she is experiencing the headache.

If she does not experience relief within 1–2 hours, refer the patient to her primary care provider for medication management.

STEP C: Respiratory Symptoms

If the patient has symptoms of an upper respiratory tract infection, she may be experiencing a sinus headache.

Recommend the patient take acetaminophen 650 mg orally every 4–6 hours as needed, not to exceed the manufacturer's recommended dosage, or other medication as agreed upon by your practice for the use of pain relief during the 1st trimester.

Consult an obstetric care provider before recommending the use of decongestants.

Refer the patient to her primary care provider if her symptoms have not improved within 3–5 days.

Instruct the patient to call her primary care provider if her symptoms worsen.

STEP D: Dull Headaches

Dull headaches, probably caused by hormonal and vascular changes, are common in early pregnancy and may peak and disappear by 14–16 weeks.

Recommend the patient take acetaminophen 650 mg orally every 4–6 hours as needed, not to exceed the manufacturer's recommended dosage, or other medication as agreed upon by your practice for the use of pain relief during the 1st trimester.

The patient's primary care provider should evaluate persistent dull headaches.

1st Trimester Nausea/Vomiting

KEY QUESTIONS

ASSESSMENT	ACTION
1. For the past 24 hours or longer, have you been unable to keep food or liquids in your stomach?	**YES** Go to Step A.
	NO Go to Question 2.
2. Did the symptoms begin with your pregnancy?	**YES** Go to Step B.
	NO Go to Question 3.
3. Do you have any pre-existing food intolerances or gastrointestinal problems?	**YES** Go to Step C.
	NO Go to Question 4.
4. Are your symptoms accompanied by fever or abdominal pain?	**YES** Go to Step D.
	NO No further action.

ACTIONS

STEP A: Food/Fluid Difficulties

Patients who cannot keep food or liquids down for 24 hours or more are at risk for dehydration and ketosis and require evaluation for hyperemesis.

Advise the patient to come to the office within 12–24 hours for urine dipstick for ketones and to assess specific gravity for dehydration.

Advise the patient to call her obstetric care provider if she has had no urine output for 12 hours while awaiting an appointment.

STEP B: Nausea/Vomiting in Pregnancy

There are many physiologic causes for nausea in pregnancy. The following are some recommendations for minimizing symptoms.

- Avoid prenatal vitamins until the nausea resolves. Try 1 tablet of an over-the-counter children's vitamin supplement per day until the nausea is gone.
- Eat small amounts but eat frequently.
- Do not allow the stomach to become too empty.
- Carry a source of complex carbohydrate (a protein source plus a carbohydrate), such as cheese and crackers, while at work or away from home.
- Consume crackers or dry toast before arising.
- Avoid fried, spicy, or fatty foods.
- Drink liquids between meals.

Patients should be instructed to notify their obstetric care provider of any of the following:

- the inability to keep food or liquids down for 24 hours or more;
- the vomiting of bile or blood;
- no urine output for 12 or more hours;
- the onset of severe abdominal pain; or
- bloody diarrhea

STEP C: Pre-existing Food Intolerance or Gastrointestinal Problem

Patients with pre-existing gastrointestinal problems, such as Crohn's disease, colitis, irritable bowel syndrome, or reflux, should have a medical evaluation and an assessment of any medication use ASAP. Ideally, these patients should have had a preconceptual evaluation, particularly to ascertain the safety of their medications and education regarding the possible course of the pre-existing illness during pregnancy.

Patients with food intolerances should have nutritional counseling.

Return to Step A or B, as appropriate.

STEP D: Fever/Abdominal Pain

Nausea and vomiting accompanied by high fever or severe abdominal pain needs immediate evaluation for acute abdominal problems, such as appendicitis. Although it may be something as simple as "the flu," more serious problems should not be dismissed! These patients should have immediate telephone consultation with their obstetric care provider or should be referred to an urgent care facility or ER.

PATIENT EDUCATION

1. Patients need to understand the usual course of nausea and vomiting in pregnancy. The onset of symptoms is rare before week 6 of pregnancy and may not magically disappear by the end of the 1st trimester.
2. A sudden absence of symptoms may indicate a need to evaluate the viability of the pregnancy.
3. It cannot be overemphasized that pre-existing serious gastrointestinal conditions that require maintenance medications warrant a medical evaluation.

1st Trimester Urinary Complaints

KEY QUESTIONS

ASSESSMENT	ACTION
1. Are you experiencing more frequent urination?	**YES** Go to Question 2.
	NO Go to Step A.
2. Do you have pubic pain or pressure, or burning on urination?	**YES** Go to Step B.
	NO Go to Question 3.
3. Do you have blood in your urine, a low backache, or flulike symptoms, such as nausea, vomiting, or a fever?	**YES** Go to Step C.
	NO Go to Question 4.
4. Do you have sickle cell disease or are you a sickle cell carrier?	**YES** Go to Step D.
	NO No further action.

ACTIONS

STEP A: Frequent Urination Without Other Symptoms

During the 1st trimester of pregnancy, women often experience increased frequency of urination. If the patient has no other symptoms, it is unlikely she has a urinary tract infection. However, women who have a history of urinary tract infections, kidney infections, sickle cell disease, or sickle cell carrier status should come to the office to give a clean-caught urine specimen for analysis, culture, and sensitivity.

STEP B: Frequent Urination With Urinary Symptoms

Increased frequency of urination with symptoms such as burning, suprapubic pressure, pain, or blood in the urine can be indicative of a urinary tract infection or other more serious problems. The patient should be instructed to come to the office to give a clean-caught urine specimen for analysis, culture, and sensitivity.

STEP C: Frequent Urination With Renal Symptoms

A patient with frequent urination and accompanying low backache, flulike symptoms, or hematuria may have a kidney infection or a more serious kidney complication. The patient should be instructed to schedule a same-day appointment with her primary care provider or a urologist.

STEP D: Sickle Cell Disease or Sickle Cell Carrier

Women who have sickle cell disease or who are sickle cell carriers are at higher risk for asymptomatic urinary tract infections. These women should be instructed to come into the office to give a clean-caught urine specimen for analysis, culture, and sensitivity.

In addition, these women should receive a urinalysis during each trimester of their pregnancy to exclude an asymptomatic urinary tract infection.

1st Trimester Vaginal Discharge

KEY QUESTIONS

ASSESSMENT	ACTION
1. Are you experiencing an increase in vaginal discharge without burning, itching, or odor?	**YES** Go to Step A.
	NO Go to Question 2.
2. Are you having vaginal burning, itching, or odor?	**YES** Go to Step B.
	NO Go to Question 3.
3. Do you have any burning or pain with urination? If so, is the pain internal, especially at the end of urination, or is it external, when the urine runs over the outside tissues?	**YES** Go to Step C.
	NO Go to Question 4.
4. Are you concerned you could have been exposed to a sexually transmitted infection?	**YES** Go to Step D.
	NO Go to Question 5.
5. Are there any lesions present?	**YES** Go to Step E. Go to Question 6.
	NO Go to Question 6.
6. Do you have a previous history of exposure to herpes?	**YES** Go to Step F.
	NO Go to Step G.

ACTIONS

STEP A: Physiologic Discharge of Pregnancy

Physiologic changes of pregnancy create a discharge that usually is thin, milk colored, and has a slight, but not unpleasant, odor. Reassure the patient that this discharge is normal and will increase during the course of the pregnancy.

Advise against douching during pregnancy. Douching can introduce air into the vagina, which is dangerous. Douching also disturbs the normal flora in the vagina and can increase susceptibility to vaginitis.

Advise the patient to call if the discharge changes in color or odor or is accompanied by itching, burning, or lesions.

STEP B: Symptoms of Vaginitis

Simple vaginitis is common in pregnancy, particularly because of an increase in yeast
infections for some women. The type of vaginitis should be diagnosed, because bacterial vaginosis has been implicated in preterm labor. Early elimination of the problem is important.

Instruct the patient to come in for evaluation within 3–5 days or sooner, if the symptoms increase.

Instruct the patient to avoid OTC products until a diagnosis is made.

Many providers will not treat vaginitis during the 1st trimester. You should know the
preference of the providers with whom you work.

STEP C: Urinary Tract Symptoms

Yeast infections can also mimic urinary tract infection (UTI) symptoms. In this case,
the burning usually occurs when the urine runs over the perineal tissues. Pain that
occurs inside, especially at the end of voiding, is more likely to be a UTI.

If the symptoms sound like a UTI, the patient should come in for evaluation ASAP.

Explain to the patient that she may be asked to give a clean-caught urine sample during her office visit.

STEP D: Possible Sexually Transmitted Infection Exposure

Sexually transmitted infections (STIs) can have a significant impact on pregnancy outcome. If the patient is found to have an STI during pregnancy, follow-up for her
partner and evaluation for reinfection are of major concern to prevent harm to the
fetus.

The patient should be instructed to come in for evaluation within 24 hours.

Explain to her that she may need to have vaginal and vulvar cultures and undergo
blood tests.

Advise the patient to avoid sexual intercourse until she undergoes evaluation.

STEP E: Vulvovaginitis Symptoms With Possible Lesions

The patient with lesions should be seen for evaluation within 24 to 48 hours.

Instruct the patient to wash her hands thoroughly after urination.

The patient should avoid applying creams or lotions to the area until she has been seen
for evaluation.

Comfort measures such as cold compresses or tepid baths may be soothing.

Advise the patient to avoid sexual intercourse until she undergoes evaluation.

STEP F: History of Herpetic Lesions

Patients with a history of herpes need to be educated about the risk if lesions are present at delivery.

Question the patient about the pattern of outbreak during this and previous pregnancies.

Your practice may or may not endorse the use of antivirals for suppression near term.

You should know your providers' opinion on this issue and discuss accordingly with
the patient.

Follow advice in Step E.

Advise the patient to come in for confirmation of the presence of a lesion if she is uncertain.

STEP G: Vulvovaginitis Symptoms, Etiology Unknown

Question the patient about recent antibiotic use or change in toilet tissue, bubble bath, or laundry detergent.

Ask if the patient previously has experienced these symptoms.

Advise the patient on comfort measures used by your providers.

Make appointment for the patient to come in for evaluation within 72 hours.

PATIENT EDUCATION

1. Vaginitis in pregnancy may have a different significance from that in a nonpregnant woman because of the potential ramifications for the developing fetus. Many patients self-diagnose these conditions and may request specific medication prescriptions based on past symptom resolution. Whether or not to treat over the telephone without seeing the patient will be at the discretion of your providers. Many offices or clinics have a policy to treat simple symptoms of yeast infections without seeing the patient. However, most providers will treat only once. If the patient experiences no improvement, she should be seen for evaluation.

2. The goal is to not miss a more serious, possibly communicable infection. If a patient is fairly certain she has been exposed to an STI, encourage her to have her partner(s) tested and to refrain from intercourse until she has been evaluated and treated. You may need to help her rehearse various scenarios before she shares the information with her partner.

3. Patients exposed to STIs early in pregnancy need full testing for possible STIs and a plan for retesting throughout their pregnancy. It is reasonable to encourage such patients to use condoms to minimize the potential for exposure.

CHAPTER 8

2nd Trimester Overview

The issue of fetal viability dominates triage concerns during the 2nd trimester of pregnancy. Depending on your setting and the proximity to neonatal intensive care facilities, the ability of a baby to survive outside of the uterus may vary considerably. Issues of recognizing and stopping preterm labor (if possible) are paramount. Understanding the importance of intervention at different points throughout the 2nd trimester is key to the successful triage of patient concerns.

The physical complaints of pregnancy increase as the pregnancy progresses, but many women feel quite well during the 2nd trimester. Early pregnancy symptoms are resolving, concerns about early miscarriage have waned, and ambivalence has lifted for most women. This is a time when many women are working, assuming full child care responsibilities, and planning for a future addition to the family. There may be little time to be "slowed down" by pregnancy complaints.

Because of the concerns of the consequences of preterm labor, all practices should establish a standard as to what is acceptable and what is not in terms of patient contractions for this point in pregnancy. Many providers educate patients to call if they have four or more contractions per hour, each lasting 45–60 seconds, with or without accompanying pain. Many practices provide patients with instructions for "first-line evaluation" of such symptoms. Common instructions include lying on the left side, consuming a quart of water, and observing for regular uterine tightening during the course of an hour.

The standard for monitoring of preterm labor in our practice is: _____
_____.

Our recommendations for evaluating symptoms at home are: _____
_____.

2nd Trimester Abdominal Pain

KEY QUESTIONS

ASSESSMENT	ACTION
1. Are you having any vaginal bleeding associated with the pain?	**YES** Go to Step A.
	NO Go to Question 2.
2. Does the pain radiate from your back to the front of your abdomen? Can you feel a sensation of uterine tightening?	**YES** Go to Step B.
	NO Go to Question 3.
3. Is the pain confined to one part of your abdomen and relieved by position change?	**YES** Go to Step C.
	NO Go to Question 4.
4. Is the pain confined to one part of your abdomen and **not** relieved by position change?	**YES** Go to Step D.
	NO Go to Question 5.
5. Is the abdominal pain accompanied by nausea, vomiting, bowel changes, fever, dysuria, lightheadedness, or dizziness?	**YES** Go to Step E.
	NO Go to Patient Education.

ACTIONS

STEP A: Vaginal Bleeding Associated With Abdominal Pain

A patient who is bleeding "like a period" needs to be seen ASAP in an appropriate facility. The patient should not drive herself. Transportation to the appropriate facility will depend on your location, the patient's location, and the availability of necessary services.

If the bleeding is "less than a period," the patient still needs to be seen ASAP to ensure that she is not experiencing preterm labor or placental problems.

Risk factors for preterm labor include:

- history of a preterm birth (prior preterm labor/birth increases the risk by 17%–37%);
- multiple gestation (10% of such pregnancies result in premature delivery);

- maternal smoking or cocaine use;
- no prior prenatal care;
- long working hours with reported fatigue;
- maternal medical or obstetric complications;
- uterine abnormalities, such as fibroids or a bicornate uterus;
- cervical incompetence; and
- DES exposure (may affect women born before 1972).

STEP B: Symptoms Consistent With Contractions

The patient may be experiencing an onset of preterm labor or an acute abdominal problem.

Symptoms of preterm labor include:

- abdominal cramps;
- abdominal pressure;
- low backache;
- increased vaginal discharge;
- pain radiating down thighs;
- bowel changes, especially diarrhea;
- vaginal spotting or bleeding; and
- leaking fluid.

Have patient time contractions. (See Patient Education for description of timing contractions.)

If the patient reports four or more contractions in an hour, each lasting 45 to 60 seconds, have patient get in a comfortable position and do the following:

- lie on left side;
- drink 1 quart of water;
- monitor contractions for 1 hour; and
- call back immediately if symptoms worsen; otherwise report in 1 hour.

If symptoms continue but do not worsen, patient should be seen within 1 to 3 hours for evaluation.

If symptoms subside, advise the patient to rest for the remainder of the day and call in the morning to report how she is feeling.

If there is **any** suspicion of preterm labor or an acute abdominal complaint, the patient should go to the labor and delivery unit or the office immediately for evaluation.

STEP C: Pain Confined to One Part of Abdomen, Relieved by Position Change

The patient may be experiencing round ligament pain.

Have the patient describe the location of pain. If the pain is in the right or left lower quadrant, this may be round ligament pain.

Advise the patient to avoid sudden position change and to support her abdomen when she coughs.

Have her call back if the symptoms increase, particularly if there is right lower quadrant pain.

If the pain is located in another region of the abdomen but still is relieved with position change, have the patient monitor her symptoms and call back if the symptoms increase or are accompanied by other symptoms. If symptoms persist beyond 24 hours, the patient should be seen for evaluation.

STEP D: Pain Confined to One Part of Abdomen, Not Relieved by Position Change

Question the patient as to area of pain.

Record the frequency, duration, and severity of the pain.

Forward a message to the patient's provider so follow-up can be made within the hour.

STEP E: Pain Associated with Other Symptoms

Remember that diarrhea may be associated with preterm labor.

Appendicitis: If the patient still has her appendix and the pain is in the right lower quadrant or the patient is experiencing bowel changes, she should be seen ASAP or sent to an ER or urgent care center for an acute abdomen evaluation.

Gallbladder Attack: If the pain is located in the right upper quadrant or to the right of the sternum, particularly if the patient has a history of gallstones, or the pain is associated with eating, the patient should be seen within 24 hours by her primary care provider or sooner if symptoms increase.

Gastrointestinal Complaints: Bowel changes, nausea, or vomiting associated with malaise or other flu-like symptoms may indicate gastritis, particularly if other family members are experiencing similar symptoms. If there are no other complications, the condition may be managed at home. (See Patient Education.)

Refer the patient to her physician or the ER if she has:

- increasing fever;
- pain localized on right side (either lower or upper right quadrant) to exclude appendicitis or portal hypertension with pregnancy-induced hypertension;
- symptoms not resolving within 12–24 hours; or
- signs of significant dehydration, including the inability to keep down any fluids (even sips of water), no urine output in the past 8 hours, or dizziness.

Urinary Tract Infection: If the patient experiences pain on urination or has unusually frequent urination, arrange for the patient to provide a urine sample for culture that day. If the patient is experiencing low-back ache or flulike symptoms, such as nausea, vomiting, or fever, she should be seen ASAP to evaluate for a kidney infection.

PATIENT EDUCATION

Monitoring for Contractions

1. Patients should be taught to monitor for contractions by doing the following.

- Place your hands lightly on each side of your abdomen.
- If the uterus tightens beneath your hands, you are contracting, whether or not you are experiencing pain.

- Time from the beginning of one contraction to the beginning of the next.
- Time the length of the contraction as the amount of time your uterus tightens.
- Call back if you are contracting four times or more in an hour, with contractions lasting 45–60 seconds; if symptoms rapidly escalate; if you are bleeding; if you are leaking fluid from the vagina; or if contractions are accompanied by bowel changes.

2. Some women experience more abdominal discomfort than do others, more contractions than do others, and more pain in general. These women will need help in establishing what is normal for them and need to feel confident they can call with symptoms any time.

Gastritis
1. Modify the diet for the next 24 hours.
   Avoid milk/milk products
   Slowly rehydrate with sips of water (2 sips of water every 5–10 minutes)
   Progress to clear liquids
   Slowly begin BRAT (bananas, rice, applesauce, and toast) diet after tolerating clear liquids.

2. Call primary care provider to schedule a same-day appointment if:
   symptoms do not begin to resolve in 12–24 hours;
   symptoms increase in intensity (more vomiting, diarrhea);
   fever begins; or
   the patient has any concerns whatsoever.

2nd Trimester Ambivalence/Depression

KEY QUESTIONS

ASSESSMENT	ACTION
1. Are you feeling ambivalent about this pregnancy or having doubts about being pregnant?	**YES** Go to Step A.
	NO Go to Question 2.
2. Are you feeling depressed or especially anxious about this pregnancy?	**YES** Go to Step B.
	NO Go to Question 3.
3. Do you have any history of depression, postpartum depression, or mental illness?	**YES** Go to Step C.
	NO Go to Question 4.
4. Are you experiencing feelings that you want to harm yourself or someone else?	**YES** Go to Step D.
	NO Return to Step B.

ACTIONS

STEP A: Ambivalence in Pregnancy

Research indicates that four of five women experience some degree of ambivalence during pregnancy. This ambivalence begins to subside the closer to term a woman approaches. Options for pregnancy termination fade in the 2nd trimester.

Even during a planned pregnancy, a woman may not feel totally sure about the concept of being pregnant.

Talking with a partner, significant other, close friend, or family member may be beneficial for some patients.

In cases of an unplanned pregnancy, it may be helpful to talk to a counselor throughout the pregnancy to keep track of emotions.

In our practice, we recommend the following counselors who may be of value in helping to sort out feelings of ambivalence and pregnancy continuation: _____
_____.

STEP B: Possible Underlying Depression or Anxiety

Major life events may unmask or precipitate depression or anxiety. If there is any question that the patient is experiencing uncontrolled mood swings, thoughts about harming herself or others, feeling out of control, or becoming withdrawn, do the following.

- Make a same-day appointment for the patient with a mental health provider, and ensure that a friend, family member, or social services worker accompanies the patient to the appointment.
- Ensure that a high-risk patient is not left alone.
- If necessary, have another person in your office call Emergency Services, and remain on the line with the patient until help arrives.
- Notify a provider in your practice of the problem and your actions.

If patient is of no danger to herself or others, do the following.

- Refer the patient to a mental health counselor within the next 3–5 days.
- Reassure the patient that she may call back at any time if symptoms worsen.

Your practice should have a system for identifying patients possibly at risk for depression early in pregnancy.

In our practice, we do the following to identify patients at risk for depression during pregnancy (and thus possibly postpartum depression): _____

_____ .

STEP C: History of Depression or Mental Illness

Patients with a history may be at greater risk with a new pregnancy.
Repeat actions in Step B.

STEP D: Desire to Harm Oneself or Others

If the patient is experiencing uncontrolled mood swings, thoughts about harming herself or others, feeling out of control, or becoming seriously withdrawn, do the following.

- Make a same-day appointment for the patient with a mental health counselor, and ensure that a friend, family member, or social services worker accompanies the patient to the appointment.
- Ensure that a high-risk patient is not left alone.
- If necessary, have another person in your office call Emergency Services, and remain on the line with the patient until help arrives.
- Notify a provider in your practice of the problem and your actions.

PATIENT EDUCATION

1. Reassuring a patient that ambivalence is common in early pregnancy may be reassurance enough that her thoughts are not abnormal. However, expressions of increasing ambivalence as the 3rd trimester approaches may signal other problems.
2. Patients with a history of depression during pregnancy or the postpartum period need education regarding the possible recurrence and to know that help is available. Avoid being judgmental. Many patients have the misconception that all feelings can be controlled by will.

2nd Trimester Backache

ASSESSMENT	ACTION
1. Do you have a pre-existing back problem?	**YES** Go to Step A. Continue to Question 2.
	NO Go to Question 2.
2. Does the pain radiate from your back to the front of your abdomen? Does the back pain "let up" at a predictable interval? Can you feel a sensation of uterine tightening associated with your backache?	**YES** Go to Step B.
	NO Go to Question 3.
3. Is the pain confined to one part of your back and relieved by position change?	**YES** Go to Step C.
	NO Go to Question 4.
4. Is the pain confined to one part of your back and **not** relieved by position change?	**YES** Go to Step D.
	NO Go to Question 5.
5. Is the back pain accompanied by nausea, vomiting, bowel changes, fever, or dysuria?	**YES** Go to Step E.
	NO Go to Patient Education.

ACTIONS

STEP A: Preexisting Back Condition

It is common for pre-existing back conditions to become aggravated during the 2nd trimester.

Determine the nature of the pre-existing problem.

Question the patient as to whether or not she has seen a health care provider regarding her condition before pregnancy.

Continue on with questions to eliminate any acute problem before encouraging the patient to call her regular health care provider if she has not done so during this pregnancy.

Refer to Patient Education.

STEP B: Backache Accompanied by Possible Contractions

This patient may be experiencing onset of preterm labor.

Have patient time the contractions. (See Patient Education for description of timing contractions.)

If patient reports four or more contractions in an hour, that last 45–60 seconds, have the patient get in a comfortable position and do the following:

- lie on left side;
- drink 1 quart of water;
- monitor contractions for 1 hour; and
- call back immediately, if symptoms worsen; otherwise report in 1 hour.

If symptoms continue but do not worsen, the patient should be seen in 1–3 hours for evaluation.

If symptoms subside, advise the patient to rest for the remainder of the day and call in the morning to report how she is feeling.

STEP C: Backache Confined to One Part of Back, Relieved by Position Change

The patient may be experiencing nerve compression or muscle spasm.

Determine the area of pain and methods that relieve the discomfort.

Attempt to pinpoint conditions that may aggravate the discomfort (such as going up and down stairs, shifting gears in car, carrying infant).

Suggest appropriate substitutions for aggravating actions.

Encourage proper body mechanics.

Refer the patient to her primary care provider for a physical therapy referral, if indicated.

See Patient Education for general measures for relief of back pain.

STEP D: Backache Confined, Unrelieved by Position Change

Question the patient regarding the area of pain.

Record the frequency, duration, and severity of the pain.

After eliminating the possibility of uterine contractions, forward a message to the patient's provider so the provider can act on the message within the hour.

STEP E: Backache Associated with Other Symptoms

Remember that diarrhea may be associated with preterm labor.

Question the patient regarding the frequency, duration, and severity of the pain.

Ask if the patient has a history of kidney stones, frequent UTIs, or has sickle cell disease or is a carrier of sickle cell.

If the patient experiences pain on urination, unusually frequent urination, and has a backache described as "mild", have her come into the office or clinic for a clean-caught urine culture.

If the patient is experiencing backache associated with flulike symptoms, nausea, vomiting, or fever, she should be seen ASAP to evaluate for a kidney infection.

PATIENT EDUCATION

1. Patients should be taught to monitor for contractions by doing the following.

   - Place your hands lightly on each side of your abdomen.
   - If your uterus tightens beneath your hands, you are contracting, whether or not you experience pain.
   - Time from the beginning of one contraction to the beginning of the next.
   - Time the length of the contraction as the amount of time your uterus feels tightened.
   - Call back if you are contracting four times or more in an hour, with contractions lasting 45 to 60 seconds; if symptoms rapidly escalate; if you are bleeding; if you are leaking fluid from the vagina; or if contractions are accompanied by bowel changes.

2. Some women experience more backache than do others. These women need help in establishing what is normal for them and need to feel confident they can call any time to report their symptoms.
3. General measures for increasing back comfort are as follows:

   - Practice good posture. Adjust as your center of gravity changes with the growing uterus.
   - Wear comfortable shoes.
   - Avoid standing for prolonged periods of time. Elevate one foot, if possible.
   - Sleep on a firm mattress.
   - Learn proper exercises for stretching back muscles.

2nd Trimester Bleeding

KEY QUESTIONS

ASSESSMENT	ACTION
1. Is there any pain associated with your bleeding?	**YES** Go to Step A. **NO** Go to Step B. Continue to next question.
2. Have you had a sonogram (ultrasound) in the 2nd trimester?	**YES** Go to Step B. **NO** Schedule a **same-day appointment** for sonogram.
3. Are you experiencing any vaginal itching, burning, odor, or other discharge?	**YES** Go to Step C. **NO** Go to Step D.

ACTIONS

STEP A: Abdominal Pain Associated With Vaginal Bleeding

A patient experiencing abdominal pain with vaginal bleeding needs to be seen ASAP in an appropriate facility. The patient should not drive herself. Transportation to the appropriate facility will depend on your location, the patient's location, and the availability of necessary services.

If the patient meets your facility's criteria for heavy bleeding, the patient needs to be seen ASAP, whether or not she is experiencing pain.

If the patient is bleeding lightly, she still needs to be evaluated that day for the possibility of preterm labor or placental problems. Question her as to the presence of contractions. If there is any question of preterm labor, the patient needs immediate evaluation.

STEP B: Painless Vaginal Bleeding

Painless vaginal bleeding in the 2nd trimester is suggestive of placenta previa until proven otherwise.

Ascertain if the patient has had a sonogram. If the answer is "no" or the sonogram cannot be located, schedule an appointment that day for the patient with a provider who can perform a sonogram to determine placental location.

STEP C: Vaginal Spotting Associated With Pain, Itching, or Odor

The patient may have a vaginal infection. She should be seen that day for a wet mount and possible vaginal culture.

STEP D: Other Possibilities

The patient may have other structural problems, such as a cervical polyp. Under **any** circumstances, the patient needs to be evaluated that day for vaginal bleeding, no matter how light. At this gestation, the chance to make a difference in outcome, because of fetal viability, should govern decision making.

PATIENT EDUCATION

1. All patients should be told that any bleeding in the 2nd trimester should be reported immediately.
2. Patients who have had a sonogram should know the location of their placenta. Placenta previa or marginal placental localization is common in the 2nd trimester. Fortunately, most of these will resolve by early in the 3rd trimester.

2nd Trimester Constipation

KEY QUESTIONS

ASSESSMENT	ACTION
1. Have your symptoms worsened during the course of your pregnancy?	**YES** Go to Step A.
	NO Go to Question 2.
2. Is the constipation accompanied by prolonged nausea, vomiting, abdominal distension, or failure to pass gas?	**YES** Go to Step B.
	NO Go to Question 3.
3. Do you have a pre-existing problem with constipation?	**YES** Go to Step C.
	NO Go to Question 4.
4. Is there blood in your stool?	**YES** Go to Step D.
	NO Return to Step A.

ACTIONS

STEP A: Pregnancy Related

Constipation is a common complaint throughout pregnancy. Causes in the 2nd trimester include continued hormonal effects. The following suggestions may be helpful:

- Increase fiber in the diet.
- Increase clear fluids by 1–2 quarts daily.
- Add stool softeners as determined by office/clinic protocols. (See list of approved stool softeners.)
- Increase exercise within limits of 2nd trimester. Keep pulse rate below 140 beats/minute.
- Change the prenatal vitamin to one that has time-released iron, or avoid iron supplementation.
- Assess calcium needs. Many patients mistakenly take more calcium supplementation than is needed.
- Avoid laxatives.

Continue on to Questions 2, 3, and 4.

STEP B: Constipation With Additional Symptoms

Ileus is uncommon in pregnancy but must not be overlooked. If the patient has additional symptoms, she should call her primary care provider immediately.
Continue on to Questions 3 and 4.

STEP C: History of Constipation

Patients with history of constipation or irritable bowel syndrome may have a worsening of symptoms.
Assess laxative and other medication use.
Encourage use of the recommendations in Step A. If the patient is a chronic abuser of laxatives or experiences no response after trying the suggestions in Step A, refer her to an obstetric care provider or gastrointestinal care provider.

STEP D: Blood in Stool

Blood in the stool may be a sign of straining or hemorrhoids but also may be a signal of a more serious medical problem. The patient should have this symptom evaluated by her obstetric care provider at her next scheduled appointment or sooner, if symptoms worsen.

PATIENT EDUCATION

1. There are many iron preparations available that are more easily absorbed for patients who are known to have anemia but are reluctant to take iron supplements because of constipation.

   Our practice recommends: _____.

2. Calcium (particularly calcium carbonate) can be constipating and can directly interfere with iron absorption.

   Our practice recommends you try: _____.

3. All minerals probably are best absorbed when obtained through consumed foods. Encourage the patient to try to meet her mineral needs through diet as well as through supplementation.

2nd Trimester Decreased Fetal Movement

KEY QUESTIONS

ASSESSMENT	ACTION
1. Did you feel fetal movement during the last 24 hours?	**YES** Go to Step A.
	NO Go to Question 2.
2. Have you felt fetal movement every day for the last week?	**YES** Go to Step B.
	NO Go to Step C.
3. Have you experienced a pregnancy loss in the past?	**YES** Go to Step D.
	NO No action.

ACTIONS

STEP A: Felt Fetal Movement in Last 24 Hours

Many patients have an unrealistic expectation of fetal movement early in the 2nd trimester. Even if they have consistently felt fetal movement, based on fetal size, a change in position may greatly decrease the sensation of fetal movement. There is no accepted standard for perception of fetal movement in the 2nd trimester.

Ask the patient when she last felt fetal movement and under what conditions she felt it.

If the patient is at less than 24 weeks' gestation, discuss the variation in fetal position and effect on fetal movement. Encourage the patient to get in a comfortable position in which she previously has felt fetal movement, make sure she's eaten or had something to drink, and wait to feel the fetal movement.

Although there is no standard, if the patient is highly anxious after a few hours and still unable to feel fetal movement, invite her in to hear the fetal heart. Many patients will not be comforted in any other way.

Patients who are highly anxious about fetal movement at this gestation need reassurance and education regarding the expectations of what movement they can feel. Patients experiencing prior losses often need more frequent visits until the time of prior loss has passed. You should discuss you practice's philosophy in dealing with these patients' needs.

Most patients at greater than 24 weeks' gestation will not be reassured unless they have confirmation of fetal viability. If such patients are unable to feel fetal movement within 2 to 3 hours of calling, they should call back and come in to hear the fetal heart.

STEP B: Has Felt Fetal Movement Every Day for A Week

Most patients who have felt fetal movement every day for at least a week will expect to feel constant fetal movement, despite that no standard exists for fetal movement at this point in pregnancy.

If the patient is at less than 24 weeks' gestation, apply Step A.

If the patient is at greater than 24 weeks' gestation, have her come in for a quick fetal heart check that day.

Ask her to call back and cancel the appointment, if she feels fetal movement in the interim.

STEP C: Inconsistent Fetal Movement

This patient is unlikely to be able to feel fetal movement "on command."

If the patient is at less than 24 weeks' gestation, reassure her that this lack of fetal movement is normal, despite what she may have read in books.

Most women experiencing pregnancy for the first time are not convinced of fetal movement until closer to 20 weeks' gestation and may not feel daily movement until approximately 24 weeks.

If this is not the patient's first pregnancy, reassure her that perceptions of fetal movement may vary from pregnancy to pregnancy.

If the patient is not reassured, she should be seen for a fetal heart check. You should discuss how to handle these patients with the providers with whom you work to offer a consistent philosophic approach for these women.

STEP D: Prior Pregnancy Loss

These patients generally will need more reassurance until the time of prior loss passes, even though no standard exists for fetal movement in the 2nd trimester. Your practice should have a plan for making these women comfortable.

PATIENT EDUCATION

1. This is one area where prior education can help to set more realistic expectations.
2. It helps to "warn" patients in the 1st trimester that their pregnancy may not follow the book!
3. Early patient classes, printed information, or one-on-one education on this issue will prevent later apprehension.
4. Patients with a history of prior loss need to know how you will reassure them along the course of this pregnancy.

2nd Trimester Fatigue

KEY QUESTIONS

ASSESSMENT

ACTION

1. Have your symptoms worsened as your pregnancy has progressed?

YES Go to Step A.

NO Go to Question 2.

2. Do you have a history of a chronic medical condition, such as anemia or thyroid or cardiac problems?

YES Go to Step B.

NO Go to Question 3.

3. Do you have extenuating circumstances that could be contributing to your fatigue, such as small children or a demanding work schedule?

YES Go to Step C.

NO No further action.

ACTIONS

STEP A: Pregnancy-Related Fatigue

There are several causes of worsening of fatigue in pregnancy. An increase in blood volume during the 2nd trimester may cause a relative anemia, which usually improves by term.

If the patient has had a recent hematocrit or hemoglobin level obtained, recommend she discuss her symptoms at her next appointment.

The following suggestions may prove useful:

- Take more frequent naps or rest periods.
- Go to bed earlier or arise later.
- Eliminate nonessential activities.
- Decrease personal expectations.
- Enlist help from family members or friends.

STEP B: Pre-existing Illnesses

Patients who have a history of a pre-existing medical condition that may be contributing to the fatigue should have that condition re-evaluated each trimester, or sooner, if the condition worsens. Pregnancy may change the amounts or types of medications the patient should be taking or may cause an alteration or worsening of the condition.

STEP C: Outside Stressors

Many patients underestimate the demands in their lives that may contribute to the already-draining adaptation to pregnancy.

Refer to Step A actions.

Evaluate resources for support.

2nd Trimester Headache

KEY QUESTIONS

ASSESSMENT	ACTION
1. Was the onset of this headache sudden and severe?	**YES** Go to Step A.
	NO Go to Question 2.
2. Is the headache accompanied by any numbness, tingling, loss of bowel or bladder control, or seizure behaviors?	**YES** Go to Step A.
	NO Go to Question 3.
3. Is the headache accompanied by visual changes?	**YES** Go to Step B.
	NO Go to Question 4.
4. Is the headache accompanied by debilitating neck stiffness or high fever?	**YES** Go to Step A.
	NO Go to Question 5.
5. Is the headache accompanied by upper respiratory tract infection symptoms (congestion, fever, cough, or facial or tooth discomfort)?	**YES** Go to Step C.
	NO Go to Question 6.
6. Is the headache dull and not debilitating in nature?	**YES** Go to Step D.
	NO No further action.

ACTIONS

STEP A: Sudden, Severe Headache

The onset of a sudden, severe headache usually is not a problem related to obstetrics and needs immediate referral to the patient's primary care provider, or ER, as appropriate. The patient should not drive herself. If the headache is accompanied by loss of sensorimotor skills, the patient or her agent should call 911. Symptoms of numbness, tingling, high fever, and debilitating neck stiffness are not usually 2nd trimester complaints and warrant medical evaluation.

STEP B: Neurological Symptoms

Question the patient regarding her history of migraine headaches. Are these headaches like the migraines that she's experienced before?

Refer the patient to an on-call provider to determine if additional neurological evaluation is warranted and to determine the safety of any medications the patient may have on hand for treatment of her migraines.

Instruct the patient to lie in a dark room and apply compresses to the area where she is experiencing the headache.

If she does not experience relief within 1–2 hours, refer the patient to her primary care provider for medication management.

STEP C: Respiratory Symptoms

If the patient has symptoms of an upper respiratory tract infection, she may be experiencing a sinus headache.

Recommend the patient take acetaminophen 650 mg orally every 4–6 hours as needed, not to exceed the manufacturer's recommended dosage, or other medication as agreed upon by your practice for the use of pain relief during the 2nd trimester.

Consult an obstetric care provider before recommending the use of decongestants.

Refer the patient to her primary care provider if she does not experience improvement within 3–5 days.

Instruct the patient to call her primary care provider if symptoms worsen.

STEP D: Dull Headaches

Dull headaches are common in early pregnancy (probably because of hormonal and vascular changes) and may peak and disappear by 14–16 weeks.

Recommend the patient take acetaminophen 650 mg orally every 4–6 hours as needed, not to exceed the manufacturer's recommended dosage, or other medication as agreed upon by your practice.

Increasing rest and decreasing stressful factors may lessen headaches.

The patient's primary care provider should evaluate persistent dull headaches.

2nd Trimester Indigestion

KEY QUESTIONS

ASSESSMENT

ACTION

1. Is the onset of your symptoms pregnancy related?

YES Go to Step A.

NO Go to Question 2.

2. Is the indigestion accompanied by prolonged nausea, vomiting, abdominal distension, or failure to pass gas?

YES Go to Step B.

NO Go to Question 3.

3. Do you have a pre-existing problem with indigestion?

YES Go to Step C.

NO No further action.

ACTIONS

STEP A: Onset Pregnancy Related

Indigestion is a common pregnancy-related problem, usually developing during the 2nd trimester and worsening near term.

The following suggestions may be helpful:

- Avoid spicy, fried, or fatty foods.
- Drink liquids between meals, instead of "washing down" food at mealtime.
- Eat small meals instead of three large meals.
- Space eating throughout the day. Avoid eating before bed.
- Change your prenatal vitamin to one with time-released iron or avoid iron supplementation.
- Try elevating your head while sleeping.
- Take antacids, as approved by your providers.

Continue on to Questions 2 and 3.

STEP B: Indigestion With Additional Symptoms

Ileus and cholecystitis are relatively uncommon in pregnancy but must not be overlooked. If the patient has additional or severe symptoms, she should call her primary care provider immediately.

Continue on to Question 3.

STEP C: History of Indigestion

Patients with a history of indigestion or reflux may have a worsening of symptoms.
Continue on with recommendations in Step A. If the patient is a chronic user of
antacids or has tried the suggestions in Step A and experienced no response, refer
her to her obstetric care provider or gastrointestinal care provider.

PATIENT EDUCATION

1. Encourage the patient to try simple methods to relieve symptoms before relying on
   antacids early in pregnancy. This is a problem that tends to worsen as the pregnancy
   progresses, so starting with the "big guns" may limit the patient's options later in
   pregnancy.
2. There are many iron preparations available that may be more easily absorbed for
   the patient who is known to be anemic but who is reluctant to take iron because of
   indigestion.

   Our practice recommends: _____.

3. Not all common antacids are recommended by all providers. Our practice recommends you try: _____.

2nd Trimester Nasal Congestion

KEY QUESTIONS

ASSESSMENT	ACTION
1. Is the nasal congestion green or yellow?	**YES** Go to Step A.
	NO Go to Question 2.
2. Do you have a fever greater than 100° F?	**YES** Go to Step A.
	NO Go to Question 3.
3. Do you have a cough, ear pain, facial pain, facial or ear pressure, or a sore throat?	**YES** Go to Step A.
	NO Go to Question 4.
4. Is the nasal congestion clear?	**YES** Go to Step B.
	NO Go to Patient Education.

ACTIONS

STEP A: Colored Nasal Congestion

Colored nasal discharge may be associated with a viral or a bacterial upper respiratory tract infection.

Other symptoms of an upper respiratory tract infection, sinus, or ear infection include fever, cough, ear or facial pain, pressure, or a sore throat. The patient should be urged to call her primary care provider for evaluation and treatment.

STEP B: Clear Nasal Congestion

The hormone progesterone rises during pregnancy. Progesterone increases and thickens nasal secretions in pregnancy. This is a normal side effect of pregnancy. See Patient Education for recommendations for dealing with increased nasal congestion during pregnancy.

PATIENT EDUCATION

Use a cool mist vaporizer. This will lessen the thickness of your secretions. Make sure you clean and dry the vaporizer, as directed by the manufacturer. This will help to prevent growth of bacteria and microorganisms in the vaporizer.

Use saline nose drops, two drops in each nostril 3–4 times/day. Avoid other types of nose drops or nasal sprays; they may be extremely irritating to the mucous membranes in your nose.

Drink lots of water (1–2 quarts more than you usually drink). Water decreases the thickness of nasal secretions and keeps the mucous membranes in your nose moist.

2nd Trimester Nausea/Vomiting

KEY QUESTIONS

ASSESSMENT	ACTION
1. During the last 24 hours or more, have you been unable to keep down food or liquids?	**YES** Go to Question 2.
	NO Go to Step A.
2. Have your symptoms continued during the course of your pregnancy?	**YES** Go to Step B.
	NO Go to Question 3.
3. Are you having any sensation of uterine tightening with the nausea and or vomiting? Is there any diarrhea associated with your symptoms?	**YES** Go to Step C.
	NO Go to Question 4.
4. Do you have any pre-existing food intolerances or gastrointestinal problems?	**YES** Go to Step D.
	NO Go to Question 5.
5. Are your symptoms accompanied by fever or spasmodic abdominal pain?	**YES** Go to Step E.
	NO No further action.

ACTIONS

STEP A: Acute Inability to Retain Food or Liquids

The patient is at risk for dehydration, which may contribute to uterine contractions.
Advise the patient to come in for evaluation of her dehydration within 12 to 24 hours.
Advise the patient to call her obstetric care provider if she has no urine output for 12 hours while awaiting an appointment.
Advise the patient to come in immediately if she experiences projectile vomiting, severe diarrhea, or other severe symptoms.

STEP B: Pregnancy-Related Symptoms

Some women have protracted nausea and vomiting throughout the course of their pregnancy. There is nothing magical for them about the end of the 1st trimester!
The patient may continue to avoid prenatal vitamins with iron. Some women take a children's vitamin daily.
Continue dietary nausea measures used during the 1st trimester.

The patient may warrant a nutrition consult, if persistent symptoms interfere with her nutritional intake or weight gain. Have her discuss this with her obstetric care provider at her next visit or sooner if indicated.

STEP C: Possible Preterm Labor Symptoms

Prostaglandins, which may cause contractions, also may cause nausea, vomiting, and diarrhea in some women.

Instruct the patient to time her contractions. (See the protocol 2nd Trimester Abdominal Pain.)

If the patient reports four or more contractions in an hour, each lasting 45 to 60 seconds, have her get in a comfortable position and do the following:

- lie on left side;
- drink 1 quart of water;
- monitor contractions for an hour; and
- call back if symptoms worsen; otherwise report in 1 hour.

If symptoms persist but do not worsen, the patient should be seen in 1–3 hours for evaluation.

If symptoms subside, advise the patient to rest for the remainder of the day, continue hydration, and call in the morning to report how she is feeling.

STEP D: Pre-existing Conditions

Patients with pre-existing serious gastrointestinal problems who are taking maintenance medication warrant a medical evaluation if they have not already had one.

Refer the patient for nutritional counseling, as indicated.

Refer the patient to the dietary measures mentioned under 2nd trimester nausea.

Have the patient call her gastrointestinal care provider, if symptoms have not been alleviated by previous treatment.

STEP E: Possible Flu or Abdominal Problem

Nausea and vomiting accompanied by temperature greater than 100.4°F need immediate evaluation.

Refer the patient immediately to an obstetric care provider, ER, or urgent care center.

PATIENT EDUCATION

1. Patients need to understand the usual course of nausea and vomiting in pregnancy, remembering that some women do not "follow the book" when it comes to symptoms.
2. It cannot be overemphasized that women with serious pre-existing gastrointestinal conditions, such as Crohn's disease, colitis, and diverticulitis, should have a medical evaluation before pregnancy. These women also may require continued gastrointestinal follow-up throughout the course of their pregnancy.
3. Women with nutritional difficulties, such as celiac disease or lactose intolerance, may have an exacerbation of their symptoms and benefit from nutritional counseling.

2nd Trimester Pelvic Pain/Pressure

KEY QUESTIONS

ASSESSMENT	ACTION
1. Are you experiencing an increase in rhythmic pelvic pressure?	**YES** Go to Step A. Continue to Question 3.
	NO Go to Step B.
2. Are you having any uterine tightening associated with the rhythmic pelvic pressure?	**YES** Go to Step A.
	NO Go to Question 3.
3. Are you having any vaginal bleeding associated with the pain?	**YES** Go to Step C.
	NO Go to Question 4.
4. Are you experiencing pelvic pressure confined to one location?	**YES** Go to Steps D and E.
	NO Go to Patient Education.

ACTIONS

STEP A: Symptoms Consistent With Contractions

If this patient is less than 36 weeks pregnant, she may be experiencing an onset of preterm labor.

Have the patient time her contractions. (See Patient Education for description of timing of contractions.)

If the patient reports four or more contractions in a hour, each lasting 45–60 seconds, have her get in a comfortable position and do the following:

- lie on left side;
- drink 1 quart of water;
- monitor her contractions for an hour; and
- call back immediately if symptoms worsen; otherwise report in 1 hour.

If the symptoms continue but do not worsen, the patient should be seen within 1–3 hours for evaluation.

If the symptoms subside, advise the patient to rest for the remainder of the day and call in the morning to report how she is feeling.

If the patient is 37 weeks to term, she may be going into labor. See the protocol 3rd Trimester Recognizing Labor.

STEP B: Nonrhythmic Pelvic Pressure

Pelvic pressure from the growing fetus is a normal symptom during the late 2nd and 3rd trimester. It may progressively increase toward term.

Advise the patient to get off her feet and rest. Symptoms should be relieved.

The patient may need to cut back on activities or work demands, if the pressure is debilitating. She should discuss this with her obstetric care provider.

The patient should report any uncomfortable change in symptoms to discuss the possibility of labor signs.

STEP C: Vaginal Bleeding Associated With Pelvic Pain and Pressure

A patient who is 36 weeks pregnant or less and who is bleeding heavily needs to be seen ASAP in an appropriate facility. The patient should not drive herself. Transportation to the appropriate facility will depend on your location, the patient's location, and the availability of necessary services.

If the bleeding is "less than a period," the patient still needs to be seen ASAP to ensure that she is not experiencing preterm labor or placental problems.

STEP D: Pressure Confined to One Part of Pelvis

The patient may be experiencing pain caused by muscle spasm or fetal position.

Have the patient describe the location of the pain.

Reassure the patient the pain usually is attributable to fetal position.

Advise the patient to avoid sudden position change and support her abdomen when coughing.

Instruct the patient to get off her feet to see if symptoms are relieved.

Instruct the patient to call back, if her symptoms increase.

If the pain is located in a region other than the abdomen but still is relieved with position change, have patient monitor her symptoms and call back if they increase or are accompanied by other symptoms. If the symptoms persist beyond 24 hours, the patient should be seen for evaluation.

STEP E: Pain Confined to One Part of Abdomen, Not Relieved by Position Change

Question the patient regarding the area of the pain.

Record the frequency, duration, and severity of the pain, particularly noting right upper quadrant pain.

Question the patient regarding any recent developing problems, such as preeclampsia.

Forward a message to the patient's provider for dispensation within 30 minutes.

PATIENT EDUCATION

1. Patients should be taught to monitor for contractions by doing the following:

   Place your hands lightly on each side of your abdomen.

   If your uterus tightens beneath your hands, you are contracting, whether or not you experience pain.

Time from the beginning of one contraction to the beginning of the next.

Time the length of the contraction as the amount of time your uterus feels tightened.

Call back, if you are contracting four times or more in 1 hour, with each lasting 45 to 60 seconds; if your symptoms rapidly escalate; if you are bleeding; if you are leaking fluid from the vagina; or if your contractions are accompanied by bowel changes.

2. Some women experience more pelvic pain and pressure than do others, more contractions than do others, and more pain in general. These women will need help in establishing what is normal for them and need to feel confident they can call with symptoms any time.

2nd Trimester Swelling

KEY QUESTIONS

ASSESSMENT	ACTION
1. Is the swelling accompanied by visual changes, headache, right upper quadrant pain, chest pain, or sharp leg pain? Or do you have a history of pregnancy-induced hypertension or chronic hypertension?	**YES** Go to Step A.
	NO Go to Question 2.
2. Is swelling occurring in the face and arms as well as in the legs?	**YES** Go to Step B.
	NO Go to Question 3.
3. Is the swelling localized to the legs?	**YES** Go to Step C.
	NO No further action.

ACTIONS

STEP A: Swelling With Other Symptoms

Swelling accompanied by headache, visual changes, right upper quadrant pain, or chest pain may be a warning sign of pregnancy-induced hypertension. The patient should be seen in the office or ER for immediate evaluation.

A history of pregnancy-induced hypertension or chronic hypertension places a pregnant woman at risk for the development of pregnancy-induced hypertension in her current pregnancy. Even without additional symptoms, such women should receive a same-day appointment for additional evaluation.

STEP B: Facial and Upper Extremity Swelling

Facial and upper extremity swelling in pregnancy may be more concerning than swelling restricted to the legs. The patient should be evaluated for pregnancy-induced hypertension within the next 24 hours.

STEP C: Uncomplicated Swelling

Swelling of the legs is a common complaint in pregnancy. Pressure by the fetus on the inferior vena cava, increased circulating blood volume, and the relaxant effects of progesterone all contribute to this symptom. See Patient Education for measures to decrease swelling.

PATIENT EDUCATION

Advise the patient to do the following for swelling:

Increase the time spent off of feet and lying on side.

Avoid the heat in warm weather.

Elevate legs above the heart level.

Drink plenty of water (1–2 quarts more than the usual fluid intake).

Avoid extra salt or MSG.

Use pregnancy support hose. If the patient is using them, make sure they have been fitted properly.

Call if additional symptoms occur or current symptoms worsen.

2nd Trimester Urinary Complaints

ASSESSMENT

	ACTION
1. Are you experiencing more frequent urination?	**YES** Go to Question 2.
	NO Go to Step A.
2. Do you have pubic pain or pressure or burning on urination?	**YES** Go to Step B.
	NO Go to Question 3.
3. Do you have blood in your urine, a low backache, or flulike symptoms, such as nausea, vomiting, or a fever?	**YES** Go to Step C.
	NO Go to Question 4.
4. Do you have sickle cell disease or are you a sickle cell carrier?	**YES** Go to Step D.
	NO No further action.

ACTIONS

STEP A: Frequent Urination Without Other Symptoms

During the 2nd trimester of pregnancy, most women do not experience increased frequency of urination. If the patient has symptoms of increased frequency of urination, she should come to the office to give a clean-caught urine specimen for analysis, culture, and sensitivity.

STEP B: Frequent Urination With Pelvic Symptoms

Increased frequency of urination with symptoms such as burning can be indicative of a urinary tract infection. However, increased frequency of urination accompanied by pelvic pain or pressure also may be a sign of premature labor. The patient should be instructed to come to the office to give a clean-caught urine specimen for analysis, culture, and sensitivity, if she has burning on urination. However, if she has pelvic pressure or pain, she also should be evaluated for preterm labor. See the protocol 2nd Trimester Pelvic Pain/Pressure to determine that the patient is not experiencing preterm labor.

STEP C: Frequent Urination With Renal Symptoms

Frequent urination with accompanying low backache, flulike symptoms, or hematuria may be signals of a kidney infection or a more serious kidney complication. The patient should be instructed to schedule a same-day appointment with either her primary care provider or a urologist.

STEP D: Sickle Cell Disease or Sickle Cell Carrier

Women who have sickle cell disease or who are sickle cell carriers are at higher risk for asymptomatic urinary tract infections. These women should be instructed to come into the office to give a clean-caught urine specimen for analysis, culture, and sensitivity.

In addition, these women should receive a urinalysis during each trimester of their pregnancy to exclude an asymptomatic urinary tract infection.

2nd Trimester Vaginal Discharge

KEY QUESTIONS

ASSESSMENT	ACTION

1. Are you experiencing an increase in vaginal discharge without burning, itching, or odor?

YES Go to Step A.
NO Go to Question 2.

2. Are you having vaginal burning, itching, or odor?

YES Go to Step B.
NO Go to Question 3.

3. Do you have any burning with urination? If so, is the pain internal, especially at the end of urination, or is it external when the urine runs over the outside tissues?

YES Go to Step C.
NO Go to Question 4.

4. Are you concerned you could have been exposed to a sexually transmitted infection?

YES Go to Step D.
NO Go to Question 5.

5. Do you have any sores in your genital area?

YES Go to Step E. Go to next question.
NO Go to Question 6.

6. Do you have a history of exposure to herpes?

YES Go to Step F.
NO Go to Step G.

ACTIONS

STEP A: Physiologic Discharge of Pregnancy

The physiologic changes of pregnancy create a discharge that usually is thin, milk colored, and has a slight, but not unpleasant, odor. Reassure the patient that this discharge is normal and will increase during the course of her pregnancy.

Advise against douching during pregnancy. Douching can introduce air into the vagina, which is dangerous.

Advise the patient to call if she experiences change in the color or odor of the discharge or itching, burning, or lesions.

An additional consideration during the 2nd trimester is the possibility of premature rupture of membranes.

Question the patient regarding the changing nature of vaginal discharge. It often is described as being more viscous than it has been during the pregnancy. It also is described as having a faintly "sweet" or "clean" aroma.

Question the patient regarding the color of the fluid. Bloody or green fluid has different significance.

Question the patient regarding associated uterine tightening or vaginal bleeding.

If there is any question of ruptured membranes, have the patient come in to be seen ASAP.

STEP B: Symptoms of Vaginitis

Simple vaginitis is common in pregnancy, particularly because of an increase in yeast infections for some women. Vaginitis diagnosed as bacterial vaginosis has been implicated in preterm labor. Early elimination of the problem is important.

Have patient come in for evaluation within 3–5 days or sooner, if symptoms increase.

Avoid the use of OTC products until a diagnosis is made.

STEP C: Urinary Tract Symptoms

Yeast infections also can mimic UTI symptoms. In this case, the burning usually occurs when urine runs over the perineal tissues. Pain that occurs inside, especially at the end of voiding, is more likely to be a UTI.

If symptoms sound like a UTI, the patient should be seen ASAP. Explain to the patient that she may be asked to give a clean-caught urine sample during her office visit.

STEP D: Possible Sexually Transmitted Infection Exposure

Sexually transmitted infections can have a significant impact on pregnancy outcome. If the patient is found to have an STI during pregnancy, follow-up for her partner and evaluation for reinfection are of major concern to prevent harm to the fetus.

The patient should be instructed to come in within 24 hours for a thorough evaluation.

Prepare her for possible vaginal and vulvar cultures as well as possible blood tests.

Advise the patient to avoid sexual intercourse until she has been evaluated.

STEP E: Vulvovaginitis Symptoms With Possible Lesions

The patient with lesions present should be seen within 24–48 hours.

Instruct the patient to wash her hands thoroughly after urination.

The patient should avoid applying creams or lotions to the area until she has been seen for evaluation.

Comfort measure such as cold compresses and tepid baths may be soothing.

Advise the patient to avoid sexual intercourse until she has been evaluated.

STEP F: History of Herpetic Lesions

Patients with a history of herpes need to be educated about the risk if lesions are present at delivery.

Question the patient regarding the pattern of outbreak during this and previous pregnancies.

Your practice may or may not endorse the use of acyclovir for suppression near term. You should know your providers' opinion on this issue and discuss accordingly with the patient.

Follow advice in Step E.

Advise patient to come in for confirmation of lesion if she is uncertain.

STEP G: Vulvovaginitis Symptoms, Etiology Unknown

Question the patient regarding recent antibiotic use or changes in toilet tissue, bubble baths, or laundry detergent.

Question the patient about the recurrence rate.

Advise the patient on comfort measures recommended by your providers.

Make an appointment for the patient to come in within 72 hours.

PATIENT EDUCATION

1. Vaginitis in a pregnant woman may have different significance than in a nonpregnant woman because of the potential ramifications for the developing fetus. Many patients self-diagnose these conditions and may request specific medication prescriptions based on past symptom resolution. Whether or not to treat over the telephone without seeing the patient is at the discretion of your providers. Many offices or clinics have a policy to treat simple symptoms of yeast infections without seeing the patient. However, most providers will treat only once. If the patient experiences no improvement, she should be seen for evaluation.

2. The goal is to not miss a more serious, possibly communicable infection. If a patient is fairly certain she has been exposed to an STI, encourage her to have her partner(s) tested and to refrain from intercourse until she has been evaluated and treated. You may need to help her rehearse various scenarios before talking with her partner.

3. Patients exposed to STIs early in pregnancy need full testing for possible STIs and a plan for retesting throughout their pregnancy. It is reasonable to encourage these patients to use condoms to minimize the potential for exposure.

2nd Trimester Visual Changes

KEY QUESTIONS

ASSESSMENT	ACTION

1. Have you had a sudden loss (central or peripheral blindness) or significant change (blurring, double vision) in your vision?

   YES Go to Step A.

   NO Go to Question 2.

2. Do you have eye pain?

   YES Go to Question 3.

   NO Go to Question 4.

3. Is the pain unilateral, intense, and did it begin suddenly?

   YES Go to Step B.

   NO Go to Question 4.

4. Is the eye red but painless and your vision unaffected?

   YES Go to Step C.

   NO Go to Question 5.

5. Is your vision changing gradually and affecting normal activities, such as reading, sewing, or driving?

   YES Go to Step D.

   NO No further action.

ACTIONS

STEP A: Sudden Loss of Vision

This patient may be experiencing a TIA or stroke, may have acute angle glaucoma, retinal detachment, or be experiencing a new onset of ocular migraine. She should be seen immediately. Refer her to the ER or have the patient call 911. Make sure the patient does not drive herself to the ER.

STEP B: Eye Pain

The patient may have iritis, acute glaucoma, cluster headache, or an unusual ocular migraine presentation. The patient should be evaluated by her primary care provider within the next 2–4 hours. Make sure patient has someone drive her to the visit.

STEP C: Unilateral, Intense, Sudden Eye Pain

This could be a spontaneous hemorrhage, conjunctivitis, acute glaucoma, or scleritis. The patient should be evaluated by her primary care provider within the next 12 to 24 hours.

STEP D: Gradual Eye Changes

Because of hormonal changes, some women find their vision has changed during pregnancy or that they are no longer able to wear their contact lenses. Most women will find they can resume contact use after pregnancy. In addition, the patient may have changing central vision and need corrective lenses or a change in her current eyewear prescription. She should see her eye care provider within the next week.

CHAPTER 9

3rd Trimester Overview

Third trimester pregnancy complaints are common because of the pressure of the growing fetus on many body organs. Changes in the center of gravity, increasing venous compression, and difficulty sleeping also are attributable to the increase in uterine size and weight. Pre-existing conditions, such as back problems, may be aggravated. During this time, patient thoughts may be dominated by a combination of growing excitement and apprehension in anticipation of labor and early child care responsibilities.

Some issues dominate telephone triage concerns at this point. The importance of continued fetal movement is a concern. Many old wives tales exist about pregnancy, and perhaps one of the most insidious is that the baby should stop moving before labor. It is true that the nature of the perception of fetal movement may change as term approaches because of the growth and descent of the fetus, as well as increasing uterine tone as labor draws near. All patients should have the expectation that the fetus will continue to move and should be educated to report the absence of movement.

The other dominant triage concern is the recognition of the onset of labor. Patients may have difficulty distinguishing between labor and normal 3rd trimester complaints. Symptoms of labor before 36 weeks' gestation warrant immediate concern. Symptoms experienced by multiparous patients may vary. You should discuss with your providers your standard for evaluating patients for labor. Typical parameters for primiparous patients from 37 weeks' gestation on are as follows.

1. Call when contractions have been 5 minutes apart for an hour.
2. Call when membranes rupture.
3. Call if bleeding occurs.

Our facility's standard for evaluating primiparous patients in labor is as follows:

_____ .

Multiparous patients often are advised to call when contractions are between 5 and 10 minutes apart for an hour, when membranes rupture, or at the onset of bloody show. Our facility's standard for evaluating multiparous patients is as follows:

_____ .

It stands to reason that any patient experiencing symptoms with more pain than anticipated should be seen in person to be evaluated.

3rd Trimester Abdominal Pain

KEY QUESTIONS

ASSESSMENT	ACTION
1. Does the pain radiate from your back to the front of your abdomen? Can you feel a sensation of uterine tightening?	**YES** Go to Step A.
	NO Go to Question 2.
2. Are you having any vaginal bleeding associated with the pain?	**YES** Go to Step B.
	NO Go to Question 3.
3. Is the pain confined to one part of your abdomen and relieved by position change?	**YES** Go to Step C.
	NO Go to Question 4.
4. Is the pain confined to one part of your abdomen and **not** relieved by position change?	**YES** Go to Step D.
	NO Go to Question 5.
5. Is the abdominal pain accompanied by nausea, vomiting, bowel changes, fever, dysuria, light-headedness, or dizziness?	**YES** Go to Step E.
	NO Go to Patient Education.

ACTIONS

STEP A: Symptoms Consistent With Contractions

If this patient is less than 36 weeks pregnant, she may be experiencing an onset of preterm labor.

Instruct the patient to time her contractions. (See Patient Education for description of timing contractions.)

If the patient reports four or more contractions in an hour, each lasting 45–60 seconds, have her get in a comfortable position and do the following:

- lie on left side;
- drink 1 quart of water;
- monitor contractions for 1 hour; and
- call back immediately if symptoms worsen; otherwise report in 1 hour.

If symptoms continue but do not worsen, the patient should be seen within 1–3 hours for evaluation.

If symptoms subside, advise the patient to rest for the remainder of the day and call in the morning to report how she is feeling.

If patient is 37 weeks pregnant to term, she may be going into labor. (See the protocol for Recognizing Labor.)

STEP B: Vaginal Bleeding Associated With Abdominal Pain

A patient 36 weeks pregnant or less who is bleeding heavily needs to be seen ASAP in an appropriate facility. The patient should not drive herself. Transportation to the appropriate facility will depend on your location, the patient's location, and the availability of necessary services.

If the bleeding is "less than a period," the patient still needs to be seen ASAP to ensure that she is not experiencing preterm labor or placental problems.

A patient 37 weeks to term who is bleeding heavily needs to be seen ASAP and should not drive herself. A patient who is bleeding lightly may be experiencing bloody show and may be going into labor. (See the protocol for Recognizing Labor.)

STEP C: Pain Confined to One Part of Abdomen, Relieved by Position Change

This patient may be experiencing pain caused by muscle spasm or fetal position.

Have the patient describe the location of the pain.

Reassure the patient it is not harmful to apply light counterpressure if it relieves pain that may be caused by fetal position or movement.

Advise the patient to avoid sudden position changes and support her abdomen when coughing.

Have her call back, if symptoms increase, particularly if she experiences right lower or upper quadrant pain.

If the pain is located in a region other than the abdomen but is relieved with position change, instruct the patient to monitor her symptoms and call back if the pain increases or is accompanied by other symptoms. If the symptoms persist beyond 24 hours, the patient should be seen for evaluation.

STEP D: Pain Confined to One Part of Abdomen, Not Relieved by Position Change

Question the patient regarding the area of the pain.

Record the frequency, duration, and severity of the pain, particularly noting right upper quadrant pain.

Question the patient regarding any recent developing problems, such as PIH.

Forward a message to the patient's care provider so that dispensation can be made within the hour.

STEP E: Pain Associated With Other Symptoms

Remember that diarrhea may be associated with preterm labor.

Appendicitis: If patient still has her appendix and the pain is in the right lower quadrant or if she is experiencing bowel changes, she should be seen ASAP or sent to an ER or urgent care center for an acute abdominal problem evaluation.

Gallbladder Attack: If the pain is located in the right upper quadrant or to the right of the sternum, particularly if the patient has a history of gallstones, or if the pain is associated with eating, the patient should be seen within 24 hours by her primary care provider or sooner if symptoms increase.

Gastrointestinal Complaints: Bowel changes, nausea, or vomiting associated with malaise or other flu-like symptoms may indicate gastritis. The patient should make arrangements to see her primary care provider only after all preterm labor symptoms have been evaluated. The patient should call back if she cannot keep liquids down for 24 hours.

HELPP Syndrome: Sudden onset of pain in the area of the liver (right upper quadrant) may be associated with the development of preeclampsia.

Urinary Tract Infection: If the patient experiences pain on urination, unusually frequent urination, arrange for the patient to provide a urine sample for culture that day. If the patient is experiencing low backache or flu-like symptoms, such as nausea, vomiting, or fever, she should be seen ASAP to evaluate for a kidney infection.

PATIENT EDUCATION

1. Patients should be taught to monitor for contractions by doing the following.

   - Place your hands lightly on each side of your abdomen.
   - If your uterus tightens beneath your hands, you are contracting, whether or not you experience pain.
   - Time from the beginning of one contraction to the beginning of the next.
   - Time the length of the contraction as the amount of time your uterus feels tightened.
   - Call back if you are contracting four times or more in an hour, each lasting 45–60 seconds; if symptoms rapidly escalate; if you are bleeding; if you are leaking fluid from the vagina; or if contractions are accompanied by bowel changes.

2. Some women experience more abdominal discomfort than do others, more contractions than do others, and more pain in general. These women will need help in establishing what is normal for them and need to feel confident they can call with symptoms any time.

3rd Trimester Ambivalence/Depression

KEY QUESTIONS

ASSESSMENT	ACTION
1. Are you feeling ambivalent about this pregnancy or having doubts about being pregnant?	**YES** Go to Step A.
	NO Go to Question 2.
2. Are you feeling depressed or especially anxious about this pregnancy?	**YES** Go to Step B.
	NO Go to Question 3.
3. Do you have any history of depression, postpartum depression, or mental illness?	**YES** Go to Step C.
	NO Go to Question 4.
4. Are you experiencing feelings that you want to harm yourself or someone else?	**YES** Go to Step D.
	NO Return to Step B.

ACTIONS

STEP A: Ambivalence in Pregnancy

Research indicates that four of five women experience some degree of ambivalence during pregnancy. Ambivalence normally subsides and fades by the 3rd trimester. However, it is not uncommon for women to have self-doubts about coping skills, integration of a new family member, or concerns about time for herself and her partner at this point in the pregnancy.

Even during a planned pregnancy, a woman may not feel totally sure about herself. Reassurance that feelings of inadequacy and of being overwhelmed are not uncommon at this point may be helpful.

Discussing the preparation for labor, delivery, and the early postpartum period may be helpful. Often it is difficult for women to identify what makes them *most* anxious or concerned at this point.

Talking with a partner, significant other, close friend, or family member may be beneficial for some patients.

It may be helpful to talk to a counselor if concerns seem overwhelming or all consuming.

In our practice, we recommend the following counselors who may be of value in helping to sort out feelings during the 3rd trimester: _____
_____ .

STEP B: Possible Underlying Depression or Anxiety

Major life events may unmask or precipitate depression or anxiety. If there is any question that the patient is experiencing uncontrolled mood swings, thoughts about harming herself or others, feeling out of control, or becoming withdrawn, do the following.

- Make a same-day appointment with a mental health provider and ensure that a friend, family member, or social services worker accompanies the patient to the appointment.
- Ensure that a high-risk patient is not left alone.
- If necessary, have another person in your office call Emergency Services and remain on the line with the patient until help arrives.
- Notify a provider in your practice of the problem and your actions.

If patient is of no danger to herself or others, do the following.

- Refer her to a mental health counselor within the next 3 to 5 days.
- Reassure the patient that she may call back at any time if her symptoms worsen.

Your practice should have a system for identifying patients who are possibly at risk for depression during pregnancy.

In our practice, we do the following to identify patients at risk for depression during pregnancy (and thus possible postpartum depression): _____
_____ .

Depression surfacing during the 3rd trimester is a **red flag** for postpartum depression!

STEP C: History of Depression or Mental Illness

Patients with a history of depression or mental illness may be at greater risk with a new pregnancy. Depression resurfacing during the 3rd trimester needs to be promptly addressed in these patients.

Follow the actions in Step B.

STEP D: Desire to Harm Oneself or Others

If the patient is experiencing uncontrolled mood swings, thoughts about harming herself or others, feeling out of control, or becoming seriously withdrawn, do the following.

- Make a same-day appointment with a mental health counselor and ensure that a friend, family member, or social services worker accompanies the patient to the appointment.
- Ensure that a high-risk patient is not left alone.
- If necessary, have another person in your office call Emergency Services and remain on the line with the patient until help arrives.
- Notify a provider in your practice of the problem and your actions.

PATIENT EDUCATION

1. Reassuring a patient that it is not uncommon to have self-doubts during the 3rd trimester may reassure her that her thoughts are not abnormal.
2. Patients with a history of depression during pregnancy or the postpartum period need to be educated as to a possible recurrence and to be told help is available. Avoid being judgmental. Many patients have the misconception that all feelings can be controlled by will.

3rd Trimester Backache

ASSESSMENT

ACTION

1. Does the pain radiate from your back to the front of your abdomen? Does the back pain "let up" at a predictable interval? Can you feel a sensation of uterine tightening associated with your backache?

   YES Go to Step A.
   Continue on next question.

   NO Go to Question 2.

2. Do you have a pre-existing back problem?

   YES Go to Step B.

   NO Go to Question 3.

3. Is the pain confined to one part of your back and relieved by position change?

   YES Go to Step C.

   NO Go to Question 4.

4. Is the pain confined to one part of your back and **not** relieved by position change?

   YES Go to Step D.

   NO Go to Question 5.

5. Is the back pain accompanied by nausea, vomiting, bowel changes, fever, or dysuria?

   YES Go to Step E.

   NO Go to Patient Education.

ACTIONS

STEP A: Backache Accompanied by Possible Contractions

Determine if the patient is at home or at work. If she is at work, recommend that she go home but not drive herself. If she is at home, determine the location of her coach or other support person.

If symptoms occur before 36 weeks, the patient may be experiencing the onset of preterm labor:

Question the patient regarding any pre-existing high-risk problems.

Question the patient regarding the presence of fetal movement.

Have the patient time the contractions. (See Patient Education for description of timing contractions.)

If the patient reports four or more contractions in an hour, each lasting 45 to 60 seconds, have the patient get in a comfortable position and do the following:

- lie on left side;
- drink 1 quart of water;
- monitor contractions for 1 hour; and
- call back immediately if symptoms worsen; otherwise report in 1 hour.

If the symptoms continue but do not worsen, the patient should be seen in 1 to 3 hours for evaluation.

If the symptoms subside, advise the patient to rest for the remainder of the day and call in the morning to report how she is feeling.

If the symptoms occur from 37 weeks to term:

Question the patient regarding any pre-existing high-risk pregnancy problems.

Question the patient regarding the presence of fetal movement.

Question the patient regarding previous instructions from her provider as to when to call if labor is suspected.

If the patient is primiparous:

Instruct her to monitor the contractions and call when they are 5 minutes apart for an hour, if her membranes rupture, or if she is bleeding.

If the patient is unusually uncomfortable or frightened, have her come in for an evaluation, even if she does not meet your criteria for early labor evaluation.

If the patient is multiparous:

Question the patient about prior pregnancies and the length of the last labor.

Instruct the patient that labor usually progresses more quickly after the first pregnancy.

If contractions are 5 to 10 minutes apart, if the membranes are ruptured, or if bloody show is present have patient come in for an evaluation.

STEP B: Pre-existing Back Condition

It is very common for pre-existing back conditions to become aggravated during the 3rd trimester.

Determine the nature of the pre-existing problem.

Ask the patient if she has seen a health care provider regarding her condition before pregnancy.

Continue with questions to eliminate any acute problem before encouraging the patient to call her regular health care provider if she has not done so this pregnancy.

Refer to Patient Education.

STEP C: Backache Confined to One Part of Back, Relieved by Position Change

The patient may be experiencing nerve compression or muscle spasm.

Determine the area of the pain and methods that relieve discomfort.

Attempt to pinpoint conditions that may aggravate discomfort (such as going up and down stairs, shifting gears in a car, or carrying an infant).

Suggest appropriate treatments for aggravating symptoms.

Encourage proper body mechanics.

Refer the patient to her primary care provider for a physical therapy referral, if indicated.

See Patient Education for general measures for relief of back pain.

STEP D: Backache Confined, Unrelieved by Position Change

Question the patient regarding the area of the pain.

Record the frequency, duration, and severity of the pain.

After eliminating the possibility of uterine contractions, forward a message to the patient's provider so that a dispensation can be made within the hour.

STEP E: Backache Associated With Other Symptoms

Remember that diarrhea may be associated with preterm labor.

Question the patient regarding the frequency, duration, and severity of the pain.

Ask if the patient has a history of kidney stones, frequent urinary tract infections, has sickle cell disease, or is a carrier of sickle cell.

If the patient experiences pain on urination, unusually frequent urination, and has a backache described as mild, have her come into the office or clinic for a clean-caught urine culture.

If the patient is experiencing backache associated with flu-like symptoms, nausea, vomiting, or fever, she should be seen ASAP to evaluate for a kidney infection.

PATIENT EDUCATION

1. Patients should be taught to monitor for contractions by doing the following.

   - Place your hands lightly on each side of your abdomen.
   - If your uterus tightens beneath your hands, you are contracting, whether or not you experience pain.
   - Time from the beginning of one contraction to the beginning of the next.
   - Time the length of the contraction as the amount of time your uterus feels tightened.
   - Call back if you are contracting four times or more in an hour, each lasting 45–60 seconds; if symptoms rapidly escalate; if you are bleeding; if you are leaking fluid from the vagina; or if contractions are accompanied by bowel changes.

2. Some women experience more backache than do others. These women need help in establishing what is normal for them and need to feel confident they can call any time to report their symptoms.

3. General measures for increasing back comfort are as follows.

   - Practice good posture. Adjust as your center of gravity changes with the growing uterus.
   - Wear comfortable shoes.
   - Avoid standing for prolonged periods of time. Elevate one foot, if possible.
   - Sleep on a firm mattress.
   - Learn proper exercises for stretching back muscles.

3rd Trimester Bleeding

KEY QUESTIONS

ASSESSMENT	ACTION
1. Is there any pain associated with the bleeding?	**YES** Go to Question 2.
	NO Go to Step A. Continue to Question 2.
2. Does the pain radiate from your back to the front of your abdomen? Does the pain "let up" at a predictable interval? Can you feel a sensation of uterine tightening associated with the pain?	**YES** Go to Step B.
	NO Schedule a **same-day appointment** for sonogram.
3. Are you experiencing any vaginal itching, burning, odor, or other discharge?	**YES** Go to Step C.
	NO No further action.

ACTIONS

STEP A: Painless Vaginal Bleeding

Painless vaginal bleeding in the 3rd trimester is suggestive of placenta previa.

Ascertain if the patient has had a sonogram. If the answer is "no" or the sonogram cannot be located, schedule an appointment that day for the patient with a provider who can perform a sonogram to determine placental location.

Most patients with a previously documented previa in the 2nd trimester will be familiar with their placental location.

STEP B: Abdominal Pain Associated With Vaginal Bleeding

A pregnant patient who is not yet at 36 weeks and who is experiencing abdominal pain with vaginal bleeding needs to be seen ASAP in an appropriate facility. The patient should not drive herself. Transportation to the appropriate facility will depend on your location, the patient's location, and the availability of necessary services.

If the patient meets your facility's criteria for heavy bleeding, the patient needs to be seen ASAP, whether or not pain is present.

If bleeding lightly, the patient still needs to be evaluated that day for the possibility of preterm labor or placental problems. Question the patient as to presence of contractions. If there is any question of preterm labor, the patient needs immediate evaluation.

If the patient is at 37 weeks to term:

If the patient meets your facility's criteria for heavy bleeding, she needs to be seen ASAP.

Light bleeding may be bloody show.

Refer to the protocol for Recognizing Labor.

STEP C: Vaginal Bleeding Associated With Pain, Itching, or Odor

The patient may have a vaginal infection. The patient should be seen that day for a wet mount and possible vaginal culture after it has been determined that she is not experiencing labor or placental problems.

PATIENT EDUCATION

1. All patients should be told that any bleeding in the 3rd trimester should be reported immediately.
2. Patients who have had a sonogram should know the location of their placenta. Placenta previa or marginal placental localization is common in the 2nd trimester. Fortunately, most of these will resolve by early in the 3rd trimester. Most patients with a previous diagnosis of placenta previa will know their last sonogram results.

3rd Trimester Constipation

KEY QUESTIONS

ASSESSMENT	ACTION
1. Have your symptoms persisted throughout pregnancy or worsened during the pregnancy?	**YES** Go to Step A.
	NO Go to Question 2.
2. Is the constipation accompanied by prolonged nausea, vomiting, abdominal distension, or failure to pass gas?	**YES** Go to Step B.
	NO Go to Question 3.
3. Do you have a pre-existing problem with constipation?	**YES** Go to Step C.
	NO Go to Question 4.
4. Is there blood in your stool?	**YES** Go to Step D.
	NO No further action.

ACTIONS

STEP A: Pregnancy Related

Constipation is a common complaint throughout pregnancy. Potential causes in the 3rd trimester include a continual hormonal effect, mechanical pressure, or a response to pain from hemorrhoids.
The following suggestions may be helpful.

- Increase fiber in the diet.
- Increase clear fluids by 1–2 quarts daily.
- Add stool softeners as determined by office/clinic protocols. (See list of approved stool softeners.)
- Increase exercise within the limits of 3rd trimester. Keep pulse rate below 140 beats/minute.
- Change your prenatal vitamin to one with time-released iron or avoid iron supplementation.
- Assess calcium needs. Many patients mistakenly take more calcium supplementation than is needed.
- Avoid laxatives.

Continue on to Questions 2, 3, and 4.

STEP B: Constipation With Additional Symptoms

Ileus is uncommon in pregnancy, but must not be overlooked. If the patient has additional symptoms, she should call her primary care provider immediately.
Continue on to Questions 3 and 4.

STEP C: History of Constipation

Patients with a history of constipation or irritable bowel syndrome may have a worsening of symptoms.
Assess laxative and other medication use.
Encourage the patient to try the recommendations in Step A. If the patient is a chronic abuser of laxatives or has tried the suggestions in Step A and experienced no response, refer her to an obstetric care provider or gastrointestinal care provider.

STEP D: Blood in Stool

Blood in the stool may be a sign of straining or hemorrhoids but also may be a signal of a more serious medical problem. The patient should have this evaluated by her obstetric care provider at her next scheduled appointment or sooner if symptoms worsen.

PATIENT EDUCATION

1. There are many iron preparations available that may be more easily absorbed for a patient who is known to have anemia but is reluctant to take iron because of constipation.

    Our practice recommends: _____.

2. Calcium (particularly calcium carbonate) can be constipating and can directly interfere with iron absorption.

    Our practice recommends: _____.

3. All minerals probably are best absorbed when obtained through foods consumed. Encourage the patient to try to eat foods that are high in needed minerals.

3rd Trimester Decreased Fetal Movement

KEY QUESTIONS

ASSESSMENT	ACTION
1. Have you felt fetal movement within the last 24 hours?	**YES** Go to Step A.
	NO Go to Step B.

ACTIONS

STEP A: Has Felt Fetal Movement Within the Last 24 Hours

Many definitions of adequate fetal movement exist for the 3rd trimester. A common one is five movements per hour when the patient is concentrating on fetal movement. Decide with your practice providers what you will accept as adequate fetal movement at this point in pregnancy.

Have the patient get in a comfortable position, one in which she usually can feel fetal movement.

Make sure she has had something to eat or drink in the last hour.

Instruct the patient to monitor for fetal movement for an hour. She should expect five movements. If the fetus moves five times in 5 minutes, she does not need to watch for an hour.

Have the patient report the results.

If fetal movement appears inadequate, have the patient come in that day for an NST. She probably will want to come in ASAP.

STEP B: No Fetal Movement in 24 Hours

This patient may be too anxious to watch for fetal movement and may need to be seen.

Ask the patient if she has been able to keep down food or drink during this time.

Do not falsely reassure the patient that the lack of ingestion of food may be the cause, but if the patient is now able to take in food or liquids, have her repeat the fetal movement monitoring described in Step A.

If the patient is unable to keep down food or liquids, it is unlikely she will feel fetal movement. Schedule her to come in for an NST and evaluation for dehydration.

PATIENT EDUCATION

1. There are benign reasons for decreased fetal movement as the patient approaches term. As the fetus descends into the pelvis, it may "lock" into position, causing a

change in sensation to a grinding in the pelvis. The fetus also may "run out of room" with increasing size and become unable to move limbs as freely. As labor approaches, the muscle tone of the uterus increases, creating a firmer surface for resistance to fetal movements.

2. Patients need to be educated about these possible causes of decreased perception of fetal movement. They also need to be warned that it is an old wives' tale that the fetus should stop moving before labor.

3. Patients need to be educated to report any decrease in fetal movement during the 3rd trimester.

4. Our practice standard for movement in the 3rd trimester is as follows: _____
_____.

3rd Trimester Headache

KEY QUESTIONS

ASSESSMENT	ACTION

1. Have you recently received a diagnosis of pregnancy-induced hypertension (PIH), preeclampsia, or toxemia?

YES Go to Step A.
NO Go to Question 2.

2. Was the onset of this headache sudden and severe?

YES Go to Step B.
NO Go to Question 3.

3. Is the headache accompanied by any numbness, tingling, loss of bowel or bladder control, or seizure behaviors? Is the headache accompanied by debilitating neck stiffness or high fever?

YES Go to Step B.
NO Go to Question 4.

4. Is the headache accompanied by visual changes?

YES Go to Step C.
NO Go to Question 5.

5. Is the headache accompanied by upper respiratory tract infection symptoms (congestion, fever, cough, or facial or tooth discomfort)?

YES Go to Step D.
NO Go to Question 6.

6. Is the headache dull and not debilitating in nature?

YES Go to Step E.
NO No further action.

ACTIONS

STEP A: Recent Diagnosis Involving Blood Pressure Elevation

Patients may use several terms to describe syndromes that include elevation of blood pressure during the 3rd trimester. Headache is not necessarily a presenting symptom with syndromes involving high blood pressure in pregnancy, but many patients believe this to be true.

If patient recently has received a diagnosis of increased blood pressure during her pregnancy, instruct her to have her blood pressure checked, even though this is not necessarily associated with the problem for which she is being followed.

STEP B: Sudden, Severe Headache

Onset of a sudden, severe headache usually is not a problem related to obstetrics and needs immediate referral to the patient's primary care provider or ER, as appropriate. The patient should not drive herself. If the headache is accompanied by loss of sensorimotor skills, the patient or her agent should call 911.

Symptoms of numbness, tingling, high fever, and debilitating neck stiffness are not usual 3rd trimester complaints and warrant medical evaluation.

STEP C: Neurological Symptoms

Ask the patient if she has a history of migraine headaches. Are these headaches like the migraines that she has experienced before?

Refer the patient to an on-call provider to determine if additional neurological evaluation is warranted and to determine safety of any medications the patient may have on hand for treatment of migraines.

Have the patient lie in a dark room and apply compresses to the area where she is experiencing the headache.

If she does not experience relief within 1–2 hours, refer the patient to her primary care provider for management.

STEP D: Respiratory Symptoms

If the patient has symptoms of an upper respiratory tract infection, she may be experiencing a sinus headache.

Recommend the patient take acetaminophen 650 mg orally every 4–6 hours as needed, not to exceed the manufacturer's recommended dosage, or other medication as agreed upon by your practice for the use of pain relief during the 3rd trimester.

Consult an obstetric care provider before recommending the use of decongestants.

Refer the patient to her primary care provider if she does not experience improvement within 3 to 5 days.

Instruct the patient to call her primary care provider if symptoms worsen.

STEP E: Dull Headaches

Dull headaches are common in late pregnancy and usually are caused by a lack of sleep and tension.

Recommend the patient take acetaminophen 650 mg orally every 4–6 hours as needed, not to exceed the manufacturer's recommended dosage, or other medication as agreed upon by your practice.

Increasing rest and decreasing stressful factors may lessen headaches.

The patient's primary care provider should evaluate persistent dull headaches.

3rd Trimester Indigestion

KEY QUESTIONS

ASSESSMENT

ACTION

1. Is the onset of your symptoms pregnancy related?

YES Go to Step A.

NO Go to Question 2.

2. Is the constipation accompanied by prolonged nausea, vomiting, abdominal distension, or failure to pass gas?

YES Go to Step B.

NO Go to Question 3.

3. Do you have a pre-existing problem with indigestion?

YES Go to Step C.

NO No further action.

ACTIONS

STEP A: Pregnancy-Related Onset

During the last 3 months of pregnancy, indigestion may be at its worst because of hormonal changes and pressure on the stomach and diaphragm from the growing fetus.

The following suggestions may be helpful:

- Avoid spicy, fried, or fatty foods.
- Drink liquids between meals, instead of "washing down" food at mealtimes.
- Eat small, frequent meals, instead of three large meals.
- Space eating throughout the day. Avoid eating just before going to bed.
- Change your prenatal vitamin to one with time-released iron or avoid iron supplementation.
- Try elevating the head while sleeping.
- Take antacids, as approved by your provider.

Continue on to Question 3.

STEP B: Indigestion With Additional Symptoms

Ileus and cholecystitis are rather uncommon during pregnancy but must not be overlooked. If the patient has additional symptoms, she should call her primary care provider immediately.

Continue on to Question 3.

STEP C: History of Indigestion

Patients with a history of indigestion or reflux may have a worsening of symptoms. Hiatal hernia may be particularly troublesome during the 3rd trimester.

Continue by suggesting the patient try the recommendations in Step A. If the patient is a chronic user of antacids or has no response after trying the suggestions in Step A, refer her to an obstetric care provider or gastrointestinal care provider.

PATIENT EDUCATION

1. Encourage the patient to try simple methods to relieve symptoms before relying on antacids. Because this is a problem that tends to worsen during pregnancy, starting with the "big guns" may limit a patient's options later in pregnancy.
2. There are many iron preparations available that may be more easily absorbed for a patient who is known to have anemia but is reluctant to take iron because of indigestion.

    Our practice recommends: _____.

3. Not all common antacids are recommended by all providers.

    Our practice recommends: _____.

3rd Trimester Inverted Nipples

ASSESSMENT	ACTION
1. Is this a new onset of an inverted nipple?	**YES** Go to Step A.
	NO Go to Question 2.
2. Are you at least 34 weeks pregnant?	**YES** Go to Step B.
	NO Go to Step C.

ACTIONS

STEP A: New-Onset Inverted Nipple

A new-onset inverted nipple may be a symptom of an underlying breast lump or other problem. The patient should be scheduled for an evaluation by an office provider within 1–2 days. If the patient is extremely anxious about this finding, schedule a same-day appointment.

STEP B: Inverted Nipples From 34 Weeks to Term

There are varying degrees of nipple inversion, from the slightly inverted to severely inverted (retracted to a level below the areola). The following measures may help with nipple inversion.

Advise the patient to wear breast cups in her bra during the day. These can be obtained at many maternity or drug stores.

Advise the patient to try the following exercises:

- Place a thumb on each side at the base of the nipple and push in firmly against the breast tissue while pulling your thumbs away from each other. Do this five times a day.
- Try rolling the nipple between the thumb and index finger for 30 to 60 seconds.
- If any of these measures cause uterine tightening or contractions, discontinue the measure.
- Advise the patient to notify her nurse when she is admitted to the labor and delivery unit that she has inverted nipples and would like to be seen by a lactation consultant after delivery.

STEP C: Inverted Nipples Before 34 Weeks

Advise patient to wait until 34 weeks before following Step B.

PATIENT EDUCATION

1. Nipple stimulation has been known to cause contractions in some women. Consequently, nipple stimulation is not recommended in women at risk for preterm labor. Advise the patient to wait until she is at least 36 weeks pregnant before instituting measures to reduce nipple inversion.
2. Nipple stimulation should not be initiated in a woman with a known placenta previa.

3rd Trimester Nausea/Vomiting

KEY QUESTIONS

ASSESSMENT	ACTION
1. During the past 24 hours or more, have you been able to keep down food or liquids?	**YES** Go to Question 2.
	NO Go to Step A.
2. Are you having any sensation of uterine tightening with the nausea or vomiting? Is there any diarrhea associated with your symptoms?	**YES** Go to Step B.
	NO Go to Question 3.
3. Have the symptoms continued throughout the course of your pregnancy?	**YES** Go to Step C.
	NO Go to Question 4.
4. Do you have any pre-existing food intolerances or gastrointestinal problems?	**YES** Go to Step D.
	NO Go to Question 5.
5. Are your symptoms accompanied by fever or spasmodic abdominal pain?	**YES** Go to Step E.
	NO No further action.

ACTIONS

STEP A: Acute Inability to Retain Food or Liquids

The patient is at risk for dehydration, which may contribute to uterine contractions. Advise the patient to come in within 12–24 hours for evaluation of her dehydration. Advise the patient to call her obstetric care provider if she has no urine output for 12 hours while awaiting an appointment.

STEP B: Symptoms Accompanying Possible Contractions

Prostaglandins, which may cause contractions, also may cause nausea, vomiting, and diarrhea in some women. If the patient is 36 weeks pregnant or less, she may be experiencing an onset of preterm labor.

Have the patient time the contractions. (See the protocol for 2nd Trimester Abdominal Pain.)

If the patient reports four or more contractions in an hour, each lasting 45–60 seconds, have her get in a comfortable position and do the following:

- lie on left side;
- drink 1 quart of water;
- monitor contractions for 1 hour; and
- call back if symptoms worsen; otherwise report in 1 hour.

If the symptoms persist but do not worsen, the patient should be seen in 1–3 hours for evaluation.

If the symptoms subside, advise the patient to rest for the remainder of the day, continue hydration, and call in the morning to report how she is feeling.

If patient is 37 weeks pregnant or more, she may be going into labor. (See the protocol for Recognizing Labor.)

STEP C: Pregnancy-Related Symptoms

Some women have protracted nausea and vomiting throughout the course of their pregnancy.

The patient may continue to avoid prenatal vitamins with iron. Some women take a children's vitamin daily.

Continue the dietary nausea measures from the 1st trimester.

The patient may warrant a nutrition consult if persistent symptoms interfere with nutritional intake or weight gain. Have her discuss this with her obstetric care provider at her next visit or sooner, if indicated.

STEP D: Pre-existing Conditions

Patients with pre-existing serious gastrointestinal problems who are taking maintenance medication warrant a medical evaluation if they have not had one.

Refer the patient for nutritional counseling as indicated.

Refer the patient to the dietary measures mentioned.

- Avoid fatty or spicy foods.
- Eat small, frequent meals.
- Complex carbohydrates (a protein source and a carbohydrate) may decrease nausea.
- Keep crackers at the bedside and eat a few before rising in the morning.

If symptoms are persistent, have the patient call her gastrointestinal care provider for reevaluation and treatment.

STEP E: Possible Flu or Acute Abdominal Problem

Nausea and vomiting accompanied by a temperature greater than 100.4°F needs immediate evaluation.

Refer the patient immediately to her obstetric care provider, the ER, or an urgent care center.

PATIENT EDUCATION

1. Patients need to understand the usual course of nausea and vomiting in pregnancy, remembering that some women do not "follow the book" when it comes to symptoms.
2. It cannot be overemphasized that women with serious pre-existing gastrointestinal conditions, such as Crohn's disease, colitis, and diverticulitis, should have a medical evaluation before pregnancy.
3. Women with nutritional difficulties, such as celiac disease or lactose intolerance, may experience an exacerbation of their symptoms and benefit from nutritional counseling.
4. Refer to Patient Education in the 3rd Trimester Abdominal Pain protocol, for guidelines on teaching the patient to monitor for contractions.

3rd Trimester Pelvic Pain/Pressure

KEY QUESTIONS

ASSESSMENT	ACTION
1. Are you experiencing an increase in rhythmic pelvic pressure?	**YES** Go to Step A. Continue to Question 3.
	NO Go to Step B.
2. Are you experiencing any uterine tightening associated with the rhythmic pelvic pressure?	**YES** Go to Step A.
	NO Go to Question 3.
3. Are you experiencing any vaginal bleeding associated with the pain?	**YES** Go to Step C.
	NO Go to Question 4.
4. Are you experiencing pelvic pressure confined to one location?	**YES** Go to Step D.
	NO Go to Patient Education.

ACTIONS

STEP A: Symptoms Consistent With Contractions

If this patient is less than 36 weeks pregnant, she may be experiencing an onset of preterm labor.

Have the patient time the contractions. (See Patient Education for a description of timing contractions.)

If the patient reports four or more contractions in an hour, each lasting 45–60 seconds, have her get in a comfortable position and do the following:

- lie on left side;
- drink 1 quart of water;
- monitor contractions for 1 hour; and
- call back immediately if symptoms worsen; otherwise report in 1 hour.

If the symptoms continue but do not worsen, the patient should be seen within 1 to 3 hours for evaluation.

If the symptoms subside, advise the patient to rest for the remainder of the day and call in the morning to report how she is feeling.

If the patient is at least 37 weeks pregnant, she may be going into labor. (See the protocol for Recognizing Labor.)

STEP B: Nonrhythmic Pelvic Pressure

Pelvic pressure from the growing fetus is a normal symptom during the 3rd trimester. It may progressively increase as term approaches.

Advise the patient to get off her feet and rest. Symptoms should be relieved.

The patient may need to cut back on activities or work demands if the pressure is debilitating. The patient should discuss this with her obstetric care provider.

The patient should report any uncomfortable change in symptoms to discuss the possibility of labor.

STEP C: Vaginal Bleeding Associated With Pelvic Pain and Pressure

A patient who is 36 weeks pregnant or less and who is bleeding heavily needs to be seen ASAP in an appropriate facility. The patient should not drive herself. Transportation to the appropriate facility will depend on your location, the patient's location, and the availability of necessary services.

If the bleeding is "less than a period," the patient still needs to be seen ASAP to ensure that she is not experiencing preterm labor or placental problems.

A patient who is at least 37 weeks pregnant and who is bleeding heavily needs to be seen ASAP and should not drive herself. The patient who is bleeding lightly may be experiencing bloody show and may be going into labor. (See the protocol for Recognizing Labor.)

STEP D: Pressure Confined to One Part of Pelvis

This patient may be experiencing pain caused by muscle spasm or fetal position.

Have the patient describe the location of the pain.

Reassure the patient such pain usually is caused by fetal position.

Advise the patient to avoid sudden position changes and to support her abdomen when she coughs.

Instruct the patient to get off her feet to see if symptoms are relieved.

Have her call back if symptoms increase.

If the pain is located in a region other than abdomen but is relieved with position change, have the patient monitor her symptoms and call back if pain is increased or accompanied by other symptoms. If the symptoms persist beyond 24 hours, the patient should be seen for evaluation.

PATIENT EDUCATION

1. Patients should be taught to monitor for contractions by doing the following:

   - Place your hands lightly on each side of your abdomen.
   - If your uterus tightens beneath your hands, you are contracting, whether or not you experience pain.
   - Time from the beginning of one contraction to the beginning of the next.
   - Time the length of the contraction as the amount of time your uterus feels tightened.

- Call back if you are contracting four times or more in an hour, each lasting 45–60 seconds; if symptoms rapidly escalate; if you are bleeding; if you are leaking fluid from the vagina; or if contractions are accompanied by bowel changes.

2. Some women experience more pelvic pain and pressure than do others, more contractions than do others, and more pain in general. These women will need help in establishing what is normal for them and need to feel confident they can call any time to report their symptoms.

3rd Trimester Precipitous Delivery

KEY QUESTIONS

ASSESSMENT	ACTION
1. Is the patient experiencing intense pressure or does she feel the presenting part of the fetus (head or feet)?	**YES** Go to Step A.
	NO Go to Question 2.
2. Is the head or other presenting part of the fetus visible?	**YES** Go to Step B.
	NO Go to Question 3.
3. Has the baby been delivered?	**YES** Go to Step C.
	NO No further action.

ACTIONS

STEP A: Intense Pressure or Viewing the Presenting Part

Advise the caller to call 911 for emergency assistance. Once emergency services have been notified, the caller should call you back for additional needed assistance.

STEP B: Visible Head or Presenting Part

If the presenting part is visible, instruct the caller to place a clean towel or cloth on the perineum. This will help to support the perineum.

Do not attempt to hold back delivery of the presenting part.

If the head is the first part to be delivered, suggest the caller use the towel placed on the perineum to gently press the baby's chin upward. This will help extend the head.

After the head is delivered, if the cord is felt around the baby's neck, it should be looped over the head. If the cord is too tight to loop over the baby's head, have the caller clamp off the cord in two places and cut between the two clamps.

Once the head has been delivered and the cord is not an issue, use a bulb syringe (if available) to suction the baby's nose and mouth. If no syringe is available, proceed.

Place hands along the sides of the baby's head and ask the mother to bear down gently. The shoulder that is facing upward should pass beneath the pubic bone.

After the top shoulder is delivered, ask the mother to pant. The baby's body should slowly be directed upward, the lower shoulder should gradually pass the perineum.

Once the shoulders have been delivered, place one hand along the shoulders and the other hand along the spine.

The baby should slowly be cradled as the delivery is completed. The patient may need to give a gentle push so that the rest of the body can be delivered. Place baby on mother's abdomen and cover with clean towels or blankets. Do not try to deliver the placenta. If it delivers itself, wrap it in a towel and keep it attached to the baby. Feel the mother's stomach for her uterus. It should now feel like a firm grapefruit at or below her belly button. Massage gently to maintain firmness.

STEP C: After the Delivery

If a clamp is available, clamp the cord. However, await the arrival of the emergency services personnel before cutting the cord.

Use a clean, dry towel to wipe off the baby.

Place the baby on the patient's chest and wrap both the mother and baby to maintain the baby's temperature. Do not separate the placenta.

If the baby is experiencing difficulty breathing, the bulb syringe can be used to help clear the baby's nose and mouth.

3rd Trimester Recognizing Labor

KEY QUESTIONS

ASSESSMENT | **ACTION**

1. Have you ever had a baby?

YES Go to Step A.
NO Go to Question 2.

2. Do you know the signs of labor, and are you less than 37 weeks pregnant?

YES Go to Question 3.
NO Go to Step B.

3. Do you know the signs of labor, and are you more than 37 weeks pregnant?

YES Go to Step C.
NO Go to Step C.

ACTIONS

STEP A: Multiparous Women

Tell the patient that the symptoms of labor she is experiencing now may be like or different than her previous labor(s).

STEP B: Early Symptoms of Preterm Labor

Early symptoms of labor may include the following:

- Low backache, which comes and goes. The backache may be localized or radiate around to the abdomen.
- Pelvic fullness or pressure. Many women will say "the baby feels like it is going to fall out."
- Low abdominal pain or cramps, which come and go at regular intervals. These may radiate down the thighs.
- Abdominal tightening, which the patient may describe as "the baby balling up."
- An increase in vaginal discharge.
- Bowel changes, typically loose stools or diarrhea.
- Bloody show, leaking fluid, or a gush of fluid.

If the patient has any of these symptoms, she should come into the office for an examination or go to the labor and delivery unit for evaluation, based on office practice. Notify the on-call provider that the patient will be arriving.

STEP C: Labor in Term Pregnancy

Labor in a term pregnancy often feels much different from preterm labor. Symptoms of labor in later pregnancy may include:

Low backache that comes and goes at fairly regular intervals. The backache may radiate around to the uterine area. The backache usually comes at shorter and shorter intervals and will not subside with changes in activity, like Braxton-Hicks contractions do.

Uterine tightening or cramping that occurs at regular intervals. These typically occur at shorter and shorter intervals and may increase in intensity with time. Unlike with Braxton-Hicks contractions, changes in activity should not make these symptoms go away.

Gushing or leaking of fluid. If this occurs, the patient should observe the fluid. If it is red, green, or brown, she should be evaluated immediately in the labor and delivery unit. Contact the on-call provider and the labor and delivery unit to tell them the patient is coming in for evaluation. If the fluid is clear and the patient is not contracting, she may stay home for 12 hours before coming to the labor and delivery unit unless:

- contractions occur every 3–5 minutes and last for 60 or more seconds and this is her first delivery;
- contractions occur every 5 minutes or less and last for 60 seconds or more and this is not her first delivery;
- she is classified as high risk; or
- she has any concerns.

3rd Trimester Ruptured Membranes

KEY QUESTIONS

ASSESSMENT	ACTION
1. Are you certain your membranes have ruptured?	**YES** Go to Question 2.
	NO Go to Step A.
2. Are you less than 37 weeks pregnant?	**YES** Go to Step A.
	NO Go to Question 3.
3. Is the fluid clear?	**YES** Go to Question 4.
	NO Go to Step B.
4. Did your membranes rupture less than 12 hours ago?	**YES** Go to Question 5.
	NO Go to Step C.
5. Are you having contractions?	**YES** Go to Step D.
	NO No further action.

ACTIONS

STEP A: Ruptured Membranes

If patient is less than 37 completed weeks, she should be seen immediately in the office or the labor and delivery unit for evaluation.

If patient is at more than 37 weeks, when membranes rupture there may be a gush of fluid or a trickle of fluid. If the patient is uncertain, she can wear a minipad or sanitary napkin for 1–2 hours. After she has worn the pad, she can see if it is wet or very moist. She also can see if it smells like urine, to exclude spontaneous urine leakage. Moist or wet pads should be interpreted as a sign of ruptured membranes, pending additional evaluation.

STEP B: Amniotic Fluid

Green, red, or brown amniotic fluid may be a matter of concern. Have the patient go to the labor and delivery unit. Contact the on-call provider and the labor and delivery unit to notify them that the patient is coming in and that her amniotic fluid was not clear.

STEP C: Prolonged Rupture of Membranes

Prolonged rupture of membranes can lead to maternal or neonatal infection. Have the patient contact the on-call provider. The provider may want you to call the labor and delivery unit to notify them that the patient is coming in and when her membranes ruptured.

STEP D: Contractions

A primiparous patient should be instructed to go to the labor and delivery unit when:

- membranes are ruptured 12 or more hours; or
- amniotic fluid is not clear; or
- contractions are occurring every 5 minutes and lasting 60 or more seconds; or the patient or nurse has any concerns.

A multiparous patient should be instructed to go to the labor and delivery unit when:

- membranes are ruptured 12 or more hours; or
- amniotic fluid is not clear; or
- contractions are occurring every 6–8 minutes and lasting 60 or more seconds; or the patient or nurse has any concerns whatsoever.

Call the provider and report the patient's status.

3rd Trimester Swelling

ASSESSMENT   **ACTION**

1. Is the swelling accompanied by visual changes, headache, right upper quadrant pain, chest pain, or sharp leg pain? Or, do you have a history of preeclampsia/pregnancy-induced hypertension (PIH) or chronic hypertension?

   YES Go to Step A.

   NO Go to Question 2.

2. Is swelling occurring in the face and arms as well as in the legs?

   YES Go to Step B.

   NO Go to Question 3.

3. Is the swelling localized to the legs?

   YES Go to Step C.

   NO No further action.

ACTIONS

STEP A: Swelling With Other Symptoms

Swelling accompanied by headache, visual changes, right upper quadrant pain, or chest pain may be a warning sign of PIH. The patient should be seen in the office or ER for immediate evaluation.

A history of PIH or chronic hypertension places a pregnant woman at risk for the development of PIH in her current pregnancy. Even if she does not have additional symptoms, such a patient should receive a same-day appointment for additional evaluation.

STEP B: Facial and Upper Extremity Swelling

Facial and upper extremity swelling in pregnancy may be more concerning than swelling restricted to the legs. The patient should be evaluated for PIH within the next 24 hours.

STEP C: Uncomplicated Swelling

Swelling of the legs is a common complaint during pregnancy. Pressure by the fetus on the inferior vena cava, increased circulating blood volume, and the relaxant effects of progesterone all contribute to this symptom. (See Patient Education for measures to decrease swelling.)

PATIENT EDUCATION

Advise the patient to do the following:

- Increase the time spent off of your feet and lying on your side.
- Avoid the heat in warm weather.
- Elevate your legs above the heart level.
- Drink plenty of water (1–2 quarts more than your usual fluid intake).
- Avoid extra salt or MSG.
- Use pregnancy support hose. If you are using them, make sure they have been fitted properly.
- Call if additional symptoms occur or current symptoms worsen.
- Avoid highly salty or processed foods.

3rd Trimester Urinary Complaints

KEY QUESTIONS

ASSESSMENT	ACTION
1. Are you experiencing more frequent urination?	**YES** Go to Question 2.
	NO Go to Step A.
2. Do you have pubic pain or pressure, or burning on urination?	**YES** Go to Step B.
	NO Go to Question 3.
3. Do you have blood in your urine, a low backache, or flu-like symptoms, such as nausea, vomiting, or a fever?	**YES** Go to Step C.
	NO Go to Question 4.
4. Do you have sickle cell disease or are you a sickle cell carrier?	**YES** Go to Step D.
	NO No further action.

ACTIONS

STEP A: Frequent Urination Without Other Symptoms

During the 3rd trimester of pregnancy, many women experience increased frequency of urination. If the patient has no additional symptoms, it is unlikely she has a urinary tract infection (UTI). However, women who have a history of UTIs or kidney infections or who have sickle cell disease or are a sickle cell carrier should come to the office to give a clean-caught urine specimen for analysis, culture, and sensitivity.

STEP B: Frequent Urination With Pelvic Symptoms

Increased frequency of urination with symptoms such as burning, can be indicative of a UTI. However, increased frequency of urination accompanied by pelvic pain or pressure also may be a sign of premature labor. The patient should be instructed to come to the office to give a clean-caught urine specimen for analysis, culture, and sensitivity if she has burning on urination. However, if she has pelvic pressure or pain, she also should be evaluated for preterm labor. See the Pelvic Pain/Pressure protocol; ensure that the patient is not experiencing preterm labor.

STEP C: Frequent Urination With Renal Symptoms

Frequent urination with accompanying low backache, flu-like symptoms, or hematuria may be symptoms of a kidney infection or a more serious kidney complication. The patient should be instructed to schedule a same-day appointment with her primary care provider or a urologist.

STEP D: Sickle Cell Disease or Sickle Cell Carrier

Women who have sickle cell disease or who are sickle cell carriers are at higher risk for asymptomatic UTIs. These women should be instructed to come into the office to give a clean-caught urine specimen for analysis, culture, and sensitivity.

In addition, these women should undergo urinalysis during each trimester of their pregnancy to exclude an asymptomatic UTI.

3rd Trimester Vaginal Discharge

KEY QUESTIONS

ASSESSMENT	ACTION
1. Are you experiencing an increase in vaginal discharge without burning, itching, or odor?	**YES** Go to Step A.
	NO Go to Question 2.
2. Are you experiencing vaginal burning, itching, or odor?	**YES** Go to Step B.
	NO Go to Question 3.
3. Do you have any burning with urination?	**YES** Go to Step C.
	NO Go to Question 4.
4. Are you concerned you could have been exposed to a sexually transmitted infection (STI)?	**YES** Go to Step D.
	NO Go to Question 5.
5. Do you have any sores in the genital area?	**YES** Go to Step E. Go to Question 6.
	NO Go to Question 6.
6. Do you have a history of exposure to herpes?	**YES** Go to Step F.
	NO Go to Step G.

ACTIONS

STEP A: Physiologic Discharge of Pregnancy

Physiologic changes of pregnancy create a discharge that usually is thin, milk colored, and has a slight, but not unpleasant odor. Reassure the patient that this discharge is normal and will increase throughout the course of her pregnancy.

Advise against douching during pregnancy. Douching can introduce air into the vagina, which is dangerous.

Advise the patient to call if the discharge changes in color or odor or is accompanied by itching, burning, or lesions.

If the patient is at 36 weeks or less, an additional consideration in the 3rd trimester is the possibility of premature rupture of membranes.

Question as to the nature of amniotic fluid. It is often described as being more viscous than leukorrhea or the physiologic discharge attributable to pregnancy. It also is described as having a faintly "sweet" or "clean" aroma.

Question the patient regarding the color of the fluid. Bloody or green fluid has different significance.

Question the patient about associated uterine tightening or vaginal bleeding.

If there is any question of ruptured membranes, have the patient come in to be seen ASAP.

If the patient is 37 weeks to term, refer to the protocol for Ruptured Membranes.

STEP B: Symptoms of Vaginitis

Simple vaginitis is common in pregnancy, particularly because of an increase in yeast infections for some women. Vaginitis diagnosed as bacterial vaginosis has been implicated in preterm labor. Early elimination of the problem is important.

Have the patient come in for evaluation within 3–5 days or sooner if the symptoms increase.

Instruct the patient to avoid using OTC products until a diagnosis is made.

You should know the preference of the providers with whom you work with regard to treatments recommended during the 3rd trimester.

STEP C: Urinary Tract Symptoms

Yeast infections also can mimic UTI symptoms. In this case, the burning usually occurs when urine runs over the perineal tissue. Pain that occurs inside, especially at the end of voiding, is more likely to be a UTI.

If the symptoms sound like a UTI, the patient should be seen ASAP. Explain that she may be asked to give a clean-caught urine sample during her office visit.

STEP D: Possible Sexually Transmitted Infection Exposure

Sexually transmitted infections can have a significant impact on pregnancy outcome. If the patient is found to have an STI during pregnancy, follow-up with her partner and evaluation for reinfection are of major concern to prevent harm to the fetus.

The patient should be instructed to come in within 24 hours for a thorough evaluation.

Explain that she may have to provide vaginal and vulvar cultures, and undergo blood tests.

Advise the patient to avoid sexual intercourse until she has been evaluated.

STEP E: Vulvovaginitis Symptoms With Possible Lesions

The patient with lesions should be seen within 24–48 hours.

Instruct the patient to wash her hands thoroughly after urination.

The patient should avoid applying creams or lotions to the area until she has been seen for evaluation.

Comfort measures, such as cold compresses or tepid baths, may be soothing.

Advise the patient to avoid sexual intercourse until she has been seen for evaluation.

STEP F: History of Herpetic Lesions

Patients with a history of herpes need to be educated regarding the risk if lesions are present at delivery.

Question the patient regarding the pattern of outbreak during present and previous pregnancies.

Your practice may or may not endorse the use of acyclovir for suppression near term. You should know your providers' opinion on this issue and discuss accordingly with the patient.

Follow the advice in Step E.

Advise the patient to come in for confirmation of lesion if she is uncertain or within 2 weeks of term.

STEP G: Vulvovaginitis Symptoms, Etiology Unknown

Question the patient about recent antibiotic use or changes in toilet tissue, bubble baths, or laundry detergent.

Question the patient about whether she's had these symptoms before and what was used to treat them.

Advise the patient on comfort measures recommended by your providers.

Make an appointment for the patient to come in within 72 hours.

PATIENT EDUCATION

1. Vaginitis in pregnancy may have a different significance because of the potential ramifications for the developing fetus. Many patients self-diagnose these conditions and may request specific medication prescriptions based on past symptom resolution. Whether or not to treat over the telephone without seeing the patient will be at the discretion of your providers. Many offices or clinics have a policy to treat simple symptoms of yeast infections without seeing the patient. However, most providers will treat only once. If the patient experiences no improvement, she should be seen for evaluation.

2. The goal is to not miss a more serious, possibly communicable infection. If a patient is fairly certain she has been exposed to an STI, encourage her to have her partner(s) tested and to refrain from intercourse until evaluated and treated. You may need to help her rehearse various scenarios before she talks with her partner.

3. Patients exposed to STIs early in pregnancy need full testing for possible STIs and a plan for retesting throughout their pregnancy. It is reasonable to encourage these patients to use condoms to minimize the potential for exposure.

3rd Trimester Visual Changes

KEY QUESTIONS

ASSESSMENT	ACTION
1. Have you had a sudden loss (central or peripheral blindness) or significant change (blurring, double vision) in your vision?	**YES** Go to Step A.
	NO Go to Question 2.
2. Do you have eye pain?	**YES** Go to Question 3.
	NO Go to Question 4.
3. Is the pain unilateral or intense, and did it begin suddenly?	**YES** Go to Step B.
	NO Go to Question 4.
4. Is the eye red but painless and your vision unaffected?	**YES** Go to Step C.
	NO Go to Question 5.
5. Is your vision changing gradually and affecting normal activities, such as reading, sewing, or driving?	**YES** Go to Step D.
	NO No further action.

ACTIONS

STEP A: Sudden Loss of Vision

This patient may be experiencing a TIA or stroke; may have acute angle glaucoma or retinal detachment; or may be experiencing a new onset of ocular migraine. She should be seen immediately. Refer her to the ER or have the patient call 911. Make sure that the patient does not drive herself to the ER.

STEP B: Eye Pain

This patient may have iritis, acute glaucoma, cluster headache, or an unusual ocular migraine presentation. The patient should be evaluated by her primary care provider within the next 2–4 hours. Make sure patient has someone drive her to the visit.

STEP C: Unilateral, Intense, Sudden Eye Pain

This could be a spontaneous hemorrhage, conjunctivitis, acute glaucoma, or scleritis. The patient should be evaluated by her primary care provider within the next 12–24 hours.

STEP D: Gradual Eye Changes

Because of hormonal changes, some women find that their vision has changed during pregnancy or that they are no longer able to wear their contact lenses. Most women will find they can resume contact use after pregnancy. In addition, the patient may have changing central vision and need corrective lenses or an increase in her current eyewear prescription. She should see her eye care provider within the next week.

Medications in Pregnancy and Lactation

Drug Name	Type of Drug	Pregnancy Risk Category	Permitted in Pregnancy?	Permitted During Lactation?	Comments
Acetaminophen	Analgesic, antipyretic	B	Yes	Yes	Safe for short-term use. Long-term use can cause severe anemia and fatal kidney disease in the newborn.
Actifed	Decongestant combination	C	No	Yes	Because this is a combination product, other one-medication products usually are better to prescribe.
Alka-Seltzer	Analgesic (buffered aspirin)	C (D in 3rd trimester)	No	Yes, American Academy of Pediatrics advises cautious use when breastfeeding.	Contains aspirin.
Amoxicillin	Antibiotic	B	Yes	Yes	Can modify bowel flora in infant and affect infant culture results. Rare allergic reaction in infant noted.
Ampicillin	Antibiotic	B	Yes	Yes	Can modify bowel flora in infant and affect infant culture results. Rare allergic reaction in infant noted.
Anusol cream	Hemorrhoidal preparation	B	Yes	Yes	

Drug	Class	Pregnancy Category			Comments
Aspirin	Analgesic	C (D in 3rd trimester)	No	Yes	Certain high-risk prenatal patients may be taking aspirin.
Bacitracin	Topical anti-infective	C	No report of congenital defects with use of drug.	No breastfeeding data available.	
Calamine lotion	Topical lotion	B	Yes	Yes	
Darvocet N-100; Darvon; Darvocet N-50; Darvon Compound (propoxyphene)	Analgesic	C (D if used for long periods)	No	Yes	Use in pregnancy associated with microcephaly, patent ductus arteriosis, cataracts, benign tumors, and clubfoot.
Dramamine	Antiemetic/antihistamine	Bm	Conflicting data. No established risk.	No breastfeeding data available.	Some providers prescribe for hyperemesis.

Pregnancy risk categories: **Category A:** Controlled studies have not demonstrated a risk to the fetus in the 1st trimester, and there is no evidence of a risk in later trimesters. Possibility of risk to fetus is remote. **Category B:** Either animal reproduction studies have not shown a fetal risk or animal studies showing an adverse risk were not demonstrated in controlled studies in women during the 1st trimester. No evidence of a risk in later trimesters. **Category Bm:** Manufacturer rated the medication. **Category C:** Either studies in animals have indicated adverse effects on the fetus or there are no controlled studies in women and animals. Should be given only if potential benefit justifies potential risk to the fetus. **Category D:** Positive evidence of human fetal risks. May be given if drug is needed in a life-threatening situation or for a serious disease in cases where safer drugs cannot be used or are ineffective. **Category X:** Human or animal studies have shown that there is evidence of fetal risk, fetal abnormalities, or both. The risk of use clearly outweighs any possible benefit. The drug is contraindicated in women who are or may become pregnant.

Continued

Medications in Pregnancy and Lactation—cont'd

Drug Name	Type of Drug	Pregnancy Risk Category	Permitted in Pregnancy?	Permitted During Lactation?	Comments
Dilantin (phenytoin)	Anticonvulsant	D	Provider needs to determine if safer drug should be prescribed. Should not discontinue use without consulting provider.	American Academy of Pediatrics considers drug to be compatible with breastfeeding.	
Emetrol	Antiemetic	B	Yes	Yes	
Entex PSE (guaifenesin/pseudoephedrine)	Decongestant	C	No	No data available.	
Erythromycin	Antibiotic	B	Yes	Yes	Can modify bowel flora in infant and affect infant culture results. Rare allergic reaction in infant noted.
Gelusil	Antacid	B	Yes	Yes	Avoid overuse, which can cause a gastric rebound effect.
Guaifenesin	Expectorant	C	Conflicting data. Likely safe in pregnancy if used moderately.	No data available.	

Kaopectate (kaolin/pectin)	Antidiarrheal	C	No reports of adverse effects, but may decrease iron absorption and cause anemia if used long term.	Yes	Counsel the patient regarding dehydration or fever. If present, schedule for same-day appointment.
KWELL (lindane)	Topical antilice/scabies preparation	Bm	Potential neurotoxicity, but not well demonstrated via the research.	Likely safe during lactation.	Because of the potential for neurological side effects, many providers prescribe pyrethrins with piperonyl butoxide (RID) during pregnancy, instead of KWELL.
Laxatives	Laxative		No	Yes	Can precipitate preterm labor.
Maalox (aluminum hydroxide/ magnesium hydroxide)	Antacid		Yes	Yes	

Pregnancy risk categories: **Category A:** Controlled studies have not demonstrated a risk to the fetus in the 1st trimester, and there is no evidence of a risk in later trimesters. Possibility of risk to fetus is remote. **Category B:** Either animal reproduction studies have not shown a fetal risk or animal studies showing an adverse risk were not demonstrated in controlled studies in women during the 1st trimester. No evidence of a risk in later trimesters. **Category Bm:** Manufacturer rated the medication. **Category C:** Either studies in animals have indicated adverse effects on the fetus or there are no controlled studies in women and animals. Should be given only if potential benefit justifies potential risk to the fetus. **Category D:** Positive evidence of human fetal risks. May be given if drug is needed in a life-threatening situation or for a serious disease in cases where safer drugs cannot be used or are ineffective. **Category X:** Human or animal studies have shown that there is evidence of fetal risk, fetal abnormalities, or both. The risk of use clearly outweighs any possible benefit. The drug is contraindicated in women who are or may become pregnant.

Continued

Medications in Pregnancy and Lactation—cont'd

Drug Name	Type of Drug	Pregnancy Risk Category	Permitted in Pregnancy?	Permitted During Lactation?	Comments
Macrobid (nitrofurantoin)	Urinary germicide	B	Yes	Yes	
Metamucil	Bulk-forming laxative	NR	Yes	Yes	
Metronidazole (Flagyl)	Antimicrobial	Bm	Controversial	Controversial	Centers for Disease Control considers use contraindicated in 1st trimester but acceptable in later pregnancy if alternative therapies have failed. Avoid single-dose therapy. American Academy of Pediatrics recommends not breastfeeding for 12–24 hours after a single dose, 2 g dose is given to a breastfeeding woman.
Milk of Magnesia	Antacid	B	Yes	Yes	Avoid overuse, which can cause gastric rebound effect.
Mylanta	Antacid	B	Yes	Yes	Avoid overuse, which can cause gastric rebound effect.
Neosporin	Topical anti-infective	C	Yes	Yes	

Penicillin benzathine, Penicillin procaine	Antibiotic	B	Yes	Yes	Can modify bowel flora in infant and affect infant culture results. Rare allergic reaction in infant noted.
Pepto-Bismol (bismuth subsalicylate)	Antidiarrheal	C	Restrict use to first half of pregnancy and only at recommended doses.	American Academy of Pediatrics recommends avoidance during lactation because of systemic salicylate absorption.	
RID (pyrethrins with piperonyl butoxide)	Antilice preparation	C	No solid data, but considered drug of choice for lice during pregnancy.	No data available.	Not effective for treatment of scabies.
Riopan	Antacid	B	Yes	Yes	Avoid overuse, which can cause gastric rebound effect.
Rocephin (ceftriaxone)	Antibiotic	Bm	Yes	Yes	

Pregnancy risk categories: **Category A:** Controlled studies have not demonstrated a risk to the fetus in the 1st trimester, and there is no evidence of a risk in later trimesters. Possibility of risk to fetus is remote. **Category B:** Either animal reproduction studies have not shown a fetal risk or animal studies showing an adverse risk were not demonstrated in controlled studies in women during the 1st trimester. No evidence of a risk in later trimesters. **Category Bm:** Manufacturer rated the medication. **Category C:** Either studies in animals have indicated adverse effects on the fetus or there are no controlled studies in women and animals. Should be given only if potential benefit justifies potential risk to the fetus. **Category D:** Positive evidence of human fetal risks. May be given if drug is needed in a life-threatening situation or for a serious disease in cases where safer drugs cannot be used or are ineffective. **Category X:** Human or animal studies have shown that there is evidence of fetal risk, fetal abnormalities, or both. The risk of use clearly outweighs any possible benefit. The drug is contraindicated in women who are or may become pregnant.

Continued

Medications in Pregnancy and Lactation—cont'd

Drug Name	Type of Drug	Pregnancy Risk Category	Permitted in Pregnancy?	Permitted During Lactation?	Comments
Sudafed (pseudoephedrine)	Sympathomimetic agent used for allergies or upper respiratory tract infections.	C	Likely safe (teratogenic in some animals, but not demonstrated in humans).	Yes	
Tagamet (cimetidine)	Inhibits gastric acid secretion.	Bm	Conflicting data. Generally thought to be safe, but one group of reviewers recommends avoidance in pregnancy.	Yes	
Tegretol (carbamazepine)	Anticonvulsant	Cm	May be associated with fetal anomalies such as spina bifida, but risks of seizure may outweigh use of drug. Patient and provider should decide jointly on choice of anticonvulsant.	Yes	American Academy of Pediatrics considers this drug safe for use during lactation.

Drug	Classification	Category			Comments
Tetracycline	Antibiotic	D	No	Yes (American Academy of Pediatrics)	Not recommended in pregnancy because of potential negative effects on fetal teeth and bones, congenital defects, maternal liver toxicity. Can modify bowel flora in infant and affect infant culture results. Rare allergic reaction in infant noted.
Tums	Antacid	B	Yes	Yes	Avoid overuse, which can cause gastric rebound effect.
Tylenol (acetaminophen)	Analgesic, antipyretic	B	Yes	Yes	
Zantac (ranitidine)	Antiulcer	Bm	Yes	Yes	

Pregnancy risk categories: **Category A:** Controlled studies have not demonstrated a risk to the fetus in the 1st trimester, and there is no evidence of a risk in later trimesters. Possibility of risk to fetus is remote. **Category B:** Either animal reproduction studies have not shown a fetal risk or animal studies showing an adverse risk were not demonstrated in controlled studies in women during the 1st trimester. No evidence of a risk in later trimesters. **Category Bm:** Manufacturer rated the medication. **Category C:** Either studies in animals have indicated adverse effects on the fetus or there are no controlled studies in women and animals. Should be given only if potential benefit justifies potential risk to the fetus. **Category D:** Positive evidence of human fetal risks. May be given if drug is needed in a life-threatening situation or for a serious disease in cases where safer drugs cannot be used or are ineffective. **Category X:** Human or animal studies have shown that there is evidence of fetal risk, fetal abnormalities, or both. The risk of use clearly outweighs any possible benefit. The drug is contraindicated in women who are or may become pregnant.

CHAPTER 10

Postpartum and Neonatal Overview

The 1st trimester of pregnancy is characterized by tremendous physical and emotional changes. So, too, is the postpartum period. Many women's health practices provide the patient with some postpartum teaching before the arrival of the baby, and most women receive postpartum teaching once they have delivered. However, with ever-shortening lengths of postpartum care, many women have difficulty absorbing and remembering this teaching. Consequently, it is common to receive calls from patients about postpartum changes and concerns.

From a telephone perspective, several issues often are encountered. Normal and abnormal bleeding during the postpartum period, postpartum infection, emotional changes associated with delivery, and questions about caring for newborn frequently arise.

The postpartum uterine discharge, or lochia, normally will transition during the first few days from lochia rubra to lochia serosa. During the next 2 weeks, lochia serosa will be replaced by lochia alba. The patient can expect the lochia to change from bright red to pink to rust-colored and finally to white-yellow. Occasionally, there is a sudden transient increase in uterine bleeding between 7 and 14 days after delivery as the placental implantation site heals. The flow of blood normally stops between 4 and 6 weeks. A protocol is provided to assist with telephone assessment of lochia.

Breast pain and nipple soreness are common postpartum symptoms. Initial breast engorgement often occurs between the 2nd and 5th postpartum day. This needs to be distinguished from postpartum mastitis, a breast infection characterized by breast pain with redness, fever, and flu-like symptoms.

Postpartum "blues" are a common psychological response to pregnancy. However, a minority of women may experience more serious psychological difficulties, often resulting in postpartum depression or psychosis. Differentiating between these reactions is an important challenge to the triage provider.

The postpartum patient frequently consults women's health providers with concerns related to the newborn. The women's health care team should answer only the most rudimentary of questions. Other questions should be referred to the patient's pediatric provider. Protocols for the most basic of neonatal questions are provided in this section of the book.

BASIC TRIAGE ASSESSMENT FORM FOR THE POSTPARTUM PERIOD

1. What date did you deliver? _____
2. Was the baby term? _____
3. What type of delivery did you have (vaginal, vaginal with vacuum or forceps assistance, or cesarean section)? _____
4. Did you have any complications at the time of delivery? _____
5. Did you have a boy or a girl? (Note: Most practices have a method for flagging charts to avoid the trauma of asking a patient who has suffered a pregnancy loss questions pertaining to the infant and infant status.) _____
6. How is the baby doing? _____
7. How are you feeding the baby (breast, bottle, or combination)? _____

Common Questions After Delivery

KEY QUESTIONS

ASSESSMENT	ACTION

1. Did you have a cesarean section delivery?

> **YES** Go to Step A.
> **NO** Go to Question 2.

2. Did you have a vaginal delivery?

> **YES** Go to Step B.
> **NO** Go to Question 3.

3. Have you begun doing postpartum exercises?

> **YES** Go to Question 4.
> **NO** Go to Step C.

4. Have you had sexual intercourse since the delivery of your infant?

> **YES** Go to Question 5.
> **NO** Go to Step D.

5. Are you using birth control measures?

> **YES** Go to Step E.
> **NO** No further action.

ACTIONS

STEP A: Activity After a Cesarean Section

The goal is to promote a speedy and safe recovery.

Cesarean section is major abdominal surgery; it may take as long as 6 months to make a complete recovery.

Begin to walk as soon as possible after delivery, keeping your back straight.

No lifting (greater than 15 pounds), carrying, or doing housework for 6 weeks.

If breastfeeding, ensure there is good support by using a pillow or the side-lying position.

Support the abdomen when coughing, laughing, or sneezing.

Wash hands frequently, especially after urinating, having a bowel movement, before and after changing diapers, and before touching the incision.

Try to keep everything to one floor in the home.

Do not drive for 6 weeks.

Drink plenty of fluids.

STEP B: Activity After a Vaginal Delivery

The goal is to promote a speedy and safe recovery.

No heavy lifting (greater than 15 pounds) for at least 2 weeks.

No stair climbing for at least 1 week.

No driving for at least 1 week.

STEP C: Exercise After Birth

Postpartum exercises are designed to assist in regaining muscle tone and body shape.

Toe stretch and pelvic floor exercises (Kegel) can be performed in bed during the immediate postpartum period.

Other exercises (such as abdominal muscle strengthening) are important and can be
added after the first postpartum visit.

STEP D: Sexual Intercourse

Sexual activity can be resumed after vaginal bleeding has stopped, the incision is healed,
and the patient is mentally ready.

To reduce the risk of infection, do not have sexual intercourse until vaginal bleeding
has stopped.

Because of hormonal changes, the patient may experience vaginal dryness.

If vaginal dryness occurs, prolonging foreplay or using a water-soluble lubricant may
add to patient comfort.

Sexual intimacy can be achieved in ways other than sexual intercourse; try expressing
love by conversation, kissing, hugging, and touching each other.

The demands of parenting are stressful on a relationship; recommend open, honest,
and frequent communication between partners.

Try having intercourse in the morning when the patient may be more rested.

Pregnancy can occur within the first 2–4 weeks after delivery, so the patient should be
sure to use contraception before resuming sexual intercourse if she wants to prevent
a pregnancy.

STEP E: Contraception

Ovulation can occur as early as 4 weeks after delivery. Do not rely on breastfeeding as
a method of reliable contraception.

Contraception ideally should be discussed with both partners during the immediate
postpartum period.

If the patient is not using contraception and is having or considering having intercourse, advise the patient to use condoms and schedule an appointment for contraceptive counseling.

Postpartum Breast Pain

KEY QUESTIONS

ASSESSMENT	ACTION

1. Do you have a temperature greater than 101°F (taken orally)?

YES Go to Step A.
NO Go to Question 2.

2. Is there any redness to your breast?

YES Go to Step A.
NO Go to Question 3.

3. Are you breastfeeding?

YES Go to Question 4.
NO Go to Step B.

4. Can you feel any lumps in your breast?

YES Go to Step C.
NO Go to Step D.

ACTIONS

STEP A: Mastitis (Breast Infection)

Mastitis is an infection of the breast that requires antibiotic therapy.

In cases in which the patient's temperature is greater than 101°F; flulike muscular aching is present; hot, tender, or red areas are present on the breast; or streaking on the breast is present, the patient should be scheduled for a same-day appointment.

The patient should continue to breastfeed while she is undergoing treatment for mastitis.

STEP B: Postpartum Breast Pain in Nonbreastfeeding Women

Engorged breasts are a common problem during the first week after delivery.
Apply cold compresses, ice packs, or cabbage leaves, as needed.
Do not pump or express breastmilk because such actions will stimulate milk production.
Do not apply heat (hot showers) or stimulate the breast.
Wear a proper fitting and supporting bra night and day for at least 2 weeks.
Take acetaminophen for pain, following the manufacturer's recommendations.

STEP C: Plugged Ducts

A plugged duct can present as a lump, redness, or tenderness to the breast.
Breastfeed on the most affected breast first.
Try to empty the affected breasts thoroughly at each feeding.

Apply warm compresses or take a warm shower before breastfeeding.

While feeding, gently massage the breast downward and toward the nipple.

Alternate the infant's feeding positions to drain all ducts.

Avoid wearing constrictive clothing or underwire nursing bras.

Plugged ducts normally disappear within 24 to 48 hours when they are properly treated.

Plugged ducts can lead to mastitis if not treated properly.

STEP D: Postpartum Breast Pain in Breastfeeding Women

Engorged breasts may make it difficult for the infant to latch on to the breast.

Manually expressing some of the milk before feeding may reduce tension in the breast.

Warm showers or a warm compress applied to the breast before feeding can facilitate the letdown reflex.

Cold compresses applied to the breasts between feedings reduce breast congestion and provide pain relief.

Wear a properly fitting and supporting nursing bra.

When breastfeeding, find a comfortable position for the mother and the infant.

Use both breasts at each feeding and feed frequently (every 2 to 3 hours).

If the infant does not breastfeed on an engorged breast, hand pump or manually express some milk to soften the breast and provide pain relief.

Massaging the breasts during feeding may lessen the plugging of milk ducts.

Take acetaminophen for pain, following the manufacturer's recommendations.

PATIENT EDUCATION

Mastitis can often be prevented by:

- proper latching when breastfeeding;
- frequent breastfeedings;
- proper care of sore, cracked, or painful nipples;
- proper rest; and
- early detection and treatment of breast lumps (plugged ducts).

Call or make an appointment with your health care provider if you have any of the following:

- severe breast pain;
- engorgement that persists beyond 72 hours without relief;
- red streaks on the breast;
- chills or flu-like symptoms;
- temperature greater than 101° F; or
- a hot, red, and tender breast with or without a lump.

Postpartum Sore or Inverted Nipples

KEY QUESTIONS

ASSESSMENT	ACTION
1. Are you experiencing nipple pain?	**YES** Go to Step A.
	NO Go to Question 2.
2. Are your nipples inverted?	**YES** Go to Step B.
	NO Go to Question 3.
3. Are you experiencing breast pain?	**YES** Go to protocol Postpartum Breast Pain.
	NO No further action.

ACTIONS

STEP A: Sore Nipples

Sore cracked nipples usually are associated with improper latching during breastfeeding.

Ensure there is a correct latch during breastfeeding.

Change breastfeeding positions.

Start breastfeeding on the less sore nipple first and switch to the other nipple when breastfeeding has slowed.

Hand express some milk before putting infant to the breast so the milk is already beginning to flow.

When removing the infant from the breast, insert your finger into the corner of the infant's mouth to break the seal.

After feeding, express some milk on the breast and air dry the nipple.

Wash breasts with water only because soap can dry the skin.

Nipple creams (lanolin) may be helpful in promoting healing.

Change breast pads frequently.

In cases of persistent nipple soreness or the sudden appearance of nipple soreness after lactation has been established, monilia infection of the nipple must be considered.

The infection may be treated with topical nystatin or clotrimazole.

The infant may have thrush or a monilia diaper rash.

STEP B: Inverted Nipples

There are varying degrees of nipple inversion, from the slightly inverted to the severely inverted (retracted to a level below the areola).

Place a thumb on each side at the base of the nipple and push in firmly against the breast tissue while pulling your thumbs away from each other. Do this five times a day.

Most infants who latch on to the breast will draw out an inverted nipple.

The patient may use an effective breast pump to draw the nipple out before breast-feeding.

Try rolling the nipple between the thumb and index finger for 1–2 minutes to draw out nipple.

Try pulling back on the breast tissue (toward the chest wall) as the infant begins to latch on; this may help the nipple to protrude.

A nipple shield should be tried only as a last resort.

Postpartum Depression/Blues

Postpartum blues are a common psychological reaction following childbirth. The symptoms of postpartum blues appear during the first week after delivery and usually are resolved by postpartum day 14. The onset of postpartum depression is usually within 6 weeks after childbirth, and symptoms last from 3–14 months. Postpartum blues are reported to occur in as many as 70% of all women, whereas postpartum depression occurs in as many as 33%. Women with a history of postpartum depression have a 50% risk of recurrence. Postpartum psychosis is characterized by a desire to harm oneself or the baby. It requires immediate attention.

KEY QUESTIONS

ASSESSMENT	ACTION
1. Are you within 14 days after delivery of your baby?	**YES** Go to Question 2.
	NO Go to Question 3.
2. Are you feeling anxious and find yourself crying for no apparent reason?	**YES** Go to Question 3.
	NO Go to Question 3.
3. Are you feeling in a low mood, fatigued, unable to concentrate, feeling hopeless, or like you can't cope with being a mother?	**YES** Go to Questions 4 and 5.
	NO Go to Step A.
4. Are you experiencing panic, confusion, insomnia, rapid mood swings, hearing voices, or feeling that someone is talking about you or wants to harm you?	**YES** Go to Question 5. Continue to Step B.
	NO Go to Question 5.
5. Do you feel like harming yourself or your baby?	**YES** Go to Step B.
	NO Go to Step C.

ACTIONS

STEP A: Treatment of Postpartum Blues

The symptoms generally are self-limiting and require no pharmacologic treatment. Reassure the mother and family that these feelings are common and usually go away without treatment, but if they persist past 2 weeks, however mildly, the patient should call back to report her symptoms.

Give her permission at the onset to call back immediately if symptoms worsen at any time.

Advise the mother to get as much rest as possible, to sleep when the baby sleeps, and to get help with housework and other child care responsibilities, if possible.

Educate her at any initial call that fatigue often is at the root of worsening symptoms and advise her not to push herself beyond reasonable limits.

Encourage the patient to eat regular meals and a well-balanced diet.

Advise the patient that mild exercise, such as walking, may be helpful.

Encourage her to plan time for some activities she enjoys and for private time with her partner.

Encourage her to continue breastfeeding if she is doing so.

All practices should have a mechanism for alerting other providers to patients experiencing severe blues.

All practices should have a mechanism for following up on patients identified early in the postpartum period as "at greater risk" for worsening postpartum problems. In our practice, we use the following system: _____

_____

STEP B: Requires Immediate Action and Referral to a Mental Health Professional

This woman could be experiencing postpartum psychosis or major postpartum depression. She requires immediate assistance.

Ask whether she is feeling like harming herself or her baby at that time (Question 5). Ask if she has thought about how she would do it. Ask whether anyone is home with her. If yes, ask her if you can talk with that person. If no, ask for the name and telephone number of a family member or friend you can reach immediately.

If it is necessary to call a family member or friend who is not at the patient's house, try to have someone else call the contact person so you can remain on the line with the patient.

If you are not able to contact a family member or other responsible person, inform a provider in your practice that an emergency situation exists. If the threat of suicide or infanticide seems immediate, have someone else in your practice call emergency services. Keep the woman on the telephone and talking until emergency services arrive. Reassure her that help is on the way.

If you are able to talk to a family member, ask them to make sure the patient is not left alone until she can see a mental health professional.

Make a same-day appointment with a mental health professional and ensure that she is accompanied by a family member or other responsible person.

Inform a provider in your practice about the problem and the actions taken.

STEP C: Requires Prompt Action and Referral to a Mental Health Professional

Even if there does not appear to be a risk of suicide or infanticide, this woman may be experiencing severe postpartum depression or psychosis and needs prompt assistance.

Refer her to a mental health professional for an appointment within a few days.

Explain to the woman and her family that the prospect for recovery is excellent, but that she will recover more quickly with treatment, which should include medication and counseling.

Make an appointment with her provider to rule out physical causes of symptoms that may resemble depression, such as anemia or hypothyroidism.

Refer her to community resources, such as support groups for new parents.

Encourage her to maintain a healthy diet and get mild/moderate exercise.

Encourage her to discuss her feelings with her partner or another significant person in her life.

Reassure her that many women have psychological problems after childbirth and that this does not mean she is a bad mother.

Encourage her to do some activities that she enjoys and to plan for some private time with her partner.

Encourage her to continue breastfeeding if she is doing so but to discuss this with her provider and pediatrician if she begins taking medication.

Encourage her to **immediately** report worsening symptoms or if she feels like harming herself, the baby, or anyone else.

Inform a provider in your practice about the problem and the actions taken.

PATIENT EDUCATION

1. Postpartum blues is a common reaction after childbirth, occurring in the first week to 10 days in as many as 70% of new mothers. The major symptoms are mild anxiety or weepiness.

2. Postpartum psychosis is a relatively rare disorder, occurring in 1 to 2 of 1000 women, with the onset often during the same time that postpartum blues is found. It may begin with confusion, insomnia, anxiety, and panic and may progress rapidly to delusions and hallucinations. Risk factors include primiparity or a personal or family history of mental illness. It may recur with subsequent pregnancies. On rare occasions, a woman may harm herself or her baby. This condition requires **immediate** attention.

3. Postpartum depression, experienced by approximately 10% of new mothers, usually has a more insidious onset, often after the third week. A gradual increase in depressed mood, with marked lack of energy and multiple physical symptoms, often is seen. Women may feel like a failure at motherhood, and suicide is a risk. Risk factors include prenatal or previous postpartum depression, poor relationship with the father of the baby, and lack of support systems. These women also need professional help.

4. Remember that a woman may not meet all of the parameters for a given diagnosis and may still be in serious trouble. Any question of threat or harm to self or baby requires immediate intervention.

Postpartum Hemorrhoids

KEY QUESTIONS

ASSESSMENT

ACTION

1. Are you experiencing a new onset of rectal bleeding or pain?

YES Go to Step A.

NO Go to Question 2.

2. Are you experiencing rectal itching, pain, or bleeding associated with your hemorrhoids?

YES Go to Step B.

NO No further action.

ACTIONS

STEP A: New Onset of Rectal Bleeding or Pain

Schedule a same-day or next-day appointment for any postpartum patient with new onset of rectal bleeding or pain.

STEP B: Treatment of Hemorrhoids

The goal is to decrease discomfort and promote healing.

Increase fluid intake; drink a minimum of six 8-ounce glasses of water per day.

Increase fiber in diet; this includes fresh fruit, vegetables, whole grain breads, and high-fiber cereals.

Fiber supplements (Metamucil) and stool softeners are recommended to prevent constipation.

Avoid straining when having a bowel movement.

Avoid prolonged sitting on the toilet.

Schedule time in your busy day to have a bowel movement; the best time is after a meal.

Clean the rectal area with soap and water after having a bowel movement.

Apply ice packs to the rectal area as necessary.

Try not to rub or wipe briskly when drying your rectal area.

Sit in a basin of water or bathtub filled with warm water for 15–20 minutes three to four times per day.

Apply cool witch hazel on the hemorrhoids.

Apply hydrocortisone ointment for itching, analgesic sprays for pain, and astringent suppositories for bleeding.

PATIENT EDUCATION

Hemorrhoids commonly occur during pregnancy and usually resolve during the first 6 months after delivery.

Postpartum Care of Incision From Episiotomy or Cesarean Section

KEY QUESTIONS

ASSESSMENT

ACTION

1. Are you experiencing increasing pain, redness, or drainage from the incision site, or do you have a temperature greater than 100° F (taken orally)?

YES Go to Step A.

NO Go to Question 2.

2. Are you able to urinate freely?

YES Go to Question 3.

NO Go to Step A.

3. Is your incision clean, dry, and intact?

YES Go to Step B.

NO Go to Step C.

ACTIONS

STEP A: Care of an Infected Incision

Make a same-day appointment for the patient if she:

- has a temperature greater than 100°F (taken orally);
- notes a sudden increase in vaginal bleeding;
- is not able to urinate freely;
- has a malodorous discharge from the incision or vagina; or
- has pus, heat, increasing tenderness, or redness surrounding the incision site.

STEP B: Care of the Episiotomy Incision

The patient may feel more comfortable while sitting and increased pain with standing and walking.

Soak the perineum in lukewarm water (sitz baths) to provide comfort and promote healing.

Apply ice packs to reduce swelling and discomfort.

Use a desk lamp with a 40-watt bulb as a heat lamp. The heat lamp should be approximately 20 inches from the perineum, and a heat lamp session should last 20 minutes.

Wash hands before and after changing sanitary pads and before and after changing diapers.

Change sanitary pads frequently.

Wear cotton underwear to promote air penetration to the wound.

Avoid bubble baths and hygiene sprays.

Avoid tampon use for 6 weeks.

Avoid constipation by drinking eight 8-ounce glasses of water per day and eating foods high in fiber.

Use nonsteroidal anti-inflammatory drugs (NSAIDs) or acetaminophen to help control pain.

STEP C: Refer Immediately Any Patient With a Cesarean Section or Episiotomy

Refer the patient to her provider immediately if the incision has separated; is draining blood; has increasing redness; has increasing tenderness; is warm to the touch; or looks "dirty" to the patient.

Postpartum Vaginal Bleeding (Lochia)

KEY QUESTIONS

ASSESSMENT	ACTION
1. Are you experiencing increasing or continuous abdominal pain?	**YES** Go to Step A.
	NO Go to Question 2.
2. Do you have a temperature greater than 100° F (taken orally)?	**YES** Go to Step A.
	NO Go to Question 3.
3. Are you passing clots more frequently, or are the clots larger than a quarter?	**YES** Go to Step A.
	NO Go to Question 4.
4. Are you changing your pad more frequently than every 2 hours?	**YES** Go to Step B.
	NO Go to Question 5.
5. Are you experiencing any dizziness or increasing fatigue?	**YES** Go to Step A.
	NO Go to Question 6.
6. Does your vaginal discharge have a foul odor?	**YES** Go to Step A.
	NO No further action.

ACTIONS

STEP A: Make A Same-Day Appointment if the Patient Has

- increasing or continuous abdominal pain;
- temperature greater than 100°F (taken orally);
- an increase in frequency or size of clots passed;
- a sudden increase in vaginal bleeding;
- pad changes more frequently than every 2 hours;
- dizziness or light-headedness; and
- malodorous vaginal discharge.

STEP B: Postpartum Bleeding

The blood seen in postpartum bleeding initially is bright red then changes from pink to brown to white.

During the first 3 days, the blood will be bright red.

Bleeding should not soil more than one pad every 2–3 hours.

The pad should be only one-third to one-half saturated and should have only a few small clots.

Do not use tampons for the first 6 weeks.

Bleeding may increase with breastfeeding because the uterus may contract more rapidly.

By 3–8 days after delivery, vaginal blood should change in color from red to pink or rust colored.

Use a perineum bottle (filled with warm water) to rinse off each time patient uses the toilet or changes her pad.

To prevent excessive vaginal bleeding, the patient should:

- massage the uterus;
- not lift anything heavy (greater than 15 lbs);
- take care only of herself and the infant for the first few weeks; and
- take daily naps, when possible.

Newborn Bottle-Feeding

ASSESSMENT	ACTION
1. Are you bottle-feeding?	**YES** Go to Question 2.
	NO See protocol for Newborn Breastfeeding.
2. Is the baby feeding every 3–4 hours?	**YES** Go to Question 3.
	NO Go to Step A.
3. Is your infant taking at least 2 ounces per feeding?	**YES** Go to Question 4.
	NO Go to Step A.
4. Is the baby having at least six wet diapers per day?	**YES** Go to Question 5.
	NO Go to Step B.
5. Is your infant vomiting?	**YES** Go to Step C.
	NO Go to Question 6.
6. Is your infant slow in finishing the bottle or showing little or no interest in feeding?	**YES** Go to Step D.
	NO No further action.

ACTIONS

STEP A: Amount and Frequency of Bottle-feedings

The amount and frequency of feedings varies with the age of the infant. An infant from birth to 1 month of age usually takes 2–4 ounces every 3–4 hours. An infant from 2–6 months of age usually takes 5–8 ounces every 4–6 hours. Many infants may eliminate the nighttime feeding between 2 and 4 months of age, although they are expected to begin feeding more frequently during the day to compensate for the missed night feeding(s).

STEP B: Assessment of Elimination

An infant with no urine output for 12 hours should be scheduled for an immediate appointment.

Urine output is a good indicator of the adequacy of formula intake and should be assessed each time a feeding problem is suspected.

Reduced frequency of bowel movements may indicate that the infant is constipated or receiving insufficient formula intake.

STEP C: Assessment of Vomiting

Spitting up is a common occurrence in infants and must be differentiated from vomiting.

An infant with projectile vomiting should be scheduled for a same-day appointment with a pediatric provider.

STEP D: When to Schedule an Appointment

The following are signs of serious illness, and a same-day appointment should be scheduled with a pediatric provider:

- Prolonged time between feedings or no interest in feeding.
- Reduced amount of formula per feeding.
- Taking a long time to finish a bottle.
- Vomiting after each feeding.
- Reduced frequency and amount of urination.
- Fever or depressed temperature.
- Increasingly yellow (jaundiced) skin.

PATIENT EDUCATION

1. It is important to have an adequate assessment of the brand, type, preparation methods, feeding time, and elimination patterns of the bottle-fed infant.
2. Infants should consume approximately 2 to 2.5 ounces per pound of body weight per day, to a total of 32 ounces per day.

Newborn Breastfeeding

KEY QUESTIONS

ASSESSMENT	ACTION
1. Are you breastfeeding?	**YES** Go to Question 2.
	NO See protocol for Newborn Bottlefeeding.
2. Is the baby feeding every 3–4 hours?	**YES** Go to Question 3.
	NO Go to Step A.
3. Is the baby having at least six wet diapers per day?	**YES** Go to Question 4.
	NO Go to Step B.
4. Is your infant vomiting?	**YES** Go to Step C.
	NO Go to Question 5.
5. Is your infant slow in finishing the bottle or showing little or no interest in feeding?	**YES** Go to Step D.
	NO No further action.

ACTIONS

STEP A: Amount and Frequency of Breastfeeding

Breastfeeding requires patience; it does not come naturally.

Infants from birth to 1 month of age will breastfeed every 2–3 hours or 8–12 times daily.

During a growth spurt, infants will feed more frequently.

Good latch-on is indicated when feedings are quiet; no popping sounds should be heard.

Air blowing out of the infant's nose and audible swallowing should be heard.

STEP B: Assessment of Elimination

An infant with no urine output for 12 hours should be scheduled for an immediate appointment.

Urine output is a good indicator of the adequacy of intake and should be assessed each time a feeding problem is suspected.

A minimum of 2–3 stools per day is expected while breastfeeding is being established in the first 2 weeks.

Reduced frequency of bowel movements may indicate that the infant is constipated or receiving insufficient formula intake.

STEP C: Assessment of Vomiting

Spitting up is a common occurrence in infants and must be differentiated from vomiting. An infant with projectile vomiting should be scheduled for a same-day appointment with a pediatric provider.

STEP D: When to Schedule an Appointment

The following are signs of serious illness, and a same-day appointment should be scheduled with a pediatric provider.

- prolonged time between feedings or no interest in feeding.
- taking a long time to finish nursing.
- vomiting after each feeding.
- reduced frequency and amount of urination.
- fever or depressed temperature.
- increasingly yellow (jaundiced) skin.

PATIENT EDUCATION

1. It is important to have an adequate assessment of feeding time, feeding frequency, and elimination patterns of the breast-fed infant.

Newborn Fussy Baby/Colic

KEY QUESTIONS

ASSESSMENT	ACTION
1. Is your infant between 1 and 3 months of age?	**YES** Go to Question 2.
	NO go to Step A.
2. Does your infant have symptoms of constipation, diarrhea, vomiting, or fever?	**YES** Go to Step B.
	NO Go to Question 3.
3. Is your infant bottle-feeding or breastfeeding well?	**YES** Go to Question 4.
	NO Go to Step B.
4. Does your infant become less fussy when held?	**YES** Go to Step C.
	NO Go to Step D.

ACTIONS

STEP A: Colic

Colic is described as unexplained paroxysmal bouts of fussing and crying that last >3 hours/day, for >3 days/week of duration, beginning around 1 month of age and usually ending by 4 months of age.
Schedule a same-day appointment.

STEP B: Fussiness Caused by an Illness

Schedule a same-day appointment for an infant that has symptoms of systemic illness.

STEP C: Treatment of Colic

Because the etiology of colic is not understood, there is no definitive treatment, try:

- holding and soothing the infant; the patient cannot spoil an infant during the first 3 months;
- cuddling in a rocking chair;
- feeding slower (bottle-feeding) and burping more often;
- rocking in a cradle;
- giving a warm bath;
- bundling up snugly for sleep;
- reducing stimuli;
- using a pacifier; or
- getting help from family, friends, or a baby-sitter.

STEP D: Urgent Treatments

Make an immediate appointment when:

- the infant cries continuously for more than 2 hours or refuses to settle;
- if the parent/guardian is afraid of losing control; or
- the infant is less than 1 month old.

PATIENT EDUCATION

1. Colic is defined as paroxysmal crying of more than 3 hours a day for at least 3 days per week in an infant between 1 and 3 months of age. Having colic as an infant does not predict a difficult temperament or future difficulties.
2. Approximately 15%–25% of infants are considered to have colic.
3. Colic is not related to gender, ethnicity, feeding method, birth weight or prematurity.
4. Patients need a support network when dealing with an extremely colicky baby.

PART III

GYNECOLOGIC PROTOCOLS

Abnormal Bleeding and Spotting Overview

Abnormal bleeding and spotting are on a continuum. Significance varies with age. However, some irregular bleeding and anovulatory bleeding are characteristics of both adolescents and women approaching menopause. Certainly causes and concerns of unusual bleeding are different at each end of the age spectrum.

Some considerations need to be taken into account when assessing a woman who reports abnormal bleeding or spotting. These basics are outlined in the Basic Triage Assessment Form for Abnormal Bleeding. You may have other basic questions that are deemed important in your practice. Please feel free to add these to this section for future reference. Some truisms must be kept in mind when evaluating these women.

1. All women of reproductive age are at risk for pregnancy if they are sexually active with male partners, even if they consistently use birth control.
2. Any spotting or bleeding in an established postmenopausal patient, unless such patient has begun a continuous dose of hormone replacement therapy (HRT) regimen in the last 6–9 months, is suspicious.
3. A sexually active woman of any age who is not monogamous, or who has a partner who is not monogamous, is at risk for STIs.

Patients have different definitions of normal. The chart "Facts on Normal Menstruation" is included in this section as a review of the parameters of onset, interval, duration, amount, and composition. Patients also vary in their descriptions of what is not normal for them. Criteria for what each office or clinic will accept as abnormal need to be established between triage nurses and providers.

Abnormal bleeding usually is described in terms of numbers of pads or tampons saturated during a certain number of hours. This is dependent on several factors, which need to be clarified with the patient and with the providers with whom you work.

1. The type of pad or tampon used (mini versus maxi; slim versus super).
2. Patient hygiene; some patients can't stand a "dirty pad". Have the patient estimate the size of the area of saturation in terms you have agreed upon with providers (ie, the size of a quarter or "soaked through to underwear").
3. Associated symptoms such as clots require a previously agreed upon classification. The classifications can be based on coins (dime, nickel, quarter), fruit (grape, plum, orange), or balls (ping-pong, golf, softball).

For the purposes of this book, the criteria for heavy, serious bleeding is defined as soaking one or more pads in 1 hour or six or more in a 12-hour period. "Soaking" is defined as saturating through a regular pad or tampon to the patient's underwear. Patients also experiencing dizziness or abdominal, rectal, or vaginal pain associated with their bleeding are considered to have a serious problem.

My office/clinic's definition of serious, heavy bleeding is: _____
_____.

BASIC TRIAGE ASSESSMENT FORM FOR ABNORMAL BLEEDING

1. How old are you? _____
2. When was your last menstrual period? _____
3. Was it normal for you? _____
4. What are the frequency, duration and amount of bleeding? _____
5. Does it have any associated symptoms, such as cramping, abdominal pain, clotting, referred pain? _____
6. How long has the problem been occurring? _____
7. Are you taking any medication(s)? _____
8. Are you taking any hormones or hormonal birth control? _____
9. Do you use any other method of birth control? _____

Facts on Normal Menstruation

Onset	Interval	Duration	Amount	Composition	Cessation
Age: 10–16 years, 95% have started by age 15 **Mean age:** 13.4 years **Precocious menstruation:** menses before age 9 years **Delayed menstruation:** menses after age 16 years	**Interval:** counted from the first day of flow 1 month to the first day of flow in the next menstrual cycle. **Average:** 27–30 days in length; 95% of cycles are from 21–45 days in length **Abnormal intervals:** less than 21 days or greater than 42 days; frequently caused by anovulation	**Average:** 3–5 days **Abnormal duration:** less than 1 day or more than 8 days	**Average:** 30–40 mL **Variability in amount:** 70–100 mL. Variability is normal **Perimenopausal women:** not unusual to see 150–200 mL.	**Primary components:** bacteria, endometrial debris, enzymes, mucous, prostaglandins, vaginal cells	**Mean Age:** 50 ½ years **Premature menopause:** Generally prior to age 40

Abnormal Bleeding in Adolescents

KEY QUESTIONS

ASSESSMENT	ACTION
1. Is this your first menstrual period?	**YES** Go to Step A.
	NO Go to Question 2.
2. Are you soaking one or more pads in 1 hour or six or more in a 12-hour period? Are you light-headed or dizzy? Do you have any abdominal, rectal, or vaginal pain associated with the bleeding?	**YES** Go to Step B.
	NO Go to Question 3.
3. Have you established any regularity to your menstrual cycle?	**YES** Go to Question 4.
	NO Go to Step C.
4. Are you sexually active?	**YES** Go to protocol Abnormal Bleeding in Women of Reproductive Age.
	NO Go to Step D.

ACTIONS

STEP A: First Menses

The first period may catch an adolescent girl off guard. The first cycle experienced does not set any pattern for coming cycles. It is not unusual for the first few cycles to be anovulatory.

Assess the patient's understanding of the menstrual cycle.

Assess the patient's readiness in terms of available supplies.

Assess any need for contraception.

STEP B: Heavy Bleeding

If the patient meets the criteria for heavy, serious bleeding, she should be instructed to come to the office immediately or go to the nearest ER. The patient should not drive herself. If there is any question of loss of sensorimotor skills, the patient or her agent should call 911.

STEP C: Bleeding in Adolescents

It is not unusual for adolescents to have irregular, often anovulatory cycles, particularly during the first year after menarche.

Determine if the patient's cycles are consistently 21 days or less or are exceeding 8 days in length.

Assess for signs of anemia, which is common in adolescents.

If the patient had regular cycles for 1 year or more and now has gone 3 months without a cycle, assess for signs of weight loss or gain, increase in athletic activity, stress from school or home, or an increase in lethargy or depression.

Schedule the patient for evaluation within 2 weeks if the answers to any of these questions are positive.

Continue to Question 4.

STEP D: Bleeding and Sexually Active

Ascertain if the answer of "no" to the question "Are you sexually active?" means (1) never have been; (2) not now; or (3) everything but vaginal penetration.

Reassure an adolescent who has never been sexually active that most of the evaluation may be able to be done via blood work or a sonogram, and a pelvic examination may not be necessary.

If the patient has been sexually active in the past, determine if the interval warrants evaluation for pregnancy.

Refer to the protocols Abnormal Bleeding in Women of Reproductive Age and 1st Trimester Bleeding, if appropriate.

PATIENT EDUCATION

1. Adolescents are impressionable and prone to exaggeration, so question thoroughly to establish normalcy for each individual.
2. It is important that adolescents understand that although much of early bleeding may be anovulatory, it is not safe to assume they cannot get pregnant if they become sexually active.
3. Adolescents are prone to habits that may alter their cycles, such as eating disorders and extreme exercise patterns. If appropriate, arrange for evaluation of these potential problems.
4. Don't miss an opportunity to counsel on contraception and STI protection.
5. Abnormal bleeding usually is described in terms of the numbers of pads or tampons saturated during a certain number of hours. Adolescents may not be good at such estimations and may need more help in describing their symptoms. Clarify with them:

   • Patient hygiene. Some patients can't stand a "dirty pad". Have the patient estimate the size of the area of saturation in terms you have agreed upon with providers (i.e., the size of a quarter or "soaked through to underwear").
   • Type of pad or tampon used (mini versus maxi; slim versus super).
   • Associated symptoms such as clots require a previously agreed upon classification. The classifications can be based on coins (dime, nickel, quarter), fruit (grape, plum, orange), or balls (ping-pong, golf, softball).

Abnormal Bleeding in Women of Reproductive Age

KEY QUESTIONS

ASSESSMENT

ACTION

1. Are you soaking one or more pads in 1 hour or six or more in a 12-hour period? Are you light-headed or dizzy? Do you have any abdominal, rectal, or vaginal pain associated with the bleeding?

   YES Go to Step A.
   NO Go to Question 2.

2. Are you sexually active?

   YES Go to Question 3.
   NO Go to Question 3.

3. Are you, or do you think you could be, pregnant?

   YES Go to Step B.
   NO Go to Question 4.

4. Do you regularly use a form of hormones, either to provide you with birth control or to control menstrual cycle symptoms?

   YES Go to Step C.
   NO Go to Step D.

5. Do you regularly use a form of barrier contraception, such as condoms?

   YES Go to Step E.
   NO Go to Step F.

ACTIONS

(Note: If the patient uses an IUD, refer to the protocol Bleeding Irregularities and Intrauterine Contraception.)

STEP A: Heavy Bleeding

If the patient meets the criteria for heavy, serious bleeding, she should be instructed to come to the office immediately or go to the nearest ER. The patient should not drive herself. If there is any question of loss of sensorimotor skills, the patient or her agent should call 911.

STEP B: Potentially Pregnant

If the patient thinks she could be pregnant, refer to the protocol 1st Trimester Bleeding for additional evaluation.

If the patient is uncertain, have her complete a home pregnancy test or come in for a blood pregnancy test.

If there is any risk for ectopic pregnancy (prior ectopic pregnancy, ruptured appendix, or abdominal surgery with adhesions), it is preferable to verify pregnancy status with a quantitative B-HCG test.

STEP C: Using Hormones, Systemic Hormonal Contraceptives

If the patient regularly uses a form of hormone therapy to regulate her cycle or for birth control and is sexually active, evaluate for the possibility of pregnancy before proceeding.

Query the patient as to the proper use of method.

If she is taking combined oral contraceptive pills (OCPs) and has missed pills, refer to the protocol Late or Missed Combined Oral Contraceptive Pills.

If she has not missed any pills, refer to the protocol Break-through Bleeding/Spotting and Systemic Hormonal Contraceptives.

If the patient is receiving Depo-Provera, refer to the protocol Bleeding and Depo-Provera.

If the patient is using her method properly, pregnancy seems unlikely, and the bleeding seems out of the ordinary for her method of birth control, continue to Step D.

Continue to Question 5.

STEP D: Timing for Evaluation

If the patient does not use a form of hormone therapy to regulate her cycle, and if her risk for pregnancy is low or nonexistent, schedule the exam when she is not bleeding if possible. This evaluation also applies if a patient is on a course of hormone therapy and the bleeding exceeds the parameters expected for her method.

If the menstrual cycles are shorter than 21 days, further apart than 3 months (unless the patient is receiving continuous dose OCPs, Depo-Provera, or Norplant), or last longer than 8 days, schedule the patient for an evaluation within 2 weeks.

Continue to Question 5.

STEP E: Barrier Methods

Patients using barrier methods without other hormonal methods may be at a slightly greater risk for pregnancy.

Determine the patient's method use and compliance.

Spermacides with condom use continues to be valuable in pregnancy prevention. However, women at high risk for HIV transmission should avoid nonoxynol-9, the chemical found in spermacide.

Reinforce the STI prevention value of condoms without spermicide.

STEP F: Sexually Transmitted Infection Risk

Patients using barrier methods without other hormonal methods may be at a slightly greater risk for pregnancy.

Ascertain the patient's STI risk by questioning her regarding whether or not she is monogamous and if she has a long-term partner or has frequent partner changes.

Schedule the patient for an examination within 3 days if her STI risk is high.

PATIENT EDUCATION

1. The possibility of pregnancy must be paramount in your mind when questioning a woman of reproductive age who is experiencing abnormal bleeding.
2. Although a woman may state she is not sexually active now, you need to establish when (if ever) she was sexually active. If she was sexually active within the last 6 months, the possibility of pregnancy still exists.
3. Use this as an opportunity to reinforce proper contraceptive use in a sexually active woman who does not desire pregnancy.
4. Abnormal bleeding usually is described in terms of the number of pads or tampons saturated during a certain number of hours. This is dependent on several factors that need to be clarified with the patient and with the providers for whom you work.

   - Type of pad or tampon used (mini versus maxi; slim versus super).
   - Patient hygiene: Some patients can't stand a "dirty" pad. Have the patient estimate the size of the area of saturation in terms you have agreed upon with the providers (i.e., the size of a quarter or "soaked through to underwear").
   - Associated symptoms such as clots require a previously agreed upon classification. The classifications can be based on coins (dime, nickel, quarter), fruit (grape, plum, orange), or balls (ping-pong, golf, softball).

5. Nonmonogamous, sexually active patients who do not use condoms are at greater risk for STIs. Patients have been counseled or treated for breakthrough bleeding while taking oral contraceptives and then have been found to have an STI.
6. The spermacide nonoxynol-9 does not provide HIV protection. It may cause vaginal erosion, and it should not be used by women at high risk for HIV infection.

Abnormal Bleeding/Spotting in Perimenopausal Women

KEY QUESTIONS

ASSESSMENT	ACTION
1. Are you soaking one or more pads in 1 hour or six or more in a 12-hour period? Are you light-headed or dizzy? Do you have any abdominal, rectal, or vaginal pain associated with the bleeding?	**YES** Go to Step A.
	NO Go to Question 2.
2. Are you sexually active?	**YES** Go to Question 3.
	NO Go to Question 3.
3. Are you, or do you think you could be pregnant?	**YES** Go to Step B.
	NO Go to Question 4.
4. Do you regularly use a form of hormones, either to provide you with birth control or to control your menstrual cycles?	**YES** Go to Step C.
	NO Go to Question 5.
5. Do you rely on another method of contraception, such as an IUD or sterilization?	**YES** Go to Step D.
	NO Go to Question 6.
6. Do you regularly use a form of barrier contraception, such as condoms?	**YES** Go to Steps D and E.
	NO Go to Steps D and F.

ACTIONS

STEP A: Serious Bleeding

If the patient meets the criteria for heavy, serious bleeding, she should be instructed to come to the office immediately or go to the nearest ER. The patient should not drive herself. If there is any question of loss of sensorimotor skills, the patient or her agent should call 911.

Remember that the amount of blood lost with menstruation during perimenopause may be two to three times more than with menstruation before menopause.

Question the patient regarding any known structural problems, such as a history of fibroids or polyps, which may routinely contribute to heavier bleeding.

Question the patient as to any known blood dyscrasias.

Intramenstrual bleeding or spotting warrants a provider consult within the next 1 to 2 weeks.

STEP B: Questionable Pregnancy

If the patient thinks she could be pregnant, refer to the protocol 1st Trimester Bleeding for additional evaluation.

If the patient is uncertain whether or not she is pregnant, have her complete a home pregnancy test or come in for a blood pregnancy test.

If there is any risk for ectopic pregnancy (prior ectopic pregnancy, ruptured appendix, or abdominal surgery with adhesions), it is preferable to verify pregnancy status with a quantitative B-HCG test.

STEP C: Hormone Use

If the patient regularly uses a form of hormone therapy to regulate her cycle or for birth control and is sexually active, evaluate for the possibility of pregnancy before proceeding.

If the patient is taking combined OCPs and has missed pills, refer to the protocol Late or Missed Combined Oral Contraceptive Pills.

If the patient has not missed pills, refer to the protocol Break-through Bleeding/Spotting and Systemic Hormonal Contraceptives.

If the patient is receiving Depo-Provera, refer to the protocol Bleeding and Depo-Provera.

If the patient is using her method properly, pregnancy seems unlikely, and the bleeding seems out of the ordinary for her method of birth control, continue to Step D.

STEP D: Low Pregnancy Risk

If the patient does not use a form of hormone therapy, and if her risk for pregnancy is low or nonexistent, evaluate for the timing of an examination. A patient receiving a course of hormone therapy in which bleeding exceeds the expected parameters for her method and one who is using an IUD or sterilization for contraception also should be evaluated in 3–5 days.

If the menstrual cycle is less than 21 days, longer than 3 months (unless the patient is using continuous dose OCPs, Depo-Provera, continuous dose NuvaRing or OthoEvra or Implanon), or lasts longer than 8 days, schedule the patient for an evaluation within 2 weeks.

If the bleeding abnormality is associated with abdominal pain, schedule an appointment within 3 to 5 days.

Explain to the patient that her risk for structural abnormalities and hormonal imbalances, leading to endometrial hyperplasia, are higher because of her age.

Continue to Question 6.

STEP E: Barrier Methods

Patients using barrier methods without other hormonal methods may be at a slightly greater risk for pregnancy, but the risk is somewhat diminished by the decrease in regular ovulatory cycles in this age group.

Determine the patient's method use and compliance.

Encourage the use of spermicide.

Reinforce the STI prevention value of condoms and note that diaphragms also may provide some protection.

STEP F: Not Using Barrier Methods

Patients not using a barrier method who are not monogamous are at greater risk for STIs and thus, abnormal bleeding. Sexually transmitted infections do not discriminate based on age!

Ascertain the patient's STI risk by questioning her regarding whether or not she and her partner are mutually monogamous and if she has a long-term partner or has frequent partner changes.

PATIENT EDUCATION

1. Educate patients regarding the expected course of menstruation in the perimenopausal years. Cycles initially may be heavier and closer together, then lighter and further apart.
2. It is not uncommon to find a patient in this age group who does not think she can get pregnant. Remind these patients that the second highest group of women with unintended pregnancies are those older than 40 years. Unwanted pregnancy is not just a teenage problem.
3. Patients who are not in a mutually monogamous relationship may need re-education regarding STI risk, particularly women who are recently separated or divorced.
4. The spermicide nonoxynol-9 does not provide HIV protection. It may cause vaginal erosion, and it should not be used by women at high risk for HIV infection.

Abnormal Bleeding/Spotting in Postmenopausal Women

KEY QUESTIONS

ASSESSMENT	ACTION
1. Are you receiving hormone therapy (HT)?	Bleeding/Spotting and Hormone Replacement Therapy.
	NO Go to Question 2.
2. Have you had a hysterectomy?	**YES** Go to Step A.
	NO Go to Question 3.
3. Are you soaking one or more pads in 1 hour or eight or more in a 12-hour period? Are you light-headed, dizzy, or passing clots? Do you have any abdominal, rectal, or vaginal pain associated with the bleeding?	**YES** Go to Step B.
	NO Go to Step C.

ACTIONS

STEP A: Patients Who Have Had a Hysterectomy

If the patient has had a hysterectomy, bleeding should be evaluated in 3–5 days, unless the patient meets the criteria for serious bleeding outlined in Question 3. In that case, proceed with the instructions in Step B.

STEP B: Heavy Bleeding

If the patient meets the criteria for heavy, serious bleeding, she should be instructed to come to the office immediately or go to the nearest ER. The patient should not drive herself. If there is any question of loss of sensorimotor skills, the patient or her agent should call 911.

STEP C: Women With a Uterus

Women who have not had a hysterectomy are at risk for endometrial hyperplasia and should be scheduled for endometrial evaluation within 72 hours.

PATIENT EDUCATION

1. It is important for patients to understand that no bleeding is normal for a post-menopausal woman who is not receiving hormone replacement therapy.
2. Patients should be instructed to call at the first sign of bleeding and not delay because the bleeding seems minimal.
3. Spotting during the first 6–9 months of continuous HT may not be abnormal. (See the protocol Bleeding/Spotting and Hormone Therapy). Patients need to understand the parameters set by the providers at your practice.

CHAPTER 12

Amenorrhea Overview

Amenorrhea is classified as primary or secondary. It is important to remember that it actually is a symptom and not a diagnosis. Primary amenorrhea refers to absence of menses by the age of 16 years, regardless of the presence or absence of normal growth or secondary sexual characteristics. It also has been used to refer to the absence of both menses and normal growth without signs of secondary sexual characteristics by the age of 14 years. Secondary amenorrhea is the cessation of menses for three cycles or more in women who have been menstruating previously.

For the purposes of this book, only secondary amenorrhea is discussed. Any young woman meeting the criteria for primary amenorrhea should be scheduled for a proper reproductive endocrinology evaluation. You should be familiar with your practice's scheduling preference for young women reporting primary amenorrhea.

Amenorrhea is a common problem, particularly as a woman begins menstruation and as she nears menopause. It also may be a common side effect of certain hormonal medications. Women on certain medications, including some contraceptives and hormone replacement therapies, may have lack of menstruation as a side effect. Low body fat, thyroid problems, and pituitary problems may result in amenorrhea too.

BASIC TRIAGE ASSESSMENT FORM FOR AMENORRHEA

1. When was your last normal menstrual period? _____
2. Do you have a history of skipping menstrual cycles? _____
3. Are you taking any hormonal medications? _____
4. Are you taking any other medications? _____
5. Is there a chance you could be pregnant? _____
6. Have you undergone any physiologic changes, such as weight loss, beginning an exercise program, or experienced unusual stress? _____
7. Do you have any pre-existing medical problems (such as a thyroid disorder or eating disorder)? _____

Secondary Amenorrhea

ASSESSMENT	ACTION
1. Are you, or do you think you could be, pregnant?	**YES** Go to Step A.
	NO Go to Step B.

ACTIONS

STEP A: Pregnancy and Risk Status

Confirm pregnancy status before proceeding. If the patient is uncertain of her pregnancy status, have her take a home pregnancy test or come in for a blood pregnancy test.

For patients desiring to continue pregnancy, assuming they have no risk factors for abnormal 1st trimester pregnancy and no medical problems, do the following:

- Schedule an initial visit with an obstetric care provider at approximately 2 months from the first missed menses.
- If the patient is uncertain of last menses, schedule an appointment within the next 2 weeks.
- Call in a prescription for prenatal vitamins if the patient is not already taking them.

If the patient has risk factors for an abnormal 1st trimester pregnancy or has medical problems, do the following:

- Notify the on-call physician if the situation is urgent. If no physician is available, have the patient seek evaluation in the ER.
- Schedule an evaluation within 24–48 hours if not at risk for problems.
- Call in a prescription for prenatal vitamins, if appropriate.

For patients desiring pregnancy termination, refer as appropriate.

STEP B: Patients Who Are Not Pregnant

For patients who are not pregnant, determine exogenous hormone use and proceed as follows:

For patients receiving Depo-Provera, Implanon, or Mirena:

- Determine the patient's method compliance.
- Reassure the patient that amenorrhea is an expected side effect.
- If the patient has been noncompliant with the timing of method administration, encourage her to take a urine pregnancy test.
- If the patient is concerned about pregnancy and has been compliant, encourage her to take a home pregnancy test for reassurance and for building confidence in her method compliance.

For patients taking oral contraceptives, NuvaRing or Ortho-Evra

- Determine the patient's method compliance.
- If the patient is using a continuous dose method, reassure her that amenorrhea is an expected side effect.
- If the patient has experienced amenorrhea for 1 month and is not using continuous dose therapy, reassure her that this may be normal.
- If the patient has experienced amenorrhea for 2 months or more and is not using continuous dose therapy, reassure her this may be normal but recommend she take a home pregnancy test.
- Determine the patient's comfort with her contraceptive method.

For perimenopausal patients not using hormonal contraception:

- Determine the length of the problem and the recurrence rate.
- Determine the patient's contraceptive use, her method compliance, and her pregnancy risk.
- If the patient has experienced amenorrhea for 1 month or more and is sexually active, encourage her to take a pregnancy test.
- If the patient has experienced amenorrhea for 3 months or more, schedule an appointment for evaluation within 2–4 weeks.

PATIENT EDUCATION

1. In cases of secondary amenorrhea, it is best to be suspicious of pregnancy in sexually active women rather than miss an opportunity for the patient to explore her options for pregnancy continuation and optimal pregnancy health.
2. It probably takes 3–4 months for endometrial hyperplasia to develop. Although this is one of our biggest concerns in perimenopausal women not using hormonal contraception, there are many other reasons for secondary amenorrhea. A thorough medical evaluation is needed for these women.

CHAPTER 13

Barrier Contraceptives Overview

Technically speaking, barrier methods comprise several categories of contraceptive options. They include the common male barrier, the male condom. They also include a variety of female vaginal barriers, including the diaphragm, cervical cap, contraceptive sponge, and female condom. Vaginal spermicides, in the various forms of suppositories, creams, jellies, films, and foams also are usually included in this category. They are not truly barriers but act in conjunction with barriers to increase effectiveness. They also can be used on their own.

With the exception of the vaginal diaphragm and cervical cap, these methods are available over the counter. This benefit provides patients with independence of action. This benefit alone is reason enough for all patients to be proficient with one of these methods, despite a possible preference for another method that has been prescribed. Any woman who has traveled and forgotten her oral contraceptives will be happy to have been previously educated in the use of condoms and spermicides.

Condoms are superior for prevention of the transmission of some STIs, which is reason enough for educating patients in proper usage. Nurses should familiarize themselves with instructing patients on when and how to use a condom. If you are unfamiliar with the techniques of this method, excellent instructions can be found in *Contraceptive Technology* (Hatcher, R.A., Trussell, J., Stewart, F., et al., 2004, pp. 347–349).

BASIC TRIAGE ASSESSMENT FORM FOR BARRIER CONTRACEPTIVE METHODS

1. Which method do you use? _____
2. Do you also use a spermicide with this method? _____
3. Are you satisfied with this method? _____
4. Are you having any problems or concerns in using this method? _____
5. Do you rely on this method for your primary mode of contraception, or do you use it as an adjunct for STI protection? _____

Allergy to Latex

KEY QUESTIONS

ASSESSMENT	ACTION

1. Are you using a latex-based contraceptive
(cervical cap, diaphragm, latex condom)?

YES Go to Step A.
NO Go to Question 2.

2. Are you experiencing shortness of breath
or wheezing?

YES Go to Step B.
NO Go to Question 3.

3. Are you experiencing a rash, vaginal or vulvar
redness, or vaginal itching?

YES Go to Step C.
NO No further action.

ACTIONS

STEP A: Using a Latex-Based Contraceptive

Some patients develop an allergic reaction to a latex method of contraception. However, some vaginal infections may mimic an allergic reaction.

Proceed to Steps B and C for appropriate questions to ask when a latex allergy is suspected.

STEP B: Wheezing or Shortness of Breath

If the patient has used a vaginal barrier made of latex and is experiencing systemic symptoms, such as shortness of breath or wheezing, she or her agent should call 911 or seek emergency care immediately.

Advise the patient **not** to drive herself to the ER.

Patients with a latex allergy should obtain and wear a medical alert bracelet.

STEP C: Symptoms of Vaginitis

Certain types of vaginitis can mimic allergic symptoms in some women. Instruct the patient to come in for evaluation within 3–5 days or sooner if symptoms are intolerable.

Instruct the patient to avoid using OTC products until a diagnosis is made.

Instruct the patient to avoid using the latex method of contraception until a definitive diagnosis is made by the provider.

Broken Condom

ASSESSMENT

ACTION

1. Did the condom break any time during intercourse or while there was penis-to-vagina contact?

YES Go to Question 2.

NO Go to Step A.

2. Do you want to avoid pregnancy?

YES Go to Step B.

NO Go to Question 3.

3. Are you trying to avoid an STI?

YES Go to Step C.

NO No further action.

ACTIONS

STEP A: Broken Condom Before/After Intercourse

Generally, there is little risk of unintended pregnancy if the condom was intact during any penile-vaginal contact. However, if the patient has any concerns about pregnancy or exposure to STIs, you should proceed to Question 2.

STEP B: Broken Condom During Intercourse

If the patient is concerned about unintended pregnancy, she should be offered emergency contraception options. Refer to the protocol Emergency Contraception.

STEP C: Sexually Transmitted Infections

All patients who experience unprotected intercourse should be offered testing for STIs. Schedule the patient for an appointment within the next 24 hours for STI testing. Explain that she may need to come back after her initial appointment for additional testing.

Trapped Diaphragm

ASSESSMENT

1. Is the diaphragm trapped in your vagina?	**ACTION**

1. Is the diaphragm trapped in your vagina?

YES Go to Step A.
NO Go to Question 2.

2. Are you concerned that the diaphragm may have become displaced during any act of intercourse during the last 24 hours?

YES Go to the protocol Emergency Contraception.
NO No action.

ACTIONS

STEP A: How to Remove a Trapped Diaphragm

Provide the patient with the following instructions:

Wash hands.

Lie on your back with your knees falling to the sides as far as possible, or place one foot on the toilet. Spread the lips of your vagina, and slide your index finger along the top of your vagina. You will feel your pubic bone. Feel directly behind your pubic bone. You may feel the rim of the diaphragm. If so, try to hook your index finger between your vagina and the rim of the diaphragm. If you can do so, apply gentle traction and slowly pull the diaphragm from your vagina.

If the first technique fails, you may have success by assuming the alternate position described. Once you are on your back or have a foot placed on the toilet, insert your index finger into your vagina while slowly bearing down. As you bear down, try to locate the rim of the diaphragm. First, try right behind your pubic bone; next, try the lower part of your vagina, in the area that is closest to your rectum. Again, once you feel the rim, try to hook your index finger around the diaphragm rim and apply gentle traction on the diaphragm while bearing down.

If these two techniques are not successful, make a same-day appointment with your gynecologic care provider for assistance with removal of the diaphragm. Remember, if it has been less than 6 hours since you last had intercourse, you should leave your diaphragm in place.

When your gynecologic care provider removes the diaphragm, try to reinsert it yourself and remove it yourself at least one time before leaving the office.

CHAPTER 14

Breast Complaints Overview

Breast complaints are highly charged issues. The increasing incidence of breast cancer with age, coupled with the high profile of this disease, creates anxiety in any woman discovering a breast problem. Often this anxiety creates real barriers in eliciting information helpful in assessment.

Although it is best not to be overly reassuring over the telephone, quick access to medical evaluation may provide the patient with the most immediate sense of relief. Most clinics and offices adopt a policy of seeing these patients within a timely fashion for anxiety's sake alone. Letting patients know that it is your facility's policy to see all patients with breast complaints promptly, and that an appointment is not being scheduled quickly because of your alarm over her symptoms, may help alleviate some concern.

It also may be helpful to outline for the woman what will take place at her appointment. Patients need to know that a physical examination may not provide all the data necessary to answer her concerns. Reassuring the patient that additional sonograms, mammograms, and surgical evaluation are commonly ordered may provide helpful information. It is extremely important that young women understand that mammography may not be the most helpful tool in their evaluation. Breast density in young women can interfere with the accuracy of mammographic data. It is not unusual for a young woman in her 20s to be referred directly to a breast surgeon for the simplest of evaluations if sonography is not conclusive. Women in this age group need to know that this measure is routine practice and not caused by alarm over her individual situation.

Common Presentation of Various Breast Nodules (see Table 14-1) is included in this section.

Table 14-1 Common Presentation of Various Breast Nodules

Usual Age at Presentation	Shape and Consistency	Tenderness and Retractability	Common Features
Simple cysts 30 to 60 years, decreasing after menopause except with HT	Round, soft, elastic, fluid filled	Often tender; no retraction	Borders well defined, very mobile, single or multiple in number
Fibroadenoma Most common in young adults, range puberty to 55 years	Round or lobular, firm	Usually nontender; no retraction	Usually very mobile and well defined
Cancer 30–90 years; common in midlife and elderly	Irregular or fixed to skin or underlying structures, firm or hard	Usually nontender (except inflammatory); retraction may be present	May be fixed or partially mobile; not often well defined

BASIC TRIAGE ASSESSMENT FORM FOR BREAST COMPLAINTS

1. How old are you? _____
2. Do you have any history of breast problems? _____
3. Are you still menstruating? _____
4. When was the first day of your last menstrual cycle? _____
5. Are you taking any hormonal medication? _____ If yes, for how long? _____
6. Have you recently stopped breastfeeding? _____
7. Have you recently had a mammogram? _____ If so, where and when? _____

Breast Discharge

KEY QUESTIONS

ASSESSMENT	ACTION
1. Do you have spontaneous nipple discharge?	**YES** Go to Question 2.
	NO Go to Question 5.
2. Is the discharge bilateral?	**YES** Go to Question 3.
	NO Go to Question 4.
3. Is the discharge milky?	**YES** Go to Step A.
	NO Go to Step C.
4. Is the discharge unilateral?	**YES** Go to Step B.
	NO Go to Question 5.
5. Do you have to manipulate your breasts to elicit discharge?	**YES** Go to Step D.
	NO No further action.

ACTIONS

STEP A: Milky Discharge

Milky discharge (galactorrhea) is common in women who are breastfeeding, have recently given birth, or who experience frequent breast stimulation (e.g., during foreplay). Galactorrhea is also a side effect of many medications (particularly psychiatric medications). Finally, galactorrhea can be indicative of a pituitary tumor.

Unless the patient has recently given birth and is breastfeeding, she should be referred to her provider for evaluation within the next 1–2 weeks.

STEP B: Unilateral Discharge

Unilateral discharge (particularly if the fluid is bloody, green, or tan) is highly suggestive of a breast problem. Refer the patient to her provider for evaluation within the next 2–3 days.

STEP C: Bloody or Discolored Discharge

Bloody or discolored discharge (whether unilateral or bilateral) is suggestive of a breast problem. Refer the patient to her provider for evaluation within the next 2–3 days.

STEP D: Discharge With Breast Stimulation

This is not an uncommon response to vigorous breast manipulation. Ask the patient to refrain from breast stimulation for the next 30 days. If the symptoms persist, instruct her to visit her provider for breast examination.

Breast Lump

KEY QUESTIONS

ASSESSMENT	ACTION
1. Have you experienced menopause?	**YES** Go to Step A.
	NO Go to Question 2.
2. Are you within 14 days of your next expected menstrual period?	**YES** Go to Step B.
	NO Go to Step C.
3. Is there any pain associated with the lump?	**YES** Go to Step D.
	NO Go to Question 4.
4. Are you taking any hormonal medication?	**YES** Go to Step E.
	NO Go to Question 5.
5. Have you had any reason to have a mammogram during the last 6 months?	**YES** Go to Step F.
	NO Go to Step F.

ACTIONS

STEP A: Postmenopausal Woman With Breast Lump

Any postmenopausal woman with a breast lump needs evaluation within 24 hours, regardless of the timing of her last mammogram or other symptoms.
Continue to Questions 3, 4, and 5 for complete assessment.

STEP B: Presumed Postovulation Lump

Determine the patient's age.
Women older than 30 years, women who have a history of breast cancer or atypical ductal hyperplasia, or those who are highly anxious should be seen within 24 hours.
Women younger than 30 years with no risk factors may be offered the opportunity to wait until after menses for examination. Cysts and fibroadenomas may increase in size before menses; however, highly anxious patients should be seen in 24–48 hours, regardless of their risks.
Continue to Questions 3, 4, and 5 for complete assessment.

STEP C: Presumed Preovulatory Lump

Cysts are less likely to appear spontaneously before ovulation. These women should not wait until after their expected ovulation because of the possible increase in anxiety and should be evaluated in 24–48 hours.
Continue to Questions 3, 4, and 5 for complete assessment.

STEP D: Associated Pain

Pain is pathologically associated with breast cysts, degenerating fibroadenomas, and inflammatory carcinoma. It also may be associated with something as simple as ingestion of caffeine or foods containing the amino acid tyrosine (bananas, yellow cheese, red wine, and nuts).

Determine any change in the patient's caffeine consumption.

Determine the patient's consumption of foods containing tyrosine.

Continue to Questions 4 and 5 for complete assessment.

STEP E: Hormonal Medications and Breast Lumps

Hormonal medications may have an effect on the development of breast masses. Determine the following:

- how long the medication has been used;
- if there has been any change in dosage or frequency of use;
- if any pills have been missed.

Continue to Question 5 for complete assessment.

STEP F: Mammogram Timing

Often, a patient is mistakenly reassured that a recent normal mammogram is a sign she does not have cancer.

Determine the timing of the patient's last mammogram (if any).

Determine the location of the facility where the patient had the last mammogram for future film comparison.

PATIENT EDUCATION

1. All patients should be taught how to perform a Breast self-examination and when to do one. Although describing a breast examination procedure over the telephone is not practical, most clinics/offices have handy "shower cards" that can be mailed to patients. The examination should be performed after, not immediately before, a menstrual period.
2. Accurately explain the oft-quoted statistic "one in eight women will have breast cancer develop." This is an age-related phenomenon and refers to one in eight women at the age of 90 years! Younger women have less of a statistical risk than do older women and need to understand this.
3. Remember that any lump in a postmenopausal woman is considered breast cancer until proven otherwise.

Breast Pain

KEY QUESTIONS

ASSESSMENT	ACTION
1. Are you taking any hormones (OCPs, HT)?	**YES** Go to Step A.
	NO Go to Question 2.
2. Are you sexually active with a male partner?	**YES** Go to Step B.
	NO Go to Question 4.
3. Are you using nonhormonal contraception regularly?	**YES** Go to Question 4.
	NO Go to Step B.
4. Is the tenderness more pronounced during the second half of the menstrual cycle, occurring almost every month before the onset of the next period (cyclic breast pain)?	**YES** Go to Step C.
	NO Go to Question 5.
5. Is the tenderness isolated to one particular area of one breast?	**YES** Go to Step D.
	NO No further action.

ACTIONS

STEP A: Taking Hormones

Hormones can cause breast tenderness during the first several months of their use.
Reassure the patient that the breast tenderness is normal and generally resolves
with time.
Refer the patient to the prescribing health care provider if the pain is an intolerable
side effect.

STEP B: Excluding Pregnancy

This woman could be pregnant. A pregnancy test is indicated.

STEP C: Cyclic Breast Pain

Cyclic breast pain is a normal response to changing hormone levels during the menstrual cycle. Reassure the patient that such pain may be normal. However, if the
pain is troublesome or worsening, she should see her provider within the next 2–4
weeks to discuss the matter.

STEP D: Breast Tenderness or Pain

This may be one of several things: a breast infection (mastitis), a breast cyst, or rarely, the early signs of an inflammatory breast cancer. To differentiate among these conditions, a provider needs to discuss signs and symptoms with the patient. Forward this call to a provider for disposition.

PATIENT EDUCATION

The following suggestions may prove helpful for women who are experiencing cyclic breast pain in whom serious breast problems have been excluded.

1. Take 400 IU daily of natural vitamin E unless patient is taking warfarin.
2. Decrease the consumption of foods and beverages with caffeine (soft drinks, chocolates, coffee, and tea).
3. Decrease foods rich in tyrosine (bananas, nuts, caffeinated food/beverages, aged cheese, red wine).
4. Wear a supportive bra.

It usually is helpful to remove offending foods or drinks one at a time to determine which one is causing the problem. Also, patients should try instituting each of these actions one at a time to more easily determine which measure is effective.

Mammography Preparation

KEY QUESTIONS

ASSESSMENT	ACTION
1. Is this your first mammogram?	**YES** Go to Step A.
	NO Go to Question 2.
2. Do you have questions about how to prepare for a mammogram?	**YES** Go to Step B.
	NO Go to Question 3.
3. Do you experience pain when breasts are manipulated or compressed?	**YES** Go to Step C.
	NO Go to Question 4.
4. Have the results of your mammogram indicated that there is an abnormal finding?	**YES** Go to Chapter 3 on counseling regarding abnormal test results.
	NO No action.

ACTIONS

STEP A: Definition of Mammography

A mammogram is a radiographic test that uses a small amount of radiation to detect very small tumors in the breasts. The goal is to detect malignant (cancerous) tumors before they are large enough to be felt. This radiographic study is also helpful in determining the nature of masses that have been discovered by the patient or her health care provider on breast examination. There are two types of mammograms:

Screening Mammogram
- This is an evaluation of the breasts of women who have no overt signs or symptoms of breast cancer. Such mammograms are done in an effort to detect a problem at a time when cure is still possible.
- Some authorities recommended that women obtain a baseline (initial) mammogram by the age of 40 years and then a mammogram every 1–2 years until the age of 50 years. After that, the patient should undergo a mammogram once a year.

Diagnostic Mammogram
- This is an evaluation of the breasts to help determine the nature of a mass or other problem that has been discovered by the patient or practitioner on breast examination.
- A radiologist often is present when diagnostic mammograms are conducted so that more views can be taken if indicated.

STEP B: How to Prepare for a Mammogram

Do not have this study conducted if you think the patient may be pregnant, unless the obstetric care provider has specifically ordered the test and the x-ray facility is aware the patient is or may be pregnant.

Advise the patient to:

- not wear powder, creams, perfumes, lotions, or underarm deodorant on the day of the test because such agents may obscure visualization and interfere with interpretation of the results;
- not wear metal objects, such as jewelry or clothing with fasteners, within the x-ray field;
- wear a top or blouse with skirt or pants because the patient must disrobe from the waist up.

STEP C: Treatment of Pain With Breast Compression

The goal is to minimize the discomfort experienced during mammography.

Instruct the patient to take a mild OTC analgesic such as acetaminophen or ibuprofen about 1 hour before the test. The patient should take this medication only if she has tolerated it in the past and it does not interfere or interact with any other medications she is taking.

If possible, the patient should have the mammogram taken 1 week after menses so that breast tenderness is minimal.

PATIENT EDUCATION

Procedure Involved for a Mammogram

- The patient sits or stands and is asked to place one breast on a flat plastic or metal holder while the arm on that side of her body is raised.
- The machine compresses that breast to remove any creases.
- During the compression, the woman is asked to hold her breath. This process is repeated so that several views of the breast can be obtained.
- There is some mild discomfort when the breast is compressed, but it lasts only a few seconds.
- The entire procedure (for both breasts) takes about 10 to 20 minutes and is performed by a mammography technician.
- A small amount of exposure to radiation occurs during a mammogram, but there is no evidence that anyone ever has or will have breast cancer develop as a result of this test.

CHAPTER 15

Emergency Contraception Overview

Emergency contraception (EC) is a term that encompasses more than the name implies. Rather than being simply a postcoital form of birth control, this method can be used, in certain circumstances, as long as 8 days after the act of unprotected intercourse in hopes of preventing pregnancy. The most common regimen is Plan B, a progestin-only product that is concentrated so that fewer pills have to be swallowed. Since August 24, 2006, Plan B has been available to U.S. women and men 18 years and older without a prescription. In some states, pharmacists can dispense Plan B to women 17 years and younger without a prescription. There is an excellent Internet site on EC that was developed by Princeton University (http://ec:princeton.edu). It contains complete, detailed information on EC. See Table 15.1.

Effectiveness rates are difficult to ascertain. All in all, the insertion of a copper-containing intrauterine device (IUD) has the highest effectiveness rate. The effectiveness rate of oral contraceptive pill (OCP) use varies based on the time in the cycle of unprotected intercourse and study variations. In general, it is usually stated that EC will prevent about 75% of the unintended pregnancies that would have resulted had no treatment been given in those circumstances.

It is important to remember that acts of unprotected intercourse do not always happen because patients were unprepared. In many cases, the condom breaks, the woman discovers that her diaphragm slipped, or the IUD string can't be felt. It is important for triage nurses to avoid being judgmental when patients call for help.

You will need to discuss with your providers how they will handle calls for this service. For example, not all practices offer IUD insertion for this purpose. For information on specific pills and dosages that can be used for EC, which patients can call for information, including the names of local providers and pharmacies where they can get assistance, refer to the Princeton Web site (http://ec.princeton.edu/questions/index.html) or the EC National Hotline (1-888-NOT-2-LATE).

BASIC TRIAGE ASSESSMENT FORM FOR EMERGENCY CONTRACEPTION

1. How long ago was the first act of unprotected intercourse? (Remember there may have been multiple exposures.) _____

2. What (if any) form of contraception were you using? _____

3. Would you like to continue using this method in the future? _____

4. If not, is there another method you would like to try? _____

Emergency Contraception with "Plan B" or Oral Contraceptives

ASSESSMENT

ACTION

1. Are you within 120 hours of having had
   unprotected intercourse?

YES Go to Step A.

NO Go to Step B.

ACTIONS

STEP A: Unprotected Intercourse Within 120 Hours

If unprotected intercourse has occurred within 120 hours, the following advice may prevent unintended pregnancy. The timing of dosing is important, so encourage patients to start as soon as possible. Although the original research for EC (and current labeling information for Plan B) was based on a time frame of 2 doses taken 12 hours apart within 72 hours, recent research has found that both Plan B pills can be taken at once, and that the time interval for Plan B and oral contraceptives can be expanded to 120 hours.

For Plan B, take both pills at once.

If using combined oral contraceptive pills, please refer to Table 15.1.

If the patient wishes to start taking oral contraceptives, use Ortho-Evra or NuvaRing, that regimen should be initiated the day after Plan B doses or the day after the second dose of oral contraceptives used as EC. Have her use a backup method of contraception for 7 days.

Refer to the Patient Education Section if nausea or vomiting occurs.

STEP B: More than 120 Hours
Since Unprotected Intercourse

If it has been more than 120 hours but less than 8 days, offer the patient EC with an IUD (see **Emergency Contraception with an IUD** protocol on page 231). This not only is the most effective type of EC, it will also provide her with a reliable method. Carefully assess her sexually transmitted disease (STD) risk if she chooses this method.

If it has been more than 8 days, advise the patient to use a backup method until her next period.

Advise the patient to expect a period within 21 days if she usually has 28- to 30-day cycles.

Once menses resumes, she should be encouraged to use a contraceptive method she will use regularly.

If the patient has no menses in 21 days, advise her to take a home pregnancy test and see a clinician if the result is positive.

If the home pregnancy test is negative and she still has no menses, advise her to continue using the backup contraceptive method, take another pregnancy test in 7–10 days, and consult a clinician even if that test result is negative.

PATIENT EDUCATION

1. If the patient is experiencing nausea, reassure her that it usually passes. If she has used oral contraceptives instead of Plan B, she might try taking her next dose with an antinausea medication as approved for use by your office or clinic protocols.

2. The patient should be advised to call back if she throws up within an hour after taking the pills. She may need to retake the dose and would be better served by doing so with antinausea medication.

3. Even though Plan B is now available without a prescription to women and men over the age of 18 in the United States, not all pharmacies may stock the drug. It would be helpful for patients to know which pharmacies in your area carry a ready supply.

4. Patients need to understand that EC is not a substitute for regularly used contraceptive measures. They are not as effective over time as other, ongoing methods of contraception. If patients find they are repeatedly failing to use a chosen method of contraception, help them choose a method with which they can succeed.

Table 15-1 Emergency Contraception With Oral Contraceptives Available in the U.S.

Brand	Company	First Dose[b]	Second Dose[b] (12 hours later)	Ethinyl Estradiol per Dose (μg)	Levonorgestrel per Dose (mg)[c]
Progestin-only pills					
Plan B[a]	Barr/Duramed	2 white pills	None[b]	0	1.5
Combined progestin and estrogen pills					
Alesse	Wyeth-Ayerst	5 pink pills	5 pink pills	100	0.50
Aviane	Barr/Duramed	5 orange pills	5 orange pills	100	0.50
Cryselle	Barr/Duramed	4 white pills	4 white pills	120	0.60
Enpresse	Barr/Duramed	4 orange pills	4 orange pills	120	0.50
Jolessa	Barr/Duramed	4 pink pills	4 pink pills	120	0.60
Lessina	Barr/Duramed	5 pink pills	5 pink pills	100	0.50
Levlen	Berlex	4 light orange pills	4 light orange pills	120	0.60
Levlite	Berlex	5 pink pills	5 pink pills	100	0.50
Levora	Watson	4 white pills	4 white pills	120	0.60
Lo/Ovral	Wyeth-Ayerst	4 white pills	4 white pills	120	0.60
Low-Ogestrel	Watson	4 white pills	4 white pills	120	0.60
Lutera	Watson	5 white pills	5 white pills	100	0.50
Lybrel	Wyeth-Ayerst	6 yellow pills	6 yellow pills	120	0.54
Nordette	Wyeth-Ayerst	4 light orange pills	4 light orange pills	120	0.60
Ogestrel	Watson	2 white pills	2 white pills	100	0.50
Ovral	Wyeth-Ayerst	2 white pills	2 white pills	100	0.50
Portia	Barr/Duramed	4 pink pills	4 pink pills	120	0.60
Quasense	Watson	4 white pills	4 white pills	120	0.60
Seasonale	Barr/Duramed	4 pink pills	4 pink pills	120	0.60
Seasonique	Barr/Duramed	4 light blue-green pills	4 light blue-green pills	120	0.60

(continued)

Table 15-1 Emergency Contraception With Oral Contraceptives Available in the U.S. *(continued)*

Brand	Company	First Dose[b]	Second Dose[b] (12 hours later)	Ethinyl Estradiol per Dose (μg)	Levonorgestrel per Dose (mg)[c]
Combined progestin and estrogen pills					
Tri-Levlen	Berlex	4 yellow pills	4 yellow pills	120	0.50
Triphasil	Wyeth-Ayerst	4 yellow pills	4 yellow pills	120	0.50
Trivora	Watson	4 pink pills	4 pink pills	120	0.50

Notes:

[a] Plan-B is the only dedicated product specifically marketed for EC. Alesse, Aviane, Cryselle, Enpresse, Jolessa, Lessina, Levlen, Levlite, Levora, Lo/Ovral, Low-Ogestrel, Lutera, Lybrel, Nordette, Ogestrel, Ovral, Portia, Quasense, Seasonale, Seasonique, Tri-Levlen, Triphasil, and Trivora have been declared safe and effective for use as EC products (ECPs) by the U.S. Food and Drug Administration. Outside the United States, more than 50 ECPs are specifically packaged, labeled, and marketed. In 50 countries, Levonorgestrel-only ECPs are available either over-the-counter or from a pharmacist without having to see a clinician. **On August 24, 2006, the FDA approved Plan B for nonprescription sale to women and men 18 and older**.

[b] The label for Plan B says to take one pill within 72 hours after unprotected intercourse, and another pill 12 hours later. However, recent research has found that both Plan B pills can be taken at the same time. Research has also shown that all of the brands listed here are effective when used within 120 hours after unprotected sex.

[c] The progestin in Cryselle, Lo/Ovral, Low-Ogestrel, Ogestrel, and Ovral is norgestrel, which contains two isomers, only one of which (levonorgestrel) is bioactive; the amount of norgestrel in each tablet is twice the amount of levonorgestrel.

(Reproduced with permission of James Trussell, Ph.D., Office of Population Research and Association of Reproductive Health Professionals, (copyright, 2007; retrieved from http://ec.princeton.edu/questions/dose.html.)

Emergency Contraception With a Copper IUD

KEY QUESTIONS

ASSESSMENT

ACTION

1. Are you within 5 days of having had unprotected intercourse?

YES Continue to Question 2.

NO Go to Step B.

2. Are you interested in a copper IUD for continued contraception?

YES Go to Step A.

NO Go to EC with Plan B or Oral Contraceptives.

ACTIONS

STEP A: Unprotected Intercourse Within 5 Days

If unprotected intercourse has occurred within 5 days, the following advice may prevent unwanted pregnancy.* The timing is important, so encourage the patient to be seen as soon as possible.

If your providers insert copper IUDs for EC, make a same-day appointment for counseling and insertion.

If your office does not provide IUD insertions for EC, local providers who are able to insert an IUD for EC can be located by calling 1-888-NOT-2-LATE.

The patient should be counseled that a copper IUD inserted for EC can be used for contraception for up to 10 years following insertion. The provider who is to insert the IUD will likely ask the patient questions concerning her suitability for an IUD. These may include the number of current sexual partners, past history of pelvic infection, past history of ectopic (tubal) pregnancy, and long-term plans for pregnancy.

STEP B: More Than 5 Days Since Unprotected Intercourse

Advise the patient to use a backup method until her next period.

Advise the patient to expect a period within 21 days.

Once menses resumes, the patient should be encouraged to use a contraceptive method she will use regularly.

If the patient does not have a menses in 21 days, advise her to take a home pregnancy test and see a clinician if the result is positive.

If the home pregnancy test result is negative and the patient still has no menses, she should continue using the backup contraceptive method, take another pregnancy test in 7–10 days, and consult a clinician even if that test result is negative.

If the patient decides to use an IUD for contraception, she should make an appointment when she experiences a normal menses for an IUD insertion.

PATIENT EDUCATION

1. To avoid excluding women who may benefit from an IUD, advise the patient that some providers may be willing to insert a copper IUD more than 5 days after she has had unprotected intercourse.
2. Women who do not desire an IUD for EC may opt to use Plan B or an oral contraceptive, since research indicates that EC using Plan B may offer some benefit on days 4 or 5 of unprotected sex, and will do no harm in the event the patient experiences a pregnancy.
3. Not all providers will insert an IUD as a method of EC. Patients can call 1-800-NOT-2-LATE to find a provider in their area who can be of assistance.
4. Patients need to understand that EC is not a substitute for regularly used contraceptive measures. EC is not as effective over time as other, ongoing methods of contraception. If the patient finds she is repeatedly failing to use a method of contraception, help her choose a method with which she can succeed. Choosing a copper IUD solves this problem.
5. Patients need to understand that this method employs *only* copper-containing IUDs and cannot be used with Mirena.

*Technically, copper IUDs can be inserted up to the time of implantation, which may be 5–7 days after ovulation. According to Dr. James Trussell, "The latest WHO guidelines allow IUDs to be inserted up to day 12 of the cycle with no restrictions and at any other time in the cycle if it is reasonable to assume she is not pregnant." For the purposes of this protocol, we are choosing to use insertion up to 5 days after unprotected intercourse, acknowledging that some providers may be more lenient. (Trussell, J., & Raymond, E. G. Emergency contraception: A last chance to prevent unintended pregnancy. Retrieved April 2008, from http://www.ec.princeton.edu.)

CHAPTER 16

Implanon Overview

Currently, there is one implantable contraceptive device available in the United States: Implanon. This system releases progesterone into the body at a constant rate. Implanon provides up to 3 years of contraception. Research indicates that Implanon is a highly effective contraceptive, with a less than 1% incidence of pregnancy among women who use Implanon for 1 year, and a less than 2% incidence in women who use this method for 2 years.

Implanon consists of one 4-cm long rod that is placed approximately 2.5–3 inches above the elbow crease at the inner side of the upper arm between the biceps and triceps. Most women elect to have the rod placed on their nondominant arm. Patients can verify the presence of Implanon by palpating both ends of the rod after it has been inserted.

The potential risks associated with Implanon are quite small, but may include difficulties with insertion or removal of the system (rare), a slightly higher chance of an ectopic pregnancy if pregnancy does occur, and the development of ovarian cysts. As with all hormonal contraceptives that contain estrogen, the FDA requires warnings regarding the incidence of high blood pressure, gallbladder problems, and rare cancerous or noncancerous liver tumors. Conventional wisdom holds that these problems occur less frequently with progesterone-only products. A small amount of weight gain may also occur (on average, users have reported increases of 2.8 pounds after 1 year and 3.7 pounds after 2 years).

It is important to exclude pregnancy before Implanon is inserted!

Implanon may be inserted when:

1. A woman has not used hormonal contraception in the past month, and is on days 1–5 of her menstrual cycle.
2. A woman is switching from a combined hormonal contraception and has taken an active contraceptive tablet within the past 7 days.
3. A woman is on a progestin-only method of contraception and has taken a pill in the last 24 hours or has used the implant or progestin-containing IUD in the last 24 hours.

4. A woman has used an injectable contraceptive and is now due for her next injection.
5. A woman has had a first-trimester pregnancy loss (abortion or miscarriage) within the past 5 days.
6. A woman has had a second-trimester pregnancy loss and is 21–28 days postpartum.
7. A woman is breastfeeding and is 4 or more weeks postpartum.

BASIC TRIAGE ASSESSMENT FORM FOR IMPLANON

1. When was your last menstrual period?_____ Was it normal? _____
2. Have you been using Implanon or are you interested in information on using it?
   _____
3. How much do you know about its side effects and risks? _____
4. Are you taking other medications? _____
5. Do you routinely use a backup method? _____
6. Stopping Implanon requires medical intervention. Are you comfortable with this?
   _____
7. Are you planning a pregnancy in the next 3 years? _____

Amenorrhea With Implanon

KEY QUESTION

ASSESSMENT	**ACTION**
1. Do you think you could be pregnant?	**YES** Go to Step A.
	NO Go to Step B.

ACTIONS

STEP A: Determine if Pregnant and Assess First-Trimester Risk Status

Research indicates that about 0.3% of women using Implanon discontinue using this method because of amenorrhea (www.IMPLANON-US.com). Although the risk of pregnancy is less than 1% over 1 year, pregnancy status will need to be confirmed. If the patient is uncertain of her pregnancy status, have her take a home pregnancy test or come in for a blood pregnancy test.

For patients who desire to continue their pregnancy, assuming they have no risk factors for abnormal first-trimester pregnancy and no medical problems, do the following:

- Schedule a same-day or next-day visit to have the Implanon rod removed.
- Schedule an initial visit with an obstetric care provider at approximately 2 months from the first missed menses.
- Call in a prescription for prenatal vitamins if the patient is not already taking them.

If the patient has risk factors for an abnormal first-trimester pregnancy (see **Protocol**) or has medical problems, do the following:

- Notify the on-call physician if the situation is urgent. If no physician is available, have the patient seek evaluation in the ER.
- Schedule an evaluation within 24–48 hours if the patient is not at risk for immediate problems.
- Call in a prescription for prenatal vitamins, refer as appropriate.

For patients desiring pregnancy termination, refer as appropriate.

STEP B: For Patients Who Are Not Pregnant

For patients who are not pregnant, proceed as follows:

- Determine the patient's method compliance. Encourage the patient to check her arm to make sure that the rod is still in place.

- Reassure the patient that amenorrhea is an expected side effect.
- If the patient has any concerns or further questions, give her an appointment within 1 week.

PATIENT EDUCATION

1. In cases of secondary amenorrhea, it is best to be suspicious of pregnancy in sexually active women rather than miss an opportunity for the patient to explore her options for pregnancy continuation and optimal pregnancy health.
2. With methods where amenorrhea can be an expected (and desirable) side effect, patients need to become confident in their chosen contraceptive. This can be difficult when irregular bleeding is also anticipated, particularly as the patient adjusts to the method.

Bleeding/Spotting with Implanon

KEY QUESTIONS

ASSESSMENT	ACTION

1. Have you been using Implanon for less than 3 years?

YES Go to Question 2.

NO Go to Step B.

2. Can you feel the Implanon rod in your arm?

YES Go to Step A.

NO Go to Step C.

3. Are you sexually active with a male partner and not using another backup method of protection, such as condoms?

YES Go to Step D.

NO No further action.

ACTIONS

STEP A: Provide General InformationAbout Appropriate Screening

Spotting is a completely normal side effect of Implanon and may continue for many days or even months. See "Patient Education." If this is undesirable to the patient, she should see her provider to discuss alternative contraceptive options.

STEP B: Patient Has Used Implanon for More Than 3 Years

Implanon is approved for 3 years of use. If it has been used longer than that, advise the patient to use a backup method until it is changed or she switches to another method. Continue to Question 2.

STEP C: Implanon Cannot Be Felt

It is unusual for the Implanon rod to become dislodged. However, if the patient cannot feel the rod or has any concerns, schedule for an appointment with 3–5 days and urge her to use a backup method of contraception (such as condoms) until she is evaluated.

STEP D: Patient Is at Risk for STI Exposure

Ascertain the likelihood of pregnancy or sexually transmitted infection (STI) exposure. Schedule her for lab work or cultures as appropriate.

Question the patient regarding medication use that may interfere with her contraceptive therapy, such as Dilantin, Tegretol, rifampin, rifabutin, griseofulvin, and some other antibiotics. The supplement St. John's wort has been found to interact with some contraceptives. If pregnancy is a possibility, have her do a sensitive urine pregnancy test at home or schedule a blood pregnancy test.

PATIENT EDUCATION

1. All patients using hormonal contraception should be instructed in a backup method. Patients at risk for STI need to be especially diligent.
2. All patients need to know that the risk of pregnancy is small.
3. Education prior to insertion is particularly important with methods that have prolonged spotting as a side effect. Acceptance is highest when patients have been appropriately counseled.
4. Patients need to be educated as to when bleeding is a serious problem. (Review protocol Abnormal Bleeding in Women of Reproductive Age on page 201 with patient.)

CHAPTER 17

Injectable Contraceptives Overview

Depo-Provera (DMPA) is the only injectable contraceptive available in the United States. It comes in two forms: intramuscular (IM) and subcutaneous (SC). Currently the IM form is available in a generic form making it much more widely used, despite the fact that the SC product can be self-administered. The risks and benefits of the different forms of DMPA are essentially the same, though the SC product is used at a lower dose. For purposes of these protocols, we will focus on the IM delivery system. Please contact the manufacturer for information on SC administration and teaching protocols for self-administration.

Depo-Provera is often the first choice of women who are not good at remembering to take oral contraceptives and who find NuvaRing and Orth-Evra undesirable. The convenience of an injection every 3 months is preferable to many women. It provides safe contraception while nursing and excellent contraception in general. However, as with all methods, proper patient selection and patient education are the keys to successful and continued use.

Patients need to know to be prepared for some predictable side effects. Bleeding irregularities are high on the list of patient complaints and are the most common reason for patients discontinuing use of the method. Amenorrhea becomes common with continued Depo-Provera use and may be a desired side effect. Another patient complaint is weight gain, which may be attributable to an actual increase in appetite rather than due to fluid retention. According to the package insert available with each Depo-Provera injection, an average weight gain of 13.8 pounds during a 4-year period of use has been reported.

There may be a delay in return to menstruation after the cessation of Depo-Provera injections, often reported as a 6- to 12-month interval, until the return of fertility. This needs to be taken into account when planning for pregnancy, and patients should be questioned as to their reproductive plans when choosing this method to allow for adequate time for return to fertility.

Long-term users of Depo-Provera need to be counseled about the potential risk for decreased bone density. There is no current standard for evaluating or treating this potential problem. Some clinicians may order bone density testing (dual energy X-ray absorptiometry [DEXA]) or estradiol levels after 2 or more years of use and may recommend estrogen supplementation if levels fall below an agreed-upon standard. It is important when ordering bone density tests in adolescents to ascertain the calibration standards for the facility you recommend. Many DEXA machines are calibrated for bone density readings in women age 20 and above and are not reliable below that age. In *Contraceptive Technology*, (2004, p.479) the authors clearly state that "calcium intake and exercise need to be addressed with each woman receiving Depo-Provera."

Some women using DMPA may complain of vaginal dryness. In such cases, the provider may recommend a small amount of estrogen cream as an "add back" to remedy this complaint.

BASIC TRIAGE ASSESSEMENT FORM FOR INJECTABLE CONTRACEPTIVES

1. When was your last menstrual period? _____ (Remind patients they may not have normal menstruation while using this method.)
2. How long have you been using Depo-Provera? _____
3. What was the date of your last injection? _____
4. Are you having any health problems at this time? _____
5. Do you use a backup method of contraception? Method type: _____

Amenorrhea With Depo-Provera Use

KEY QUESTIONS

ASSESSMENT	ACTION
1. Do you think you could be pregnant?	**YES** Go to Step A.
	NO Go to Question 2.
2. Are you late for your Depo-Provera shot?	**YES** Go to the protocol Late for Depo-Provera Injection.
	NO Go to Question 3.
3. Have you been using Depo-Provera for more than 3 months?	**YES** Go to Step B.
	NO Go to Step B.

ACTIONS

STEP A: Pregnancy Possible

Confirm pregnancy status before proceeding. If the patient is uncertain of her pregnancy status, have her take a home pregnancy test or come in for a blood pregnancy test.

For patients desiring to continue pregnancy, assuming they have no risk factors for abnormal 1st trimester pregnancy and no medical problems, do the following:

- Because the patient probably will be uncertain of the date of her last menses, she should be scheduled for an initial visit with an obstetric care provider or at least have a sonogram to confirm dates; either should occur within 1 week.
- Call in a prescription for prenatal vitamins if the patient is not already taking them.

If the patient has a risk factor for an abnormal 1st trimester pregnancy (prior ectopic pregnancy, prior abdominal surgery or ruptured appendix, or repeated miscarriages) or has medical problems, do the following:

- Notify an on-call physician if the situation is urgent. If no physician is available and the patient has symptoms accompanied by abdominal pain, have the patient seek evaluation in the ER.
- Schedule an evaluation within 24–48 hours if no problems are noted by the patient.
- Call in a prescription for prenatal vitamins, if appropriate.

For patients desiring pregnancy termination, refer as appropriate.

STEP B: Pregnancy Unlikely

Determine the patient's method compliance.

Reassure her that amenorrhea is an expected side effect.

If the patient has been noncompliant with the timing of method administration, encourage her to have a sensitive urine pregnancy test.

If the patient is concerned about the possibility of a pregnancy and has been compliant, encourage her to take a home pregnancy test for reassurance and for building confidence in her method compliance.

Determine the patient's comfort with the method.

PATIENT EDUCATION

1. Although pregnancy is unlikely in a patient compliant with her Depo-Provera regimen, it is best to be suspicious of pregnancy in a sexually active woman rather than miss an opportunity for the patient to explore her options for pregnancy continuation and optimal pregnancy health.
2. Patients using Depo-Provera need to be comfortable with this expected side effect. Those who are not should consider switching to a different method at a convenient time.
3. Use this opportunity to encourage consistent condom use in women at risk for STIs.

Bleeding and Depo-Provera Use

KEY QUESTIONS

ASSESSMENT

ACTION

1. Are you in your first 3 months of Depo-Provera use?

YES Go to Step A.
NO Go to Question 2.

2. Have you used Depo-Provera for more than 3 months?

YES Go to Question 3.
NO No action.

3. Are you soaking one or more pads in 1 hour or six or more in a 12-hour period? Are you light-headed or dizzy? Do you have any abdominal, rectal, or vaginal pain associated with the bleeding?

YES Go to protocol Abnormal Bleeding in Women of Reproductive Age.
NO Go to Question 4.

4. Would you characterize the bleeding as irregular spotting, bleeding as a period, or bleeding frequently but not excessively?

YES Go to Step B and continue to next question.
NO Go to Question 5.

5. Are you sexually active?

YES Go to Step C.
NO Go to Step B.

6. Are you, or do you think you could be, pregnant?

YES Go to Step D.
NO Go to Question 7.

7. Was the result of your last Pap smear normal?

YES No further action.
NO Go to Step E.

ACTIONS

STEP A: First 3 Months of Depo-Provera Use

Use this as an opportunity to educate the patient about this expected side effect of Depo-Provera. Bleeding is the most common reason for discontinuing use of the method.

Assess how much the patient is bleeding and refer her if it meets the criteria for excessive bleeding in your practice.

Reassure the patient that menstrual changes are normal with this method.

Have the patient speak to the provider if she is troubled by the symptoms.

STEP B: Irregular But Not Excessive Bleeding/Spotting

Irregular bleeding or spotting is common during the first several months of therapy and may reappear after bouts of amenorrhea.

Reassure the patient this is an expected side effect of the method and amenorrhea may eventually occur.

Assess bleeding in terms of duration. Patients may become anemic with prolonged but not excessive bleeding. Refer the patient accordingly.

Continue to Question 5 to determine other possible harmful causes of the bleeding.

STEP C: Patient Is Sexually Active

Use this as an opportunity to reinforce consistent condom use if the patient is not monogamous.

Assess the patient's potential for STI exposure.

Schedule an appointment for screening within 3 to 5 days if the assessment is suggestive of STI exposure.

Query the patient about the timing and normalcy of her last Pap smear. Schedule an appointment within the next month, if appropriate.

STEP D: Pregnancy Is A Possibility

If the patient thinks she could be pregnant, refer to protocol on 1st Trimester Bleeding for additional evaluation.

If the patient is uncertain of her pregnancy status, have her take a sensitive urine pregnancy test or come in for a blood test.

If there is any risk of ectopic pregnancy (prior ectopic pregnancy, ruptured appendix, or abdominal surgery with adhesions), it is preferable to verify the patient's pregnancy status with a quantitative B-HCG test.

STEP E: Prior Abnormal Pap Smear Result

Remember that abnormal bleeding is one sign of cervical cancer.

Ascertain the timing of the patient's last Pap smear and schedule her for another, as appropriate.

PATIENT EDUCATION

1. Do not underestimate the patient's response to the irregular bleeding associated with this method. Bleeding is the most common reason for patients discontinuing use of the method.
2. Take this opportunity to educate or reeducate the patient about this common side effect.
3. Emphasize STI protection and the importance of regular Pap smears.

Depression and Depo-Provera Use

KEY QUESTIONS

ASSESSMENT | ACTION

1. Did your depressed mood begin after you started on the Depo-Provera regimen?

YES Go to Step A.
NO Go to Step B.

2. Do you have a history of depression or bipolar disorder?

YES Go to Question 3.
NO Go to Question 4.

3. If you have a current prescription for antidepressant medication, are you taking it?

YES Go to Step C.
NO Go to Step C.

4. If you do not have a history of depression, have you had a recent onset of sadness, depressed mood, withdrawal, sleep disturbances (insomnia or daytime somnolence), change in appetite, or loss of energy (fatigue)?

YES Go to Step A.
NO Not applicable.

5. Do you feel like harming yourself or others? Do you have a suicide plan?

YES Go to Step D.
NO No further action.

ACTIONS

STEP A: Depression That Begins With Depo-Provera Use

Depression may be a side effect of Depo-Provera use and can be severe for some people. This may be a new onset of depression, and whether or not it is related to Depo-Provera use, it requires thorough evaluation. Depression is particularly troublesome because the method cannot be reversed while the shot is delivering active hormone.

If the patient suspects Depo-Provera is the underlying cause, have her speak with her obstetric/gynecologic care provider within 12–24 hours.

The patient should consider evaluation with a mental health professional within 7–10 days.

The patient should be instructed to consider another method of birth control, when her next shot is due.

STEP B: Pre-existing Depression

This patient may have pre-existing depression, which could be aggravated by her Depo-Provera use.

Refer the patient to her obstetric/gynecologic care provider if she thinks the method of contraception has aggravated her condition.

Refer the patient to a mental health professional within 7–10 days.

Continue to Question 3 regarding medication use patterns.

STEP C: Depression History and Medication Use

This patient needs follow-up care by her mental health provider or referral to a mental health professional if she is currently not receiving regular care.

Ask the patient if she thinks Depo-Provera may be adversely influencing her moods.

If so, instruct her to consider consulting her obstetric/gynecologic care provider to discuss alternative methods of contraception.

If the patient has discontinued taking any prescribed medication for depression, bipolar disorder, or other mood disorder, encourage her to be in touch with the prescribing provider.

STEP D: Suicidal Thoughts or Actions

This patient may be suicidal and requires immediate referral for appropriate evaluation.

Try to keep the patient on the telephone if her symptoms are severe.

Have another health care provider or agent of the patient call 911 while you keep the patient on the line, if possible.

You should have suicide outreach hotline telephone numbers close at hand.

PATIENT EDUCATION

1. It is appropriate and necessary that new users of Depo-Provera be screened for history of depression and educated at the time of initiation about the possibility of their condition worsening with the use of Depo-Provera.
2. You must be prepared for this type of call by having hotline or emergency referral telephone numbers close at hand. Although serious calls indicative of suicidal thoughts may be rare, they certainly are not the time to be searching for telephone numbers for appropriate referral and help.

Late for Depo-Provera Injection

KEY QUESTIONS

ASSESSMENT	ACTION
1. Are you within 11–13 weeks of your last Depo-Provera injection or have you had a period in the last 5 days?	**YES** Go to Step A.
	NO Go to Question 2.
2. Have you had unprotected intercourse since your last menstrual period?	**YES** Go to Question 3.
	NO Go to Step B.
3. Has the unprotected intercourse been within the last 72 hours?	**YES** Go to Step C.
	NO Go to Question 4.
4. Do you want to receive your Depo-Provera shot as soon as possible?	**YES** Go to Step D.
	NO Go to Step E.

ACTIONS

STEP A: Within Depo-Provera Time Limits

This patient is not late for her shot.
Advise the patient to come in for a Depo-Provera injection now.

STEP B: No Unprotected Intercourse

Advise the patient to come in for a Depo-Provera injection now.
She must use a backup contraceptive method for 7 days.
If it has been 14 weeks or more since her last Depo-Provera injection, she should take a urine pregnancy test first.

STEP C: Excluding Pregnancy

Advise the patient to take a urine pregnancy test.
If the pregnancy test results are negative, offer her emergency contraception (see protocol Emergency Contraception page 227).
If the pregnancy test results are positive, counsel the patient regarding her options. Continue to Question 4.

STEP D: Potential Pregnancy

Advise the patient that although the urine pregnancy test may not be conclusive, there is no evidence to suggest that the Depo-Provera would affect a fetus.

If the patient accepts emergency contraception and wants her Depo-Provera injection now, advise her to come in for a Depo-Provera injection and use a backup method of contraception for the next 7 days.

Advise the patient to see her care provider if any signs or symptoms of pregnancy develop.

If she desires, she may take another pregnancy test 21–28 days later for confirmation because she may not experience any menstrual bleeding after taking the emergency contraception.

If the patient is beyond the usual window of opportunity for emergency contraception and has a negative UCG test result, proceed with the Depo-Provera injection.

STEP E: Reinstitution of Depo-Provera Therapy

Offer a barrier method of contraception for 2 weeks or until menses starts.

If menses starts within 2 weeks, advise the patient to come in within 5 days of menses for her Depo-Provera injection.

If the patient has no menses within 14 days with consistent barrier method use, advise her to take another urine pregnancy test.

If the pregnancy test result is negative, she should come in for her Depo-Provera injection. She should use a back-up contraceptive method for 7 days after the injection.

PATIENT EDUCATION

1. Patients need to understand that there is no data to indicate a risk to a developing fetus, if Depo-Provera is administered early in pregnancy.
2. Patients need access to immediate counseling regarding options should a pregnancy test result be positive.
3. We should not be punitive in our approach to patients. Make sure they understand their chosen method and what to do should an error in administration or timing of method use occur.

Pain or Redness at the Depo-Provera Injection Site

KEY QUESTIONS

ASSESSMENT

ACTION

1. Was your Depo-Provera injection given within the last 12 hours?

YES Go to Step A.

NO Go to Question 2.

2. Was your Depo-Provera injection given more than 12 hours ago?

YES Go to Step B.

NO No further action.

3. Has this happened with a previous Depo-Provera injection?

YES Go to Step C.

NO No further action.

ACTIONS

STEP A: Depo-Provera Injection Within Last 12 Hours

Rubbing the injection site within the first several hours may decrease the method's effectiveness and increase pain.

Advise the patient not to rub the injection site.

Advise the patient to apply a cold compress to the area.

Advise the patient to take an anti-inflammatory agent (ibuprofen or naproxen) per the manufacturer's recommended dose if such agents are not contraindicated by allergies or gastrointestinal disturbances.

Instruct the patient to call back if symptoms worsen.

Schedule an appointment within 24 hours if the patient's pain radiates down the arm or leg.

STEP B: Depo-Provera Injection More Than 12 Hours Ago

Inflammation lasting longer than 12 hours may indicate infection at the injection site.

Schedule an appointment for the patient to be seen within 24 hours to determine if cellulitis has developed or antibiotics should be prescribed.

If the patient's pain persists, particularly if it radiates down the arm or leg, have her come in within 24 hours for evaluation of nerve damage.

STEP C: Recurrence of Pain or Redness at Site

Some clinicians suspect that recurring redness at the injection site may be a sign of potential allergic reaction.

Have the patient discuss her symptoms with the prescribing provider.

Educate the patient about other methods appropriate for her.

PATIENT EDUCATION

1. Allergic reactions are rare. Anaphylactic reactions have been reported immediately following injection.
2. Educate the patient at the time of the initial injection not to disrupt the site of administration. Remind the patient at each injection of this simple but important point.

Weight Gain and Depo-Provera Use

KEY QUESTIONS

ASSESSMENT	ACTION
1. Have you been gaining weight steadily since you started the Depo-Provera regimen?	**YES** Go to Step A.
	NO Go to Question 2.
2. Did you have a pre-existing weight problem?	**YES** Go to Step B.
	NO Go to Question 3.
3. Have you had a sudden weight increase of 5 pounds or more?	**YES** Go to Step C.
	NO No further action.

ACTIONS

STEP A: Gradual Weight Gain Since Depo-Provera Initiation

Weight gain with Depo-Provera use probably is attributable to an increase in appetite, and not fluid retention, despite reports of patients feeling bloated.

Query the patient regarding changes in eating or exercise habits.

Recommend that the patient decrease food amounts and exercise at least three times per week.

Recommend that the patient increase her water consumption to 8–10, 8-ounce glasses daily.

If the patient is dissatisfied with method, discuss options for switching methods when her next injection is due.

If the weight gain continues despite patient efforts, she should see her provider for an evaluation to eliminate medical problems, such as an underactive thyroid.

STEP B: Pre-existing Weight Concerns

Women with pre-existing weight problems may have an unacceptable weight increase while on a Depo-Provera regimen.

Go to Step A for recommendations.

Advise patients to seek counseling, such as is provided by Overeaters Anonymous or Weight Watchers, for support while on a Depo-Provera regimen.

STEP C: Sudden Gain of 5 or More Pounds

This type of gain is more likely to be transient fluid retention, or rarely, symptoms of a more serious problem.

Query the patient regarding any increase in sodium intake or addition of a new medication that may have edema as a side effect.

Advise the patient to increase her water intake during the next 24 hours.

If the weight gain persists or other symptoms are present, the patient should call back to talk with her provider.

PATIENT EDUCATION

1. Weight gain is a major side effect of Depo-Provera, and patients should be told of the expected gain that occurs over time. According to the package insert enclosed with Depo-Provera (which patients probably don't see), the average gain is as follows: 5.4 pounds in year 1, 8.1 pounds after year 2, and 13.8 pounds after year 4.
2. Patients should understand that it is believed that an actual increase in appetite occurs, which causes the weight gain. This appetite increase may be difficult for some patients to manage.

CHAPTER 18

Intrauterine Contraception Overview

The inclusion of progesterone in IUDs has given rise to the term "intrauterine system" (IUS). Currently two products are available in the United States: ParaGard (Cu T 380A), and Mirena (LNg 20-IUD). Of these, ParaGard is the only true IUD; the other is a system that releases progesterone into the uterus at a constant rate. Both Para Gard and Mirena can provide long-term contraception.

Intrauterine contraception definitely is underused in this country for several reasons. Probably the most prominent cause is misunderstanding about the potential risks. Severe pelvic infections can be a result of IUD use. However, proper selection of candidates for this method will greatly reduce the potential for problems. Risk factors for pelvic infection directly parallel a woman's risk for STI exposure. Women at low STI risk, who have borne children, and who may be looking for a method with potential for long-term contraception, may find this a convenient, and over time, cost-effective method.

These methods have other advantages. Copper IUDs have been inserted postcoitally for emergency contraception. The progesterone-releasing IUDs decrease menstrual symptoms, and they may have other beneficial uses, such as decreasing symptoms of fibroids, adenomyosis, and providing progestin support during HRT.

Even if your office or clinic does not insert intrauterine contraception, you need to be familiar with triaging patient complaints. Because of the long-term approval for some of these methods (10 years for ParaGard and 5 years for Mirena), it is not uncommon for a patient to present herself at a facility other than the facility where it initially was inserted.

The following acronym often is used to educate patients to early warning signs of problems with these devices and systems:

P, Late period (pregnancy), abnormal spotting or bleeding;
A, Abdominal pain, pain with intercourse;
I, Infection exposure (STIs), abnormal discharge;
N, Not feeling well, fever, chills;
S, String missing, shorter or longer.

BASIC TRIAGE ASSESSMENT FORM FOR INTRAUTERINE CONTRACEPTION

1. What type of IUD or IUS do you have? _____
2. How long has it been in place? _____
3. When was your last menstrual period, and are your menstrual periods regular for you? _____
4. Have you had any change in menstrual symptoms recently? _____
5. Have you experienced any pelvic pain or vaginal discharge lately? _____

Abdominal Pain/Cramping and Intrauterine Contraception

KEY QUESTIONS

ASSESSMENT	ACTION
1. Was your IUD or IUS inserted within the last 24 hours?	**YES** Go to Step A.
	NO Go to Question 2.
2. Is this your first menstrual cycle after insertion?	**YES** Go to Step B.
	NO Go to Question 3.
3. Is the pain severe in nature, accompanied by cramping or bleeding, or not related to any anticipated menstruation?	**YES** Go to Step C.
	NO Go to Question 4.
4. Is the pain mild to moderate, with or without cramping or bleeding, and not related to anticipated menstruation?	**YES** Go to Question 5.
	NO No action.
5. Have you had a change in sexual partners, or do you think you could have been exposed to an STI?	**YES** Go to Step D.
	NO Go to Question 5.
6. Do you have any reason to suspect you could be pregnant?	**YES** Go to Step E.
	NO Go to Steps D and E.

ACTIONS

STEP A: Recent Insertion of Intrauterine Device/Intrauterine System

Cramping and pain after insertion should resolve rapidly, usually within the first 1–2 hours. Pain that persists and increases, particularly with abdominal tenderness, warrants evaluation.

Mild pain may be treated with acetaminophen 1000 mg every 4 hours or NSAIDs per the manufacturer's recommendation or as preferred by your office/clinic.

Ask the patient to feel for the string. If it is not present, the patient should be seen ASAP to rule out the possibility of perforation of the uterus or device expulsion.

The patient should monitor her symptoms and check for fever. She should call back if her temperature is greater than 100.4° F or there is an increase in symptoms.

STEP B: First Menses After Insertion

An increase in cramping at the time of menstruation may be expected, particularly with the first cycle. Cramping will decrease over time with Mirena.

See instructions in Step A.

Instruct the patient to call back if symptoms persist beyond menses.

STEP C: Severe Pain

The potential serious complications are uterine perforation, infection, or pregnancy. The patient needs immediate referral. See her within a few hours at your facility or refer her to an ER. The patient should not drive herself.

STEPS D and E: Mild to Moderate Pain, Possible Sexually Transmitted Infection, Possible Pregnancy

All IUD/IUS users with mild to moderate pain need to be considered at risk for infection, perforation, partial expulsion of the device, or pregnancy.

Have the patient feel for the string. If it is not present, is lengthened, or if hard plastic is palpable, the patient should be seen ASAP.

If the string is unchanged, the patient should be seen for evaluation within 24–48 hours.

Instruct the patient to call back if symptoms increase or if her temperature is greater than 100.4° F.

The patient may take a sensitive urine pregnancy test if she wishes; suggest that serial quantitative blood pregnancy tests or an ultrasound may be necessary to eliminate the possibility of ectopic pregnancy.

The patient should avoid sexual intercourse until she has been evaluated.

PATIENT EDUCATION

1. All patients choosing this method need to know the warning signs of possible severe infection or expulsion of the device.
2. Patients need to be taught at the time of insertion how to feel for their device's string. They should be reminded to locate it if problems arise.
3. Use the opportunity to remind of the need for backup methods for STI protection. Patients at high risk for STIs should receive education to help them choose a more appropriate method.
4. Patients who may not be at risk for STIs are still at risk for infection from endogenous bacteria.
5. All sexually active women with IUDs/IUSs need to consider the possibility of pregnancy, as is true with the use of any form of birth control.

Amenorrhea With Intrauterine Contraception

Initiate the Basic Triage Assessment Form for Intrauterine Contraception.

KEY QUESTIONS

ASSESSMENT	ACTION
1. Was your last menstrual period normal?	**YES** Go to Question 2.
	NO Go to Step A.
2. Do you think you could be pregnant?	**YES** Go to Step A.
	NO Go to Question 3.
3. Are you experiencing any abdominal pain or bloating?	**YES** Go to Step B.
	NO Go to Step C.

ACTIONS

STEP A: Abnormal Menses

Amenorrhea is an expected side effect of Mirena

Confirm the patient's pregnancy status before proceeding. Have the patient take a home pregnancy test or come in for a blood pregnancy test.

For patients desiring to continue the pregnancy, have them be seen within 24 hours to discuss the advisability of removing the IUD.

Call in a prescription for prenatal vitamins for patients desiring to continue pregnancy.

If the patient has risk factors for an abnormal 1st trimester pregnancy (prior ectopic pregnancy, history ruptured appendix or abdominal surgery, or repeated miscarriages) or has medical problems, do the following:

- Notify the on-call physician if the patient's symptoms are urgent. If no physician is available, have the patient seek evaluation in the ER.
- Schedule an appointment within 24 hours if the patient's symptoms do not appear urgent.
- Call in a prescription for prenatal vitamins, if appropriate.
- For patients desiring pregnancy termination, refer as appropriate.

STEP B: Pregnancy Unlikely, Pain Present

Unless the patient is not sexually active, pregnancy must be your first suspicion if using ParaGard. See Step A.

If the patient has a negative pregnancy test result, a history of her last menses being normal, and no risk factors, see her within 24 hours. Sonogram equipment should be available at your facility or preparations should be made for the patient to have a sonogram performed elsewhere in a timely fashion.

If the patient has any prior risk factors, see her the same day or have her go to an ER.

Reinforce that amenorrhea is anticipated after several months use of Mirena.

STEP C: Pregnancy Unlikely, No Pain Present

Unless the patient is not sexually active, pregnancy must be your first suspicion if using ParaGard. See Step A.

If the patient has a negative pregnancy test result, a history of her last menses being normal, and no risk factors, see her within 48–72 hours.

If the patient has any prior risk factors, see her within 24 hours.

Counsel the patient to call immediately if any symptoms of abdominal pain, bloating, referred pain, or bleeding develop.

PATIENT EDUCATION

1. Pregnancy is risky with an IUD in place. Data exist for older IUD models that indicate a pregnancy loss rate of approximately 50% with an IUD in place. The loss rate with early removal is approximately 25%.
2. Patients should be counseled at the time of IUD insertion of the risk of severe intrauterine infection if an IUD is left in place with a pregnancy intact.
3. A woman desiring a pregnancy termination should have the IUD removed at the time of abortion.
4. The ectopic pregnancy rate with an IUD in place is approximately 5%.

Bleeding Irregularities and Intrauterine Contraception

KEY QUESTIONS

ASSESSMENT	ACTION
1. Was your IUD/IUS inserted within the last 24 hours?	**YES** Go to Step A.
	NO Go to Question 2.
2. Is this your first menstrual cycle since the insertion?	**YES** Go to Step B.
	NO Go to Question 3.
3. Are you soaking one or more pads in 1 hour or six or more in a 12-hour period? Are you light-headed or dizzy? Do you have any abdominal, rectal, or vaginal pain associated with the bleeding?	**YES** Go to the protocol Abnormal Bleeding in Women of Reproductive Age.
	NO Go to Question 4.
4. Would you characterize the bleeding as irregular, spotting or bleeding as a period, or bleeding frequently but not excessively?	**YES** Go to Step C and continue to Question 5.
	NO Go to Step D.
5. Are you sexually active?	**YES** Go to Step E.
	NO Go to Step C.

ACTIONS

STEP A: Recent Insertion

Any bleeding after insertion should be minimal and limited. Bleeding heavier than normal menses that continues beyond 1–2 hours needs immediate evaluation for possible perforation.

STEP B: First Menses After Insertion

It is not uncommon for bleeding to be heaviest in the first 1–3 months after insertion. Reassure the patient that this may be normal and may subside with time.
Ask the patient to feel for her string. If it is not present, the patient should be seen in 24–48 hours to rule out expulsion of the device.

The patient should monitor her symptoms and check for fever. She should call back if she experiences abdominal pain or cramping or has a temperature greater than 100.4° F and should be seen ASAP.

The patient should avoid sexual intercourse if she is experiencing symptoms.

If the bleeding subsides and the string still cannot be felt, the patient should use a backup method until evaluated.

If bleeding subsides with menses and the string is in place, have the patient take ibuprofen 400 mg three times a day for the first 3 days of the next cycle and call to report her response.

STEP C: Irregular Bleeding, Spotting, Not Excessive

If using Mirena, reinforce that spotting and irregular bleeding may occur in the first 6–9 months of use.

Even minor bleeding or spotting may indicate infection, pregnancy, or dysfunctional uterine bleeding from other causes.

Have the patient feel for the string. If it is not present, is lengthened, or if hard plastic is palpable, the patient should be given a same-day appointment.

If the string is unchanged and no other symptoms are present, see the patient within 24–48 hours.

Instruct the patient to call back if symptoms increase, if they are accompanied by abdominal pain or cramping, or if her temperature is greater than 100.4° F.

If these symptoms are present when the patient calls, have the patient evaluated ASAP.

The patient should avoid sexual intercourse until she has been evaluated.

STEP D: Patient's Symptoms Not Characterized by Steps Above

Even the most minimal of complaints in the realm of irregular bleeding need to be taken seriously when an IUD/IUS is in place. The patient needs to be evaluated for pelvic infection, pregnancy, partial expulsion, cervicitis, and dysfunctional uterine bleeding of other causes. She may not take her symptoms as seriously as you do.

Instruct the patient as in Step C.

STEP E: Patient Is Sexually Active

All sexually active patients with an IUD/IUS need to be considered at risk for possible infection or pregnancy when bleeding of any amount is present at a time other than the anticipated menstruation.

Question the patient regarding the normalcy of her last menstrual period if using ParaGard. She may be experiencing amenorrhea with Mirena.

Question the patient about her routine use of back-up methods.

Have her check for the string if she has not done so.

If the string is not present, the patient should avoid sexual intercourse or use a back-up method.

If the last menstrual period was not normal, the patient may wish to take a sensitive urine pregnancy test.

Advise the patient to avoid sexual intercourse if any adverse symptoms are present.

Schedule an appointment for the patient within 24–48 hours and instruct her to call to be seen ASAP if symptoms of abdominal pain or cramping, excessive bleeding, or fever develop.

PATIENT EDUCATION

1. Patients using this method need thorough instruction on the potential significance of even minimal bleeding. The patient's reproductive future may be at stake.
2. Patients in the perimenopausal age group, who may be experiencing heavier bleeding, may be better candidates for intrauterine contraception that contains a progesterone-delivery system. The normal causes of bleeding in this age group need to be considered.

Lost String and Intrauterine Contraception

KEY QUESTIONS

ASSESSMENT	ACTION
1. Have you previously tried to feel your string and been able to locate it?	**YES** Go to Question 2.
	NO Go to Step A.
2. Was your IUD/IUS inserted within the last 24 hours?	**YES** Go to Step B.
	NO Go to Question 3.
3. Is this after your first menstrual cycle since insertion?	**YES** Go to Step C.
	NO Go to Question 4.
4. Did you feel your string after your last menstrual period?	**YES** Go to Question 5.
	NO Go to Step D.
5. If you previously were able to feel your string, did you notice a change in the string's length before you were unable to feel it?	**YES** Go to Step E.
	NO Go to Step F.

ACTIONS

STEP A: Patient Has Never Felt String

Some patients are squeamish about feeling for their string. If the patient has never tried to feel for it before, she may need instruction in how to do so.

Have the patient position herself over a toilet or at a chair/stool where she can place one leg up, as if inserting a tampon.

Instruct her that her cervix will feel tough in comparison to vaginal tissue, akin to touching the end of her nose.

The string may be felt coming out of the cervical os (opening).

If she cannot feel the string through the os, she should sweep her finger behind and then around her cervix because the string may be adhering to the vaginal mucosa.

If the patient cannot feel the string, schedule an appointment for her to come in for evaluation within 48–72 hours.

Have her call back if symptoms of pain, severe cramping, bleeding, or fever develop and see her ASAP.

Advise her to avoid sexual intercourse in the presence of any other accompanying symptoms.

If the patient has no adverse symptoms and plans to have intercourse, instruct her to use a condom or other backup method.

STEP B: Recent Insertion

Some clinicians counsel that expulsion may be more likely in the first 24 hours.

Follow the instructions in Step A.

STEP C: First Menses After Insertion

Some clinicians routinely schedule patients for a recheck after the first menstrual period because many anticipate this to be a time when expulsion may happen.

Follow the instructions in Step A.

STEP D: String Not Felt After Last Menstrual Period

This patient may not be used to feeling for her string or may have been lax in checking on a regular basis. Pregnancy is a possibility.

Question the patient regarding the normalcy of her last menstrual period.

Question the patient regarding her routine use of back-up methods.

Repeat the instructions in Step A if the patient is unfamiliar with checking for her string.

Instruct her to use a backup method until seen.

Advise her to avoid intercourse if she has any adverse symptoms.

If the patient's last menstrual period was not normal, she may wish to take a sensitive urine pregnancy test.

Schedule an appointment in 48–72 hours and instruct the patient to call to be seen ASAP if other symptoms develop.

STEP E: Change in String Length at Last Check

This may be a clue that the device is beginning to be expelled. Pregnancy is a possibility.

Follow the instructions in Step D.

STEP F: String Appropriately Felt After LMP

If the patient is diligent about checking her string, and her last check was after her last menstrual period, with no problems found, it is likely this is a more recent problem. Pregnancy still is possible but probably is too early to diagnose.

Schedule an appointment for the patient within 48–72 hours for evaluation.

Have the patient use a back-up method if she plans to have intercourse before she is evaluated.

Advise the patient to call back to be seen ASAP if adverse symptoms develop.

PATIENT EDUCATION

1. All patients choosing this method need to be proficient in locating their string. Use the instructions in Step A to educate patients who are unfamiliar with the technique.
2. Patients need to be able to use a backup method in case they cannot locate their string.

CHAPTER 19

Hormone Therapy Overview

Hormone therapy (HT or still referred to as hormone replacement therapy [HRT] by some) is an issue that becomes more complex on a daily basis. The Women's Health Initiative (WHI) results, published in 2002, turned the conventional wisdom on this issue upside down. The number of women taking hormones for menopausal symptoms plummeted after the initial release of study data. However, with time and more analysis, the tide is turning. While caution still exists on this topic, it is imperative that triage nurses educate themselves as to what we know is true— *as well as what we don't know*—about this complicated issue.

HT refers to the prescribing of estrogen, progesterone, or a combination of both. The hormones may be given continuously, meaning that same doses of both estrogen and progesterone are used daily. The desired result with this regimen is amenorrhea. They may also be used in a cyclic fashion, with estrogen given throughout the month, and progesterone used to counteract the buildup of the uterine lining by taking it for part of the cycle. This results in a withdrawal bleed for most women.

The various hormones come in an array of delivery systems: pills, patches, topicals, rings and—rarely—injections. A patient may use one or a combination of delivery systems, based on her preference or response to HT. Other hormones are occasionally added. In traditionally manufactured HT, the only hormone currently included is testosterone. So-called "bioidentical hormones", used in compounded products, are currently under scrutiny by the FDA. They are beyond the scope of this text but may be utilized by practitioners with whom you work.

In 2004, the FDA created new guidelines for the labeling of HT products, stating that they are effective for treating "moderate to severe hot flashes and night sweats, moderate to severe vaginal dryness and prevention of osteoporosis associated with menopause" (February 10, 2004, FDA Bulletin). The FDA specifically emphasized that the lowest effective dose should be used for the shortest period of time. In the case of vaginal dryness, local therapy should be considered first (e.g., creams, suppositories, rings). When used for the treatment of osteoporosis, women treated with HT should be at significant risk and inappropriate candidates for alternative therapies.

However, the FDA guidelines do not tell the entire story. Many studies continue to show benefits of HT in areas the FDA does not recognize, and some experts conclude that the "timing and initiation of hormone therapy is the main determinant of balance of benefits and risks" (Lynne T. Shuster, MD, presentation "HRT/The Pendulum Swings" given at Women's Health Update, the Mayo Clinic, April 17–19, 2008). The findings of these clinical trials demonstrate that healthy women, who are early in menopause, have many fewer risks than were originally reported in the WHI study. In fact, research indicates that if started at the onset of menopause or early in its course, HT may be associated with a reduction of risk for cardiovascular disease, osteoporosis and possibly dementia.

Some other important information for our patients to know is that although HT is not thought to cause breast cancer it may promote the growth of breast cancers that are already present. The risk is higher for women who use estrogen plus progesterone. In the WHI study, women who took estrogen alone did not show an increased risk of breast cancer, while women in the trial who took both estrogen and progesterone showed a slight increased risk. Another important point of clarification is that clinical trials have shown that transdermal estrogen appears to have little effect on venous thrombolic events (blood clots).

The potential benefits of HT have not yet been totally thwarted by the FDA labeling guidelines and the fear that persists since the WHI media frenzy. But we need to "stay tuned" with unbiased ears. As triage nurses, our goal is to stay abreast of developing research, guidelines and conventional thought. This is not an easy task. The two resources listed below can be of help to you and to the patients you advise. They are reliable and filled with measured, critical analysis:

North American Menopause Society (NAMS) www.menopause.org (be certain to emphasize the ".org" portion of the address)
Food and Drug Administration www.fda.gov/women/menopause/

In summary, there is perhaps no more controversial topic in women's health than the subject of hormone replacement therapy. Many women desire to take HT due to symptoms and sometimes for "health reasons" that are not totally substantiated. As educators, our goal is to help the women we serve make informed choices. We need to recognize that "quality of life" is also an important measure of health which may conflict with conventional wisdom. We need to be as factual and non-judgmental as possible in advising patients on this controversial topic.

BASIC TRIAGE ASSESSMENT FORM FOR HORMONE THERAPY

1) What hormone regimen are you following?
   a.) Estrogen only (confirm that patient has had a hysterectomy or has provider approval)
   b.) Estrogen and progesterone
2) How are you taking your estrogen?
   a.) Day 1 through day 25
   b.) Every day
   c.) Other _____.

3) What dose and what brand of estrogen are you taking? Brand _____
   Dose _____
   a.) Oral product _____
   b.) Patch _____
   c.) Combined estrogen and progesterone oral _____
   d.) Combined estrogen and progesterone patch _____
   e.) Other _____
4) How are you taking your progesterone?
   a.) Cyclically, days _____ of the month (example: days 1–12;
      Days 15 to 25.)
   b.) Continuously (every day)
   c.) Other _____
5) What dose and what brand of progesterone are you taking? Brand _____
   Dose _____
   a.) Oral product _____
   b.) Combined estrogen and progesterone oral _____
   c.) Combined estrogen and progesterone patch _____
   d.) Other _____
6) Are you taking any other hormones?
   a.) Androgens _____
   b.) Thyroid _____
   c.) Other _____
7) Are you taking any other medications?
   Drug _____ Dose _____ Duration _____

Abdominal Pain and Hormone Therapy

KEY QUESTIONS

ASSESSMENT	ACTION

1. Is the pain severe in nature and did it start recently (in the past 24–48 hours)?

YES Go to Step A.

NO Go to Question 2.

2. Is the pain mild/moderate in nature or been present longer than 24 to 48 hours?

YES Go to Step B.

NO Go to Question 3.

3. Is the abdominal pain recent and accompanied by nausea, vomiting, diarrhea, or fever?

YES Go to Step C.

NO No further action.

ACTIONS

STEP A: Severe Pain

The patient may have an acute abdominal problem or vascular condition; immediate referral to a primary care provider is indicated. The patient or her agent should call 911. The patient should not drive herself.

STEP B: Mild/Moderate Pain

The patient may have an acute abdominal condition and needs evaluation, but the disease process may be milder. Refer the patient to a primary care provider within 24 hours.

STEP C: Nausea, Vomiting, Diarrhea, or Fever

The patient may have gastroenteritis. If she has no other complications, the condition may be managed with the patient at home (see Patient Education).

A referral to the patient's primary care provider or closest ER is appropriate when:
Evolving appendicitis is possible; instruct the patient to call back if she experiences
  • increasing fever;
  • pain localizing in the right lower quadrant; or
  • symptoms not resolving within 12–24 hours.

Another disease condition is present (cardiovascular, pregnancy, diabetes, cancer, HIV).

The patient is very elderly and
- unable to communicate;
- you are unable to adequately assess the patient's condition on the telephone; or
- the patient is living alone.

Signs of significant dehydration are evident.
- The patient is unable to keep down any fluids (not even sips of water).
- The patient has not voided in the last 8 hours.
- The patient reports dizziness.

PATIENT EDUCATION

1. The patient with gastroenteritis symptoms should be instructed to modify her diet for the next 24–48 hours. She should:
   - avoid milk and milk products;
   - slowly rehydrate with sips of water (two sips every 5–10 minutes); and
   - begin the BRAT diet (bananas, rice, applesauce, toast) after she has tolerated clear liquids.
2. Diarrhea often is the last symptom to resolve. Reassure the patient that this symptom may persist for several days after nausea and vomiting subside.
3. The patient should call back if:
   - symptoms do not begin to resolve within 1–2 days;
   - symptoms increase in intensity (more vomiting/nausea); or fever develops.

Acne and Hormone Therapy

KEY QUESTIONS

ASSESSMENT	ACTION
1. Have you recently started HT?	**YES** Go to Step A. **NO** Go to Question 2.
2. Have your skin care practices changed recently (using different soaps, new makeup, sunscreen, or moisturizers, or washing with a different frequency)?	**YES** Go to Step B. **NO** Go to Question 3.
3. Is this a rash with papules/pustules over the central portion of the face? Does your face flush after eating hot/spicy foods or after drinking alcohol?	**YES** Go to Step C. **NO** Go to Question 4.
4. Is the rash erythematous, flat, or slightly raised, appearing over the cheeks or the bridge of the nose (butterfly pattern)?	**YES** Go to Step D. **NO** Go to Question 5.
5. Do you have a single lesion that has become asymmetrical, has irregular borders, or has changed color or increased in size (ABCD)?	**YES** Go to Step E. **NO** Go to Question 5.
6. Do you have scattered small papules or pustules with a few additional whiteheads or blackheads?	**YES** Go to Step A. **NO** Have patient describe symptoms.

ACTIONS

STEP A: Recent Start of Hormone Therapy

Skin changes consistent with mild acne may occur at initiation or restart of HT. They may occur, rarely, at a later time in use.

Reassure the patient that this is a transient side effect.

Refer to Patient Education for methods to minimize or decrease the acne.

If the acne is severe or unresponsive to usual treatments, refer the patient to a dermatologist.

STEP B: Change in Skin Care Practices

The patient may have come into contact with an allergenic agent, and this could be dermatitis.

Instruct the patient to stop using the offending agent.

For severe reactions, the patient should be referred to a provider within 24–48 hours.

If the patient experiences no improvement in 7 days, she should see a care provider.

STEP C: Facial Redness

This may be rosacea, an acneform disorder in older adults characterized by vascular dilatation of the central face.

The condition is common in women older than 30 years.

It is more common in fair-complected women of Northern European descent.

The condition is characterized by a "rosy cheek" appearance.

Rosacea commonly requires topical antibiotic therapy.

Refer the patient to a dermatologist or her primary care provider within 2–4 weeks.

STEP D: Butterfly Pattern

This may be a skin change associated with systemic lupus erythematosus, a systemic immune system condition.

Confirmation of this diagnosis is difficult.

Skin signs are "classic" but often are absent.

Early diagnosis is helpful, so skin signs that are apparent assist in the prompt recognition of the disease.

Refer the patient to her primary care provider within 7 days.

STEP E: ABCD Lesion

This could be skin cancer.

Refer the patient to a primary care provider or dermatologist within 7 days.

PATIENT EDUCATION

1. Instruct the patient in methods to decrease mild to moderate acne.
2. Wash affected areas twice a day with a washcloth and noncreamy soap.
3. Consider using cleansers such as Cetaphil lotion or benzoyl peroxide 10% acne wash.
4. Avoid picking at lesions.
5. Avoid oil-based cosmetics and facial creams such as Vaseline, Oil of Olay, or baby oil.
6. For dryness, may use Moisturel or Nutraderm.

Amenorrhea, Abnormal Bleeding and Adjustment to HT

KEY QUESTIONS

ASSESSMENT	ACTION
1. Are you taking estrogen only pills?	**YES** Go to Question 2.
	NO Go to Question 3.
2. Have you had a hysterectomy?	**YES** Go to Step A.
	NO Go to Step B.
3. Are you using continuous, combined HT (both progesterone and estrogen daily)?	**YES** Go to Step C.
	NO Go to Question 4.
4. Are you using cyclic therapy (stopping progesterone use occasionally)?	**YES** Go to Step D.
	NO Go to Question 5.
5. Are you taking another form of HT (shots, bio-equivalent therapy, "natural" hormones)?	**YES** Refer to provider.
	NO No further action.

ACTIONS

STEP A: Bleeding After Hysterectomy

Women who have had a hysterectomy are not expected to bleed! Reassure the patient and tell her to report any vaginal bleeding immediately.
If bleeding, see in 24–48 hours.

STEP B: Abnormal Bleeding

If the patient has not had a hysterectomy, she is at risk for endometrial hyperplasia and should be scheduled for endometrial evaluation within 72 hours.
Patients who do not tolerate progesterone may be routinely followed up for potential hyperplasia.

STEP C: Continuous Combined Hormone Replacement Therapy

Amenorrhea is a desired side effect of continuous dose HT but may take months to be established.

Reassure the patient that amenorrhea is normal with continuous HT.

If the patient remains anxious about this side effect, refer her to her OB/GYN care provider.

Break through bleeding may occur with continuous combined use for 6–9 months.

STEP D: Cyclic Therapy

After several years of cyclic therapy, it is not uncommon for periods to stop completely. However, periods do not usually stop suddenly. Amenorrhea is normal for some women using cyclic HT, even at the time of initial administration. These women usually have a plan with their provider for occasional evaluation for endometrial hyperplasia.

Reassure the patient.

If the patient routinely has had absence of withdrawal bleeding and has not spoken with her provider about this, have her speak with her provider about the advisability of routine screening for endometrial hyperplasia.

If pregnancy is a possibility, perform a urine pregnancy test. Do not forget that recently menopausal women can become pregnant.

PATIENT EDUCATION

1. Make certain the patient understands the expectations of episodes of bleeding and amenorrhea with her particular method of HT. There are many forms of potential therapy, and patients are easily confused.
2. If there is any question about the patient's regimen, refer her to the provider who is prescribing her HT.

Bleeding/Spotting and Hormone Therapy

KEY QUESTIONS

ASSESSMENT	ACTION
1. What type of HT are you on?	
Estrogen only	Go to Question 2.
Cyclic estrogen and progesterone	Go to Step C.
Continuous dose estrogen and progesterone	Go to Step D.
Other	Go to Step E.
2. If estrogen only, have you had a hysterectomy?	**YES** Go to Step A.
	NO Go to Step B.

ACTIONS

STEP A: Hysterectomy

If the patient had a hysterectomy, bleeding should be evaluated in 3–5 days.
The bleeding likely is coming from the vagina.
Patients may confuse rectal bleeding on underwear or tissue with vaginal bleeding.

STEP B: No Hysterectomy

If the patient has not had a hysterectomy, she is at risk for endometrial hyperplasia and
    should be scheduled for endometrial evaluation within 72 hours.
Patients who do not tolerate progesterone may be routinely followed up for potential
    hyperplasia.

STEP C: Cyclic Therapy

If the patient is taking cyclic estrogen and progesterone, and her bleeding is out of
    phase, initiate the Basic Triage Assessment Form for Hormone Therapy.
If the patient is taking the cyclic dose correctly and has been taking it for at least 6–9
    months without problems, she should be scheduled for a clinical evaluation within
    2 weeks.
If patient has been taking the cyclic dose correctly for 6 to 9 months and the problem
    has persisted longer than one cycle, she should be evaluated within 3–5 days.
If the patient is not taking the cyclic dosage correctly, instruct her on the proper dosage
    and have her call back if the problem persists beyond her next cycle.

If you can't figure out how she's taking the cyclic dosage or how it was prescribed, have her contact the prescriber within 24–48 hours.

STEP D: Continuous Dose Hormone Therapy

If the patient is taking continuous dose HT and is bleeding erratically, initiate the Basic Triage Assessment Form for Hormone Therapy.

If the patient has been taking the dosage correctly for less than 6–9 months, explain that the bleeding/spotting can be expected. If it continues two more cycles, she should see her care provider for clinical evaluation.

If the patient has been taking the dosage correctly for longer than 6–9 months, she should be seen for clinical evaluation in 3–5 days.

STEP E: Other Forms of Hormones

The patient is taking another form of hormone (such as added testosterone, injectable hormones, or topical hormones).

Refer the patient to the prescriber within 24–48 hours unless specific protocols exist within your facility for other hormone preparations.

PATIENT EDUCATION

1. It is important for patients to understand how common bleeding/spotting can be during the first several months of continuous, combined HT.
2. A certain percentage of women do not have withdrawal bleeding from a progestin. Those women need to establish a plan with their provider for being evaluated for hyperplasia, just as the woman with an intact uterus who elects not to take a progestin with estrogen needs a plan.

Chest Pain and Hormone Therapy

KEY QUESTIONS

ASSESSMENT	ACTION
1. Is the pain recent in onset (within 1–2 hours), described as "pressure" or "crushing" in nature, accompanied by shortness of breath, unrelieved by rest, or radiating into the left arm or jaw? (If the patient answers "yes" to any one of these questions, this is a positive response.)	**YES** Go to Step A. **NO** Go to Question 2.
2. Is the pain intermittent, associated with activity, relieved by rest, or described with any of the terms used in Question 1?	**YES** Go to Step B. **NO** Go to Question 3.
3. Is the pain localized to the chest/lung, sudden in onset, or accompanied by severe shortness of breath or significant anxiety?	**YES** Go to Step C. **NO** Go to Question 4.
4. Has the chest pain evolved more gradually than that described? Does the pain/discomfort increase with inspiration?	**YES** Go to Step D. **NO** Go to Question 5.
5. Can the patient point to a specific painful spot on the chest wall? Does it hurt when this area is palpated? Does the pain increase with specific movement?	**YES** Go to Step E. **NO** Go to Question 6.
6. Is the pain described as "indigestion" or "burning" in the chest, particularly after meals? Does the patient report increased gas or belching?	**YES** Go to Step F. **NO** Go to Question 7.
7. Is the pain localized to the breast? (All of the above complaints have been ruled out?)	**YES** Go to protocol Breast Pain and HRT. **NO** No further action.

ACTIONS

STEP A: Severe Pain

This may be a myocardial infarction (heart attack). Immediate evaluation is required. The patient or her agent should call 911.

Instruct the patient to take 325 mg aspirin while she waits for transport.

STEP B: Pain During Activity

This may be angina (coronary artery disease). Urgent evaluation is required.

Instruct the patient to call her primary care provider immediately for instructions or go to the ER for evaluation. The patient should not drive herself.

Instruct the patient to take 325 mg aspirin.

STEP C: Respiratory Symptoms

This may be a pulmonary embolus or severe asthma. Immediate evaluation is required. The patient or her agent should call 911.

STEP D: Gradual Onset and Pain With Inspiration

This may be pulmonary in origin (pneumonia, emphysema, or pleurisy). Evaluation within the next 12 to 24 hours is required.

STEP E: Point-Specific Pain

This may be a chest wall problem (costochondritis or shingles). Evaluation within the next 5 to 7 days by a primary care provider is recommended.

Advise the patient to take anti-inflammatory drugs (ibuprofen or naproxen).

She should use anti-inflammatory drugs only if no allergies or contraindications to these agents are evident (such as no history of gastrointestinal bleeding).

The patient can apply ice packs or heat to the affected area.

If a rash develops along the painful chest wall area, shingles should be considered as a diagnosis.

Once the rash develops, the patient needs to be seen by a care provider within 24 to 48 hours for possible antiviral therapy.

STEP F: Pain Associated With Meals

This may be GERD (acid indigestion). Evaluation within the next 7–10 days by a primary care provider is recommended. Refer the patient to the ER if she has taken antacids (Tums, Rolaids, Maalox, Mylanta) and experienced no relief (she may be experiencing evolving myocardial infarction). If the patient agrees, she should go to the ER. She should not drive herself.

PATIENT EDUCATION

1. Patients on HT need to be educated as to the possibility of blood clots.
2. All patients should have a plan for calling for emergency help if they are home alone.

Breast Pain and Hormone Therapy

KEY QUESTIONS

ASSESSMENT	ACTION
1. Is the breast pain bilateral?	**YES** Go to Step A.
	NO Go to Question 2.
2. Is the breast pain unilateral?	**YES** Go to Question 3.
	NO No action.
3. Is the pain isolated to one particular area of the breast?	**YES** Go to Step B.
	NO Go to Step B.
4. Did you recently start HT (within the last 3 months)?	**YES** Go to Step C.
	NO Go to Question 5.
5. Did you recently restart HT after several months' absence, or has your dosage changed?	**YES** Go to Step D.
	NO Go to Question 6.
6. Could this pain be chest wall or muscular pain (myocardial infarction, pulmonary embolus, costochondritis, or pulled muscle.)?	**YES** Go to protocol Chest Pain and Hormone Therapy.
	NO No further action.

ACTIONS

STEP A: Bilateral Breast Pain

Both estrogen and progesterone have been implicated in breast pain associated with HT. Pain associated with hormone use usually is bilateral in nature.

Initiate the Basic Triage Assessment Form for Breast Complaints.

Question the patient regarding her consumption of caffeine and foods containing the amino acid tyrosine (bananas, nuts, red wine, and yellow cheese).

Ask the patient if her bra size has changed.

Determine when the patient last had a mammogram.

Go to Step C.

STEP B: Unilateral Breast Pain

Unilateral breast pain is rarely caused by HT use. Other causes need to be investigated, such as breast cysts, fibroadenoma, and breast cancer.

Query the patient as to whether or not she has felt a lump.

Query the patient as to where she is in her menstrual cycle if still cycling.

Have the patient come in within 24–48 hours for a physical evaluation. Prepare her that she may need a mammogram, even if she has recently had one.

STEP C: Recent HT Start

Reassure the patient that hormones can cause breast tenderness during the first few months of use.

Recommend a good supportive bra.

Recommend the patient avoid activities that cause aggravation of symptoms (for example, she should walk, instead of jogging).

Recommend the patient decrease caffeine and tyrosine consumption.

If the patient's symptoms are intolerable, refer her to her provider for other recommendations or alteration in HT.

STEP D: Hormone Replacement Therapy Restart or Dosage Change

The patient may experience an adjustment period of 1–3 months with a restart of HT or a change in dosage, particularly an increase in estrogen or a switch to a different progesterone.

Return to Step C for supportive actions.

PATIENT EDUCATION

1. One of the keys to successful use of HT is understanding the expected problems and usual course of action. Educating the patient about the possible nature of her pain, particularly in the case of recent HT starts with bilateral pain, may help her tolerate the symptoms until her body adjusts to the hormone dosage.

2. Particular attention must be given to patients with unilateral pain who may be at risk for breast problems of a more serious nature. Refer to the Breast Complaints Section for approaches in dealing with women who have additional concerns.

3. Fear of breast cancer is high in patients in this age group. Be sure to ask the patient the date of her last mammogram.

Depression and Hormone Therapy

KEY QUESTIONS

ASSESSMENT

ACTION

1. Did the depressed mood begin gradually after HT began?

YES Go to Step A.

NO Go to Step B.

2. Do you have a history of depression or bipolar disorder?

YES Go to Question 3.

NO Go to Question 4.

3. If you have a current prescription for antidepressant medication, are you taking it?

YES Go to Step C.

NO Go to Step C.

4. Do you have no history of depression, but a recent onset of sadness, depressed mood, withdrawal, sleep disturbances (insomnia or daytime somnolence), change in appetite, or loss of energy (fatigue)?

YES Go to Step A.

NO Not applicable.

5. Do you feel like harming yourself or others? Do you have a suicide plan?

YES Go to Step D.

NO Go to Step A.

ACTIONS

STEP A: Depression on Initiation or Hormone Replacement Therapy

Depression may be a side effect of oral hormone therapy, but it generally is milder than with oral contraceptives because of the decrease in dosage. The exception may be progesterone, which may be high in some HT regimens. This may be a new onset of depression, and whether or not it is related to HT use, it requires thorough evaluation.

If the patient suspects HT is the underlying cause, have her speak with her OB/GYN provider within 12–24 hours.

The patient should consider evaluation with a mental health care professional within 7–10 days.

STEP B: Pre-existing Depression

This patient may have pre-existing depression, which could be aggravated by the HT.

Refer the patient to her OB/GYN provider if the patient thinks HT has aggravated her condition.

Refer the patient to a mental health care professional within 7–10 days.

Continue to Question 3, regarding medication use patterns.

STEP C: Depression History, Medication Use

This patient needs follow-up care by her mental health care provider or referral to a mental health care professional if she is not receiving regular care.

Ask the patient if HT may be adversely influencing her moods. If so, instruct her to consider consulting her OB/GYN provider to discuss alternative type/delivery method of hormones.

If the patient has discontinued taking any prescribed medication for depression, bipolar disorder, or other mood disorder, encourage her to be in touch with the prescribing provider.

STEP D: Suicidal Thoughts or Actions

This patient may be suicidal and requires immediate referral for appropriate evaluation.

Try to keep patient on the telephone if her symptoms are severe.

Have another health care provider or agent of the patient call 911 while you keep the patient on the line, if possible.

You should have suicide outreach hotline telephone numbers close at hand.

PATIENT EDUCATION

1. It is appropriate and necessary that patients new to HT be screened for history of depression. Depression is a part of menopause for some women. Although HT may help some women in terms of mood elevation, the potential for other causes or multiple causes of depression should be addressed.
2. You must be prepared for this type of call by having hotline or emergency referral telephone numbers close at hand. Although serious calls indicative of suicidal thoughts may be rare, they certainly are not the time to be searching for telephone numbers for appropriate referral and help.

Eye and Visual Changes and Hormone Therapy

KEY QUESTIONS

ASSESSMENT	ACTION
1. Have you had a sudden loss (central or peripheral blindness) or significant change (blurring, double vision) in your vision?	**YES** Go to Step A.
	NO Go to Question 2.
2. Do you have eye pain?	**YES** Go to Question 3.
	NO Go to Question 4.
3. Is the pain unilateral, intense, and did it begin suddenly?	**YES** Go to Step B.
	NO Go to Question 4.
4. Is the eye red but painless and your vision unaffected?	**YES** Go to Step C.
	NO Go to Question 5.
5. Is your vision changing gradually and affecting normal activities such as reading, sewing, or driving?	**YES** Go to Step D.
	NO No further action.

ACTIONS

STEP A: Severe Symptoms

This patient may be experiencing a transient ischemic attack (stroke); may have acute angle glaucoma, retinal detachment, or macular degeneration; or may be experiencing a new onset of ocular migraine. The patient needs to be seen immediately; refer her to the ER or have her call 911.

STEP B: Eye Pain

This patient may have iritis, cluster headache, or an unusual ocular migraine presentation. She needs to be evaluated by her primary care provider within the next 2–4 hours.

STEP C: Red Eye

This could be a spontaneous hemorrhage, conjunctivitis, or scleritis. This symptom should be evaluated by the patient's primary care provider within the next 12 to 24 hours.

STEP D: Gradual Change in Vision

This patient may have cataracts or gradually developing macular degeneration. She needs to see her primary care provider within the next week.

Gastrointestinal Complaints: Nausea/Vomiting and Hormone Therapy

KEY QUESTIONS

ASSESSMENT	ACTION
1. Have you been on HT for less than 1 year, have a male partner, and are not using any form of contraception?	**YES** Go to Step A.
	NO Go to Question 2.
2. Is the emesis dark black (like coffee grounds) or bloody? Have you noted black tarry stools?	**YES** Go to Step B.
	NO Go to Question 3.
3. Is the nausea/vomiting intermittent, associated with certain foods (fatty, greasy, spicy), and accompanied by pain (right upper quadrant or shoulder)?	**YES** Go to Step C.
	NO Go to Question 4.
4. Did the nausea/vomiting start within the past 24 hours, and is it accompanied by diarrhea and mild/moderate abdominal pain?	**YES** Go to Step D.
	NO Go to Question 5.
5. Did the nausea start with initiation or change in HT?	**YES** Go to Step E.
	NO No further action.

ACTIONS

STEP A: Unprotected Intercourse

This patient may be pregnant. Have her take a pregnancy test.

STEP B: Colored Emesis

This may be gastrointestinal bleeding (either esophageal varices or a bleeding ulcer). The patient should go immediately to the ER or call 911.

STEP C: Gastrointestinal Symptoms With Food

This may be gallbladder disease. Encourage the patient to eat a bland diet and see her primary care provider for evaluation within the next 24–48 hours.

STEP D: Nausea, Vomiting, and Diarrhea

The patient may have gastroenteritis. If she has no other complications, her condition may be managed with the patient at home (see Patient Education).

The patient should be referred to a physician or ER when:

Evolving appendicitis is possible; instruct the patient to call back if she experiences
- increasing fever or;
- pain localizing in the right lower quadrant, or
- her symptoms do not resolve during the next 12–24 hours.

Another disease condition is present (cardiovascular, pregnancy, diabetes, cancer, HIV). The patient is elderly and
- unable to communicate;
- her condition cannot be adequately assessed over the telephone; or she
- lives alone.

Signs of significant dehydration are evident.
- The patient is unable to keep down any fluids (not even sips of water).
- The patient has not voided in the past 8 hours.
- The patient reports dizziness.

STEP E: Nausea Associated with HT Dosing

Have patient try changing timing of oral dosing or take with food.
If associated with transdermal use, may try lowering the dose.
Advise she speak with her OB/GYN provider.

PATIENT EDUCATION

1. Nausea with HT dosing initiation or change is usually mild and transient. Severe GI symptoms are usually not due to HT and further evaluation is warranted.
2. The patient should modify her diet for the next 24–48 hours. She should:
   - avoid milk and milk products;
   - slowly rehydrate with sips of water (two sips every 5–10 minutes); and
   - begin the BRAT (bananas, rice, applesauce, toast) diet after she has tolerated clear liquids.
3. Diarrhea often is the last symptom to resolve. Reassure the patient that this symptom may persist for several days after nausea and vomiting subside. Instruct the patient to call back if:
   - symptoms do not begin to resolve within 1–2 days;
   - symptoms increase in intensity (more vomiting/nausea); or
   - fever develops.

Hair Growth or Loss and Hormone Therapy

KEY QUESTIONS

ASSESSMENT	ACTION
1. Is hair loss a problem?	**YES** Go to Step A.
	NO Go to Question 2.
2. Is hair excess a problem?	**YES** Go to Question 3.
	NO Go to Question 3.
3. Are you taking Estratest (an HT that contains estrogen and testosterone) or another testosterone preparation (oral, patch, or topical)?	**YES** Go to Step B.
	NO Go to Step C.

ACTIONS

STEP A: Hair Loss

This could be thyroid disease or an androgen imbalance causing male pattern baldness. Refer the patient to her primary care or OB/GYN care provider.

Women older than 50 years are at high risk for thyroid disorders. Routine screening is appropriate in this population.

STEP B: Excess Hair

This patient's testosterone levels may be too high, resulting in androgen excess.

The testosterone in the patient's HT regimen may need to be decreased or eliminated. Instruct the patient to consult her OB/GYN care provider or primary care provider regarding possible adjustment of medication.

STEP C: Taking a Testosterone Preparation

The patient may experience transient growth in hair; however, she may have androgen excess (adrenal gland dysfunction, Cushing disease, or an androgen-secreting tumor). Refer the patient to her primary care provider.

Headache and Hormone Therapy

KEY QUESTIONS

ASSESSMENT

ACTION

1. Did the headache begin within the last 1–2 hours, and is it described as being the worst headache she's ever had in her life?

YES Go to Step A.

NO Go to Question 2.

2. Is the headache accompanied by visual changes?

YES Go to Step B.

NO Go to Question 3.

3. Is the headache accompanied by any numbness, tingling, loss of bowel or bladder control, or seizure?

YES Go to Step A.

NO Go to Question 4.

4. Is the headache accompanied by neck stiffness?

YES Go to Step C.

NO Go to Question 5.

5. Do you have upper respiratory tract infection symptoms (such as congestion, fever, or cough)?

YES Go to Step D.

NO No further action.

ACTIONS

STEP A: Severe Headache

This may be an aneurysm or an evolving cerebrovascular accident. Call 911 for immediate evaluation.

STEP B: Visual Changes

This patient may have cluster headache or an unusual ocular migraine presentation. She needs to be evaluated by her primary care provider within the next 2–4 hours.

STEP C: Neck Stiffness

This patient may have spinal meningitis. She should be evaluated by her primary care provider within the next 2–4 hours.

STEP D: Respiratory Tract Symptoms

This patient may have a sinus headache. Suggest she take ibuprofen or naproxen if such agents are not contraindicated by allergies or gastrointestinal disturbances. If her symptoms persist or worsen, she should be evaluated by her primary care provider within the next 2–4 days.

Hot Flashes/Sweats and Hormone Therapy

KEY QUESTIONS

ASSESSMENT

ACTION

1. Did you have a recent hysterectomy (within the past 6 months)?

YES Go to Step A.
NO Go to Question 2.

2. Has your HT dose changed recently (particularly if decreased), or have you missed any pills or stopped taking them?

YES Go to Step B.
NO Go to Question 3.

3. Has your environment changed (summertime, working out of doors, working in warm or humid surroundings)?

YES Go to Step C.
NO No further action.

ACTIONS

STEP A: Recent Hysterectomy

Women who have had a recent hysterectomy, particularly young women of reproductive age, have more problems with vasomotor instability. "Normal" doses of HT (0.625 conjugated ethinyl estradiol or 1 mg estradiol) may be inadequate, at least for the first 12–18 months. Refer the patient to her provider for management of these symptoms.

STEP B: Recent Change in Hormone Replacement Therapy

Dose changes may result in an increase in hot flash symptoms.
If the patient's dose was decreased, reassure her that this side effect is temporary and will resolve once hormone levels stabilize.
If the patient has discontinued medication use, she should discuss this with her provider.
If she has missed only a few pills, reassure her that when she restarts her HT, these symptoms should resolve.

STEP C: Environmental Change

This is not an unusual problem. Discuss the Patient Education measures. If symptoms persist and are interfering with activities, refer the patient to her provider. An increase in HT dose may be indicated.

PATIENT EDUCATION

1. Lifestyle and dietary changes can help manage vasomotor instability. Offer the following suggestions.
2. Limit the following dietary items (particularly just before bedtime):
   • spicy foods;
   • red wine; and
   • high-fat foods.
3. Consider wearing loose clothing, particularly during the hot summer months. Cotton is cooler than nylon.
4. Stress management plays a role. Many women notice a change in vasomotor symptoms with changes in anxiety or stress levels.
5. Alternative therapies such as acupuncture, herbal supplements, and massage have helped some women. Despite lack of sufficient data on effectiveness, most providers tell women despite possible placebo effect, anything lessening symptoms may be a blessing!

Leg Cramps and Hormone Therapy

ASSESSMENT	ACTION
1. Do you have unilateral pain and have you been immobile recently (recent surgery or sitting for prolonged periods in a car or airplane)?	**YES** Go to Step A.
	NO Go to Question 2.
2. Is the pain unilateral and localized in your calf?	**YES** Go to Step A.
	NO Go to Question 3.
3. Do you have unilateral leg swelling?	**YES** Go to Step A.
	NO Go to Question 4.
4. Does the pain increase with walking? Is it relieved with rest?	**YES** Go to Step B.
	NO Go to Question 5.
5. Is the pain bilateral, worse when reclining at night, and keeping you from sleeping?	**YES** Go to Step C.
	NO Go to Question 6.
6. Does this feel like a "charley horse" (sharp leg cramp that commonly awakens people during sleep)? Is it related to a recent increase in activity?	**YES** Go to Step D.
	NO No further action.

ACTIONS

STEP A: Immobility, Unilateral Pain

This patient may have a deep vein thrombosis. Refer her immediately to her primary care provider (within 12–24 hours).

She should stop HT immediately until further evaluation.

STEP B: Pain Increases With Walking and Is Relieved by Rest

This patient may have intermittent claudication. Refer her to her primary care provider within the next week.

STEP C: Nighttime Pain

This may be restless leg syndrome. Refer the patient to her primary care provider within the next 1–2 weeks.

STEP D: Charley Horse

This may be muscle fatigue or cramping.

Offer some management suggestions.

If the pain is a charley horse, the patient can try:

- gentle stretching,
- massage, and
- hot packs.

If the pain is muscle strain/fatigue, the patient can take anti-inflammatory drugs, if such agents are not contraindicated.

If the pain persists, the patient should see her primary care provider within the next 1–2 weeks.

Review patient's calcium intake.

Libido Decrease and Hormone Therapy

KEY QUESTIONS

ASSESSMENT	ACTION
1. Did this change in libido begin concurrently with HT use?	**YES** Go to Step A.
	NO Go to Question 2.
2. Is this decrease in libido associated with a depressed mood?	**YES** Go to Step B.
	NO Go to Question 3.
3. Is this change in libido associated with painful intercourse?	**YES** Go to Step C.
	NO No further action.

ACTIONS

STEP A: Decreased Libido Associated With Start of Hormone Replacement Therapy

Instruct the patient to consult with her OB/GYN care provider. The patient may need a change of HT (sex hormone-binding globulins may be affected by menopause and HT, resulting in changes in libido).

STEP B: Depressed Mood

Libido changes (particularly decreased libido) often are associated with relationship problems. They also can be associated with cumulative life stressors. Encourage the patient to see a psychiatric/mental health care provider or her primary care provider to discuss these issues.

Possible causes include:
- depression;
- marital/relationship discord; or
- significant emotional stress (such as an ill child, elderly parents, or financial stressors).

STEP C: Dyspareunia

Dyspareunia is a common complaint among women. It often is caused by low vaginal
estrogen levels, vaginal infection, vaginal lesions, or more complex pelvic floor
complications (such as vulvar vestibulitis).

If this is a chronic problem, refer the patient to her OB/GYN care provider within the
next 2–4 weeks.

If this is an acute problem, refer the patient to her OB/GYN care provider within the
next 2–4 days.

PATIENT EDUCATION

1. Research has shown that the over-the-counter product Replens, if used consistently
   for 3 months, may be as helpful as estrogen in relieving dyspareunia due to vaginal
   dryness. It will not alter cytology.
2. A good resource for patients experiencing decreased libido is the book Reclaiming
   Desire: 4 Keys to Finding Your Lost Libido by Andrew Goldstein, MD & Marianne
   Brandon, PhD. New York: Rodale, 2004.

Missed or Late Pills, Patch or Topicals and Hormone Therapy

KEY QUESTIONS

ASSESSMENT	ACTION
1. Have you had a hysterectomy?	**YES** Go to Step A.
	NO Go to Question 2.
2. Are you taking estrogen and progesterone as separate tablets/patches/topicals?	**YES** Go to Question 3.
	NO Go to Question 5.
3. Have you missed any estrogen tablets/patches/topicals?	**YES** Go to Step B.
	NO Go to Question 4.
4. Have you missed any progesterone tablets/patches/topicals?	**YES** Go to Step C.
	NO Go to Question 5.
5. Are you taking a combined tablet or patch (such as CombiPatch or Prempro)?	**YES** Go to Step D.
	NO No further action.

ACTIONS

STEP A: Patients Who Have Had a Hysterectomy

Women without a uterus usually take estrogen only. Missing an occasional estrogen dose is not a problem.

Deliberate discontinuation of estrogen therapy for extended periods of time is not recommended (for instance, taking estrogen during the summer months to manage hot flashes and discontinuing its use during the cooler winter months). Such practices have a cumulative negative effect on bone density and should be avoided.

STEP B: Missed Estrogen Dose(s)

Missing an estrogen dose is not a particular problem. Reassure the patient and encourage her to start taking the medication again and take it consistently.

Instruct her regarding methods that help to increase compliance, including taking the pills at night during her bedtime routine or in the morning with breakfast.

STEP C: Missed Progesterone Tablet(s)

Missing progesterone tablets is a matter of concern. The risk of endometrial hyperplasia and uterine cancer increases the more the uterus is exposed to unopposed estrogen. The patient needs to be **strongly** encouraged to take progesterone regularly as prescribed.

If she is reluctant to take it as prescribed, she needs to discuss her reservations with her OB/GYN care provider.

Potential options for management include:

- changing the progesterone formulation (e.g., from medroxyprogesterone acetate to micronized progesterone);
- changing the route of administration; or
- performing regular endometrial evaluations.

STEP D: Missed Combined Hormone Therapy

Missing a combined HT product is not a particular concern, as long as the misses occur only intermittently. However, if HT is missed or forgotten regularly, it is not providing the patient with the full anticipated benefits. She should schedule an appointment with her provider within the next 2–4 weeks to discuss reasons for her intermittent use.

PATIENT EDUCATION

A woman who has not had a hysterectomy is likely to experience spotting if she does not take her HT as directed. This may cause her to undergo more evaluative testing to rule out hyperplasia or uterine cancer.

Weight Gain and Hormone Therapy

ASSESSMENT	ACTION
1. Did you start taking HT recently (within the past 3 months)?	**YES** Go to Question 2.
	NO Go to Question 2.
2. Is the weight gain associated with foot, ankle, or leg swelling or shortness of breath?	**YES** Go to Step A.
	NO Go to Question 3.
3. Have you gained more than 5 pounds in the past 7 to 10 days?	**YES** Go to Step B.
	NO Go to Question 4.
4. Do you think you might be pregnant?	**YES** Go to Step C.
	NO Go to Question 5.
5. If pregnancy has been excluded, and your weight has increased slowly, has your activity level decreased or your nutritional habits changed significantly? (Are you eating more processed/convenience foods? Do you have more life stressors, such as an altered living situation [divorcing, homeless]?)	**YES** Go to Step D.
	NO Go to Question 6.
6. Has your weight increased slowly during the past 3–6 months?	**YES** Go to Step E.
	NO No further action.

ACTIONS

STEP A: Foot, Ankle, or Leg Swelling or Shortness of Breath

This may be a significant adverse effect of HT. This patient may have a thromboembolic disorder (deep vein thrombosis or pulmonary embolus). This patient needs to be evaluated by her primary care provider within the next 2–4 hours. If she has shortness of breath, she needs to be seen immediately (may need to call 911). She should stop HT until further medical evaluation.

STEP B: Rapid Weight Gain Not Accompanied by Other Symptoms

This may be an adverse effect of HT and should be evaluated by the OB/GYN care provider or the primary care provider within the next 1–2 days.

If additional symptoms develop, the patient may need to be seen sooner.

STEP C: Potential Pregnancy

Pregnancy should be considered in women who have not had menopause confirmed by laboratory testing or those who have not had a hysterectomy. A pregnancy test is indicated.

Inquire as to whether the patient has other symptoms of pregnancy, such as breast tenderness, fatigue, or missed or abnormal menses.

STEP D: Changes in Diet or Activity

Decrease in activity or changes in nutritional intake may result in an increase in body weight.

Advise the patient to monitor her activities and caloric intake.

The patient may need to consult a dietitian or seek stress management counseling.

STEP E: Continued Weight Gain

If activity levels and caloric intake are stable and the patient continues to gain weight, recommend that she undergo evaluation by her primary care provider. Such symptoms may be an early sign of an underactive thyroid.

PATIENT EDUCATION

Occasionally, women may experience bloating for the first three cycles of HT. After you have ruled out the other causes for weight gain, reassure the patient that this is normal and usually subsides with time.

If this is a significant problem, suggest the patient talk with her provider and consider changing the type or route of HT.

The patient also may elect to discontinue HT because of this side effect and select another method of managing menopausal symptoms. The patient also may elect to manage low estrogen effects with lifestyle modifications, such as taking calcium 1000 mg/day, vitamin D IU/day, performing weight-bearing exercise for at least 30 minutes three times/week, and undergoing bone densitometry and lipid testing every 2–3 years, as directed by the patient's primary care provider.

CHAPTER 20

Natural Family Planning Overview

Naturally family planning (NFP) typically refers to methods that seek to either prevent or achieve a pregnancy. Modern NFP methods use a variety of physiologic changes that occur during a woman's menstrual cycle to assist the couple in daily fertility awareness. These physiologic changes include the length of the woman's menstrual cycle, changes in basal body temperature (BBT), and cervical mucous changes. Some women also may use additional body changes, such as discomfort at time of ovulation (mittelschmerz), or breast tenderness before menstruation to predict fertility.

Natural family planning has been found to be acceptable to many couples for a variety of reasons. Some couples elect to use NFP because of religious beliefs; other couples use NFP to avoid the use of medications or contraceptive devices; still others feel that NFP involves both partners in sexual decision making and use of a method. Others use NFP practices to assist with conception. Regardless, with proper instruction NFP has proven to be highly acceptable and successful.

Most providers strongly recommend that the patient and her partner enroll in an NFP class or complete an NFP home study course before using this method. There are a number of organizations that assist couples with this method. One such group is The Couple to Couple League, which maintains a website with information on NFP classes (grouped by area code), instructions are in English and Spanish, and a home study course is also available. Their website can be found at http://www.ccli.org. Other NFP resources are listed in Appendix A.

Although it is impractical and unwise for a triage nurse to do extensive NFP counseling over the telephone, it is important that the triage nurse know a bit about how patients are using NFP and the valuable community resources that are available. For this reason, this book contains an NFP protocol.

Natural Family Planning to Achieve or Avoid a Pregnancy

Natural family planning typically refers to methods that seek to either prevent or achieve a pregnancy based on daily fertility awareness. Most providers strongly recommend that the patient enroll in an NFP class or do an NFP home-study course before using this method for contraception (see resources in Appendix A for NFP information). This protocol provides an overview of some of the parameters used to determine fertility.

KEY QUESTIONS

ASSESSMENT

ACTION

1. Are you attempting to avoid a pregnancy?

YES Go to Step A.

NO Go to Question 2.

2. Are you attempting to achieve a pregnancy?

YES Go to Step B.

NO No further action.

ACTIONS

STEP A: Avoidance of Pregnancy

Estimations of the patient's fertile period are based on calendar calculations, variations in basal body temperature, changes in cervical mucous, or a combination of these methods.

Calendar Calculations: Assuming a woman has an absolutely regular 28-day cycle, the fertile period lasts from days 10 through 17 of the month. Day 1 begins on the first day of the patient's menstrual period. For women who do not have regular 28-day cycles, additional days are added to the fertile period based on the shortest and longest menstrual cycles she experiences. For example, if the patient has a menstrual period every 28 days ± 3 days, she would be considered to be fertile from days 7 (10 − 3) through 20 (17 + 3). During the fertile period, the couple avoids sexual intercourse.

Basal Body Temperature: An increase in BBT of 0.5° to 1° F indicates ovulation. When determining BBT, the patient needs to make sure she has a special BBT thermometer. She should take her temperature before arising each morning because activity affects BBT. She also should avoid using an electric blanket because she may have trouble with BBT accuracy. Couples avoid intercourse from the start of menses until 2 to 3 days after the temperature rise.

Cervical Mucous: The presence of thin, "stretchy," clear mucous also is an indication of ovulation. When this stretchy, clear mucous is present, the couple abstains from intercourse until 4–5 days after it disappears. During the "safe" period, cervical mucous should appear milky or opaque.

STEP B: Achieving a Pregnancy

Estimations of the patient's fertile period are based on calendar calculations, variations in BBT, changes in cervical mucous, or a combination of these methods.

Calendar Calculations: Assuming a woman has an absolutely regular 28-day cycle, the fertile period lasts from days 10 through 17 of the month. Day 1 begins on the first day of the patient's menstrual period. For women who do not have regular 28-day cycles, additional days are added to the fertile period based on the shortest and longest menstrual cycles she experiences. For example, if the patient has a menstrual period every 28 days ± 3 days, she would be considered to be fertile from days 7 (10 − 3) through 20 (17 + 3).

Basal Body Temperature: An increase in BBT of 0.5° to 1° F indicates ovulation. When determining BBT, the patient needs to make sure she has a special BBT thermometer. She should take her temperature before arising each morning because activity affects BBT. She also should avoid using an electric blanket because she may have trouble with BBT accuracy. Couples attempting to become pregnant should time daily intercourse from the start of menses until at least 2 to 3 days after the temperature rise.

Cervical Mucous: The presence of thin, "stretchy," clear mucous also is an indication of ovulation. When this stretchy, clear mucous is present, the couple has daily intercourse 4 to 5 days after it appears.

CHAPTER 21

Pelvic Complaints Overview

The pelvic complaints discussed in this section concern devices placed (or misplaced) in the vaginal area, such as pessaries or tampons, and vaginal discharge and lesions. Often when a patient has complaints in this region, they are vague and overlapping. Careful questioning is needed to determine the true nature of the complaint.

Far too many vulvar and vaginal infections are managed over the telephone. The reasons are patients often have symptoms they've had before and are self-diagnosing, providers have only so much time and many such complaints are dismissed as minor, and there are a host of available over-the-counter products worth trying. In reality, it is hard **not** to treat these complaints via telephone, for the sake of convenience alone.

However, there are compelling reasons to delay such treatment. Serious infections, some of them communicable, can be missed. Patient symptoms may be exacerbated by inappropriate treatments. Superinfection with simple and common body bacteria may occur. It can be better to offer patients some comfort measures for relief until they can be seen and their conditions adequately diagnosed. Your clinic or office practice philosophy often dictates what direction you take.

The biggest challenge in this arena is not letting a potential sexually transmitted infection (STI) go undiagnosed and thus missing an opportunity for proper treatment at a critical time. It is important to determine patients who may be at greatest risk for STIs. This also is a good opportunity to educate them about the signs and symptoms of potential problems. A chart of STI presenting symptoms, incubation periods, usual course of the disease, and important facts and implications is included here.

It is important to remember that urinary symptoms and vulvovaginitis symptoms may overlap. Yeast infections can affect the urethra and bladder, causing the familiar triad of dysuria, urgency, and frequency. Patients also may mistake the discomfort of urine irritating a vulvar lesion as symptoms of abnormal urination.

Some tried and true remedies may keep patients comfortable until they can be adequately evaluated. Some suggestions of common home remedies are zinc oxide, oatmeal bath products, cold compresses, bags of frozen vegetables secured in an outer wrapper, and even vegetable shortening! You should discuss with the providers with whom you work what comfort measures will be suggested to patients until they can be seen.

Comfort measures we recommend in our clinic/office are:

_____

_____

_____

_____.

Abnormal Cervical Pap Smear

KEY QUESTIONS

ASSESSMENT

ACTION

1. Is the Pap smear unsatisfactory for evaluation?

YES Go to Step A.

NO Go to Question 2.

2. Does the Pap smear report read "epithelial cell abnormality"?

YES Go to Step B.

NO Continue to Question 3.

3. Does the Pap smear report read "atypical squamous cells of undetermined significance (ASCUS)"?

YES Go to Question 4 and Step C.

NO Go to Question 5.

4. Was the HPV test positive?

YES Go to Step E.

NO Go to Step D.

5. Does the Pap smear report low-grade squamous intraepithelial lesion (LGSIL) or higher?

YES Go to Step E.

NO Continue to Question 6.

6. Does the Pap smear report atypical glandular cells of unknown significance (AGCUS)?

YES Go to Step F.

NO Go to Step G.

ACTIONS

STEP A: Unsatisfactory Smear

There are multiple reasons for unsatisfactory smears. Since the Pap test requires a sample of cervical squamous and endocervical cells, anything that reduces the quality of that sample, such as blood, infection, recent intercourse, or vaginal medication, may contribute to an unsatisfactory smear. Poor sampling technique on the part of the clinician and lab error can also produce an unsatisfactory result.

A Pap smear that is "unsatisfactory for evaluation" must be repeated under optimal sampling conditions as described above as soon as those conditions can be met.

STEP B: Epithelial Cell Abnormalities

This is an abnormal Pap smear. All abnormal Pap smears require follow-up with further testing. The abnormality should be further defined as one of the classifications in the following steps.

STEP C: ASCUS Pap Smear

An ASCUS test is considered a "borderline" abnormal test. This means that abnormal cells were seen on the smear, but they did not meet the criteria for dysplasia (precancerous cells). A DNA test for high-risk HPV may be ordered automatically ("reflex" test) at the time the pathologist determines the Pap to be ASCUS. It may also be ordered on request. You should know which of the labs that your office uses does DNA testing for high-risk HPV. High-risk types of HPV are associated with most cases of cervical cancer. Thus the presence of high-risk HPV raises the suspicion for dysplasia.

STEP D: ASCUS, Negative HPV

The Pap smear may be repeated in 1 year (normal interval).

STEP E: ASCUS/Positive HPV, LGSIL, or Higher*

All reports with squamous cell abnormalities of ASCUS (positive HPV) or higher require diagnostic testing. The primary diagnostic test is colposcopy (see Colposcopy protocol for further information).

STEP F: AGCUS Pap Smear

All reports with a reading of glandular cell abnormalities require further diagnostic testing. This may include colposcopy and endometrial biopsy (EMB; see Endometrial Biopsy protocol).
The ordering clinician will determine the course of action.

STEP G: Other Comments on Pap Smear

Some Pap reports may contain comments on the adequacy of the specimen, lack of endocervical cells, atrophic pattern, etc. How these comments are handled needs to be decided upon with your providers and may need to be individualized based on the patient's health and Pap history.

PATIENT EDUCATION

1. Take the opportunity to provide general information about the Pap smear screening test for cervical cancer. Advise that the Pap smear is only a screening test for cervical cancer. The test evaluates skin cells obtained from the uterine cervix. An abnormal test does not mean that the patient has cancer. Rather, it serves to narrow the number of women who require additional, potentially more invasive tests and/or treatment. Cervical cancer is not symptomatic until it is advanced. The purpose of the Pap smear is to detect asymptomatic premalignant and malignant lesions early.
2. Acquiring a good specimen is key to a meaningful Pap smear. The test should be scheduled at the midcycle when possible, and the patient should be instructed not to put anything in her vagina for 24–48 hours before the test (no tampons, douching, creams, gels, or intercourse).

*Pap Smears are reported according to the 2001 Bethesda System.

3. The conventional Pap smear does not diagnose vaginal or cervical infections. However, the newer generation of Pap smears (ThinPrep, SurePap, etc.) can be used to diagnose chlamydia and GC infections. If the patient thinks she may have vaginitis, the Pap smear should be postponed, the infection treated, and the Pap should be rescheduled until symptoms have subsided and the vagina is clear of any medications.

4. The fear of potential cancer may make some patients unable to adequately take in the information you are providing. Make sure you stress that the Pap smear is only a screening test and further testing is needed for a diagnosis. Provide ample time for questions and make sure the patient knows how to reach you should more questions arise.

5. Every office/clinic should have a system for documenting follow-up for abnormal Pap smears and for tracking all Pap smears performed.

Colposcopy

ASSESSMENT

ACTION

1. Is the colposcopy being ordered as a follow-up
   to an abnormal Pap smear?

   YES Go to Step A.
   NO Go to Question 2.

2. Is the colposcopy being ordered to evaluate a
   visible vulvar lesion?

   YES Go to Step B.

ACTIONS

STEP A: Colposcopy for Diagnosis of Cervical Dysplasia

Cervical colposcopy is a diagnostic test for cervical cancer. It is the test that follows up
   an abnormal Pap smear. The purpose of colposcopy is to determine whether premalignant or malignant cells are present on the cervix. Cervical dysplasia (precancerous cells) cannot be detected by the naked eye. During colposcopy, the trained
   clinician (colposcopist) views the cervix and vagina under magnification with a
   binocular lens and filtered light (the colposcope). A dilute vinegar solution (acetic
   acid) is placed on the cervix and helps to highlight skin changes on the cervix. This
   allows the colposcopist to discern normal from abnormal tissue. Abnormal-appearing
   tissue can be sampled by punch biopsy. Biopsy provides a small sample of tissue for
   further laboratory examination to determine whether it is normal or abnormal, and, if
   abnormal, how deeply it extends into the layers of tissue. An additional biopsy, called
   endocervical curettage (ECC), samples tissue from the inner cervical lining, an area
   that the clinician cannot visualize.

Precolposcopy instructions:
The client should be instructed to schedule her colposcopy when she is not menstruating. COLPOSCOPY CANNOT BE PERFORMED IF THE PATIENT IS MENSTRUAT-
   ING. Menstruating clients must be rescheduled. The procedure takes about 15 minutes and is performed in the office. The patient is placed in the lithotomy position
   (the same position used for Pap smears). The patient should expect some discomfort
   or cramping during and shortly after biopsies are obtained. If the colposcopist ordered
   any preprocedure medications (such as ibuprofen), the client should take it half hour
   before the colposcopy.

Postcolposcopy instructions:
You may return to normal activities after colposcopy.
Expect some bloody, brownish, or "coffee-grounds" discharge for several days.
Do not insert anything vaginally for 5–7 days.

Results (pathology) will be available in 1–2 weeks. The colposcopist's impression plus the biopsy results determine colposcopy follow-up (observation via Pap/colposcopy versus treatment).

Call the office if there is heavy bleeding (like a period), fever, or purulent discharge.

STEP B: Vulvar Colposcopy

Vulvar colposcopy is undertaken for further evaluation of visible external genital lesions. Speculum insertion is not required. The external genitalia are examined under magnification with the colposcope. Abnormal-appearing skin may be biopsied. Local anesthesia may be utilized. The procedure can be scheduled at any time during the patient's cycle. Post procedure, the patient can expect some discomfort and oozing of serosanguinous (pinkish tinged, watery) fluid at the biopsy site. Silver nitrate, applied to the biopsy site to control bleeding, will leave a black stain on the skin that will clear when healed.

It may be wise to advise the patient to schedule vulvar colposcopy and possible biopsy when she anticipates 24–48 hours of limited to light activity. She should be advised to avoid wearing tight-fitting clothing and avoid intercourse or strenuous exercise during this initial period.

Instruct her to call if any frank bleeding occurs that does not stop with pressure to the area. She should apply pressure with a sterile gauze pad for 2–5 minutes.

PATIENT EDUCATION

1. Not every colposcopy ends in biopsy! Patients need to understand that the colposcopy may provide reassurance that the Pap smear was "overcalled."
2. The patient needs to have a plan for receiving her results and a clear understanding of what the plan will be for follow-up once the results are received.
3. The patient may need support while anxiously awaiting these results. Having realistic expectations about when the results will be available may help.

Common Questions Regarding Sexually Transmitted Infections*

Characteristic	Presenting Symptoms	Incubation Period	Mode of Transmission	Usual Course of the Disease	Important Facts
• Bacterial vaginosis	Homogenous white/gray noninflammatory discharge. Patient may report fishy odor, particularly noticeable after intercourse or during menses.	N/A	Associated with multiple partners but can occur in nonsexually active women.	Clinical syndrome resulting from replacement of normal peroxide-producing lactobacillus with increased number of anerobes. Can lead to preterm labor, premature rupture of membranes, endometritis, PID, or vaginal cuff cellulitis.	May occur as an acute or episodic problem; can resolve spontaneously; may become persistent.
• Chancroid (Hemophilus ducreyi)	Initial lesion consists of a small papule with surrounding erythema; covered with gray/yellow necrotic exudate. Ulcer is painful, has ragged edge, is friable (bleeds when touched with swab).	3–7 days, with a range of 10 days.	Sexual	Healing occurs in 2 or more weeks.	Often a cofactor with HIV; 10% may be coinfected with HSV or T. pallidum (syphilis).

Continued

Common Questions Regarding Sexually Transmitted Infections*—cont'd

Characteristic	Presenting Symptoms	Incubation Period	Mode of Transmission	Usual Course of the Disease	Important Facts
• Chlamydia	Mucopurulent discharge. May see cervicitis, bartholinitis, proctitis; PID symptoms; urethritis; spotting/bleeding; dysuria/increased frequency; dyspareunia; fever/malaise.	6–14 days	Sexual intercourse	Can lead to ectopic pregnancy, PID, infertility (male and female).	Often women have no symptoms. Occurs in 15%–20% of sexually active individuals; 20%–40% of people with gonorrhea have concomitant chlamydia.
• Genital herpes (HSV type I, HSV type II)	Primary outbreak: symptoms may be severe. Patient may experience itching, burning, or tingling. Lesions may begin as vesicles or pustules and progress through ulcer stage. Initial lesions may be extensive. Flulike symptoms peak in 3–4 days. Dysuria, urinary retention may occur. Inguinal adenopathy and sacral paresthesia may be complaints. Subsequent outbreak: patient may experience a prodrome, characterized by itching, burning, or tingling before occurrence of lesions. Painful, localized vesicles or small clusters of vesicles may appear. External dysuria may be a complaint. Less extensive systemic symptoms.	Primary outbreak: 2–10 days is usual incubation; up to 21 days reported. Subsequent outbreak: prodrome typically occurs 1–2 days before outbreak.	1. Mucosal contact with HSV secretions. 2. Asymptomatic viral shedding. 3. Human reservoir. 4. Fomite or aerosol transmission is unlikely.	Primary outbreak: lesions start healing in 1–2 weeks. Complete healing takes 3–4 weeks. Viral shedding lasts 11–14 days.	Genital lesion maybe type I or type II. Many patients with recurrent lesions benefit from episodic or suppressive therapy.

Disease (Organism)	Signs/Symptoms	Incubation	Transmission	Sequelae	Notes
• Gonorrhea (*Neisseria gonorrhoeae*)	Cervicitis, urethritis, Skene's or Bartholin's abscess, or rectal or pharyngeal symptoms. Some may report back or abdominal pain or cramping. May state symptoms are worse postmenstrually. Disseminated: asymmetrically arthralgic, septic arthritis, perinephritis, endocarditis.	3–5 days	Sexual; fomite transmission rare; 80%–90% transmission male to female with single act of intercourse.	Serious sequelae: PID in 15%–20% of infected women. Ectopic pregnancy greater after infection. Disseminated infection.	600,000 cases yearly; 20% of women with gonorrhea are coinfected with chlamydia.
• Granuloma inguinale (*Calymmatobacterium granulomatis* also called donovanosis)	Painless, progressive ulcerative lesion. No regional lymphadenopathy.	1–4 weeks (to 6 months); difficult to determine, but probably averages 3–40 days.	Many cases appear not to be sexually transmitted, but 80% do appear in the genital region.	Tissue destruction can appear 2–10 years after infection. Extragenital lesions may occur from self-inoculation.	Rare in the United States

Continued

Common Questions Regarding Sexually Transmitted Infections*—cont'd

Characteristic	Presenting Symptoms	Incubation Period	Mode of Transmission	Usual Course of the Disease	Important Facts
• Hepatitis A	Some patients, particularly children, may be asymptomatic. Nausea and vomiting, with resultant dehydration, may be seen. Hospitalization may be needed for patients who become dehydrated because of nausea and vomiting.	Approximately 28 days, range is 15–50 days.	Primarily transmitted by the fecal-oral route, by either person-to-person contact or consumption of contaminated food or water. Use of illegal drugs, foreign travel, and men having sex with men have also been identified as modes of transmission.	Usually a self-limiting disease. CDC estimates 10%–15% of patients may experience a relapse of symptoms during the 6 months after acute illness. Acute liver failure is rare.	Those with hepatitis typically receive symptomatic care. Hospitalization may be warranted in cases of liver failure or severe dehydration. Medications that are metabolized by the liver are used cautiously in patients with hepatitis A. Usually not considered sexually transmitted.
• Hepatitis B	Only half of these patients will be symptomatic. About 1% of cases result in liver failure and death. Risk of chronic infection is inversely related to age.	Incubation from time of exposure to onset of symptoms averages 6 weeks to 6 months.	Blood and other body fluids (semen, vaginal secretions, wound exudates).	Can be self-limited or chronic. Among those with chronic HBV, the risk of premature death due to cirrhosis or hepatocellular CA is 15%–25%.	Vaccination (both single-antigen vaccine and combination vaccine) is available and recommended. Those who are exposed to hepatitis B should receive a single IM dose of Ig (0.02 mL/kg) as soon as possible, but not more than 2 weeks after exposure. All pregnant women receiving STD services should be tested for HBsAg. Those who are HBsAg-positive should be reported to state/local perinatal hepatitis prevention programs.

Those who are HB-Ags positive should be referred to an infectious-disease specialist for counseling and monitoring. Sex partners should be counseled on measures to diminish exposure risk. Also, patients should be advised to use protection with sex partners (condoms); cover cuts and skin lesions to prevent spread of infectious secretions or blood; refrain from donating blood or blood products, organs, or other tissues; and refrain from using household or personal items (toothbrushes, razors, etc). Limiting alcohol or medications that are metabolized through the liver is helpful.

Continued

Common Questions Regarding Sexually Transmitted Infections*—cont'd

Characteristic	Presenting Symptoms	Incubation Period	Mode of Transmission	Usual Course of the Disease	Important Facts
• Hepatitis C	Patients are often asymptomatic or have mild flu-like symptoms.	HCV RNA can be detected in blood within 1–3 weeks after exposure. Average time from exposure to seroconversion (anti-HCV) is 8–9 weeks.	Often transmitted through large or repeated percutaneous exposure to infected blood (transfusion, drug injection). Also seen in occupational, perinatal, and sexual exposures.	Chronic HCB develops in 60%–85% of those infected; 60%–70% of those with chronic HCV will have evidence of active liver disease.	Most common bloodborne infection in the United States. HCV testing recommended as a routine screening measure, but not recommended for pregnant women who do not have a known HCV risk factor. To protect the liver, HCV patients should be counseled to avoid alcohol; not take new medications until cleared by the provider; not donate blood, organs, or tissues; and cover cuts and sores to reduce the risk of spreading the infection. Those with one long-term, steady partner do not need to change sexual practices. Referral of a chronic infectious disease specialist may be warranted for those who experience chronic liver disease.

• HIV	Many patients may be asymptomatic for quite awhile. Those who present will typically have symptoms of immunodeficiency (opportunistic infections, weight loss, etc.).	Variable. CDC recommends HIV testing as a routine part of medical care, and that all patients 13–64 years old should receive HIV screening unless established diagnostic yield is <1 per 1,000 patients screened.	Can be transmitted percutaneously and by intercourse (both heterosexual and homosexual), pregnancy, and breastfeeding.	In untreated patients, time between infection and development of AIDS can be from a few months to 17 years (median: 10 years).	Providing important pretest information and securing informed consent for testing are critical. The CDC recommends universal HIV screening preconceptually (if possible) or early in pregnancy, since antiretroviral medications, C/S delivery, and avoidance of breastfeeding have been associated with diminished rates of mother-to-fetus/baby transmission.

Continued

Common Questions Regarding Sexually Transmitted Infections*—cont'd

Characteristic	Presenting Symptoms	Incubation Period	Mode of Transmission	Usual Course of the Disease	Important Facts
• Human Papilloma virus (HPV)	May be totally asymptomatic. External HPV lesions may present as multiple or single pink/brown soft papules on genitalia, or sharply demarcated white flat plaques on the cervix. Fleshy papules may become a confluent cauliflower-like mass.	Precise time from exposure to overt lesions is quite variable and depends of the type of HPV virus, the patient's immune status, and other factors.	Sexual intercourse or skin-to-skin contact. Route of transmission from mother to infant is not well understood.	Course of the disease varies tremendously with host immune response and type of HPV virus exposure.	Approximately 100 HPV types have been identified, and more than 40 of these infect the genital area. On average, 70% of cervical cancers worldwide are caused by HPV types 16 and 18 (DHHS Advisory Committee on Immunization Practices, 2007). HPV vaccine (Gardisil) is now available in the U.S. It targets HPV types 6, 11, 16, and 18. The CDC (2007) recommends that all women 13–26 years of age be vaccinated, but the vaccine can be given to girls age 9 and older. The vaccine is given in three doses, with administration of dose 2 two months after the first dose, and dose 3–4 months after the second dose.
• Lympho-granuloma venereum (caused by any of 3 L serotypes of *Chlamydia trachomatis*)	Primary: painless papule; ulcer (rare). Secondary: tender lymphadenopathy, fistulas and strictures in peri-anal/perirectal area; inguinal bulboes.	1–3 weeks; lymphadenopathy occurs 7–30 days after lesion.	Sexual	Ulceration is a minor feature of this disease.	Epidemiology in the United States is basically unknown; largest number of cases clustered in New York City.

Organism	Signs/Symptoms	Transmission	Incubation	Comments
• Syphilis (*Treponema pallidum*)	Tertiary: progressive anal symptoms with constitutional effect. Primary: papule or chancre 10–50 days after exposure. Painless ulcer. Inguinal or cervical adenopathy 7–10 days after lesions. No systemic symptoms. Secondary: onset 3–6 weeks after primary infection. May overlap with primary infection. Patient may have no symptoms or may have lymphadenopathy or systemic symptoms. Flulike symptoms in 50% of cases. Maculopapular rash may occur (80%). May have condyloma lata, which resemble warts. Alopecia may occur.	Sexual	Mean incubation is 3 weeks in primary cases.	Chancre occurs at site of inoculation and disappears in 2–6 weeks unless superinfected. Secondary symptoms may appear as long as 10 weeks after primary chancre, if initially untreated. Often a co-factor with HIV infection.
• Trichomoniasis	Commonly include diffuse, malodorous, yellow-green vaginal discharge with vulvar irritation. Men may present with complaint of mild penile irritation. Some patients may be asymptomatic.	Typically transmitted through sexual contact, although fomite transmission (e.g., inanimate objects such as wet towels) have been implicated.	1–4 weeks	If untreated, patient may experience development of diffuse, malodorous, yellow-green vaginal discharge and/or vulvar irritation. Associated with increased risk of HIV susceptibility, prematurity, low birth weight. Metronidazole given as a single 2 gram treatment is safe in pregnancy (Category B). Women who are breastfeeding can reduce their baby's exposure by withholding breastfeeding (and pumping) for 12–24 hours after last dose of metronidazole.

Common Questions Regarding Sexually Transmitted Infections*—cont'd

Characteristic	Presenting Symptoms	Incubation Period	Mode of Transmission	Usual Course of the Disease	Important Facts
	Latent: gumma occurs on skin, bone, liver, brain, and heart. Cardiovascular symptoms: aortic aneurysm, aortic insufficiency. Coronary artery disease (uncommon) 5–10 years after infection. Tertiary: rare (neurologic).			Latent: appears 2–10 years after infection. Tertiary: appears 2–35 years after infection.	
Vaginitis: • Vulvovaginal candidiasis (*C. albicans; C. tropicalis; C. glabrata*)	Curdy, white discharge; pruritus; erythema; vaginal soreness; vulvar burning; external dysuria; dyspareunia.	N/A	Causative substances: antibiotic use; stress; steroids, altered immune status; 15% of men harbor yeast in seminal fluid.	May be self-limited or progress.	5% of women experience recurrent episodes. Rarely considered sexually transmitted.

*Information extracted from the CDC's Sexually Transmitted Disease Guidelines (2006). These are available on the Web at: http://www.cdc.gov/std/treatment/2006/rr5511.pdf.

The CDC (2006) has published revised recommendations for HIB testing of adults, adolescents and pregnant women. These are available online at: http://www.cdc.gov/mmwr/preview/mmwrhtml/rr5514a1.htm

The CDC has published excellent information on HBsAg-positive pregnant women and their infants. This information is available on the Web at: http://www.cdc.gov/mmwr/PDF/rr/rr5426.pdf.

Centers for Disease Control and Prevention (CDC), Division of Sexually Transmitted Disease Prevention: National Immunization Program (NIP), HPV vaccine information statement sheet (VIS) (2007). Retrieved May 17, 2008, from http://www.cdc.gov/std/hpv.

Department of Health and Human Services (HHS), Advisory Committee on Immunization Practices (ACIP): Quadrivalent Human Papillomavirus Vaccine Recommendations (2007). Retrieved May 17, 2008, from http://www.cdc.gov/mmwr/preview/mmwrhtml/rr56e312a1.htm.

Cryosurgery

KEY QUESTIONS

ASSESSMENT

ACTION

1. Are you experiencing a vaginal discharge?

YES Go to Step A.

NO Go to Question 2.

2. Do you have an oral temperature greater than 100°F?

YES Go to Step B.

NO Go to Question 3.

3. Are you having vaginal bleeding that is heavier than a menstrual period?

YES Go to Step C.

NO Go to Question 4.

4. Are you experiencing a foul vaginal odor?

YES Go to Step D.

NO No further action.

ACTIONS

STEP A: Vaginal Discharge

Patients often experience a thick, gray or brown discharge after cryosurgery. The thick, mucous-laden discharge after cryosurgery occurs as frozen cervical cells slough.
If the discharge is accompanied by a foul odor, instruct the patient to take her temperature. If she has an oral temperature greater than 100°F or the vaginal discharge smells foul or fishy, schedule a same-day appointment to evaluate the patient for infection.
Complete questions 2–4 for a thorough assessment.

STEP B: Fever

Temperature rarely exceeds 100°F after cryosurgery.
An oral temperature greater than 100°F may indicate an infection. The patient should receive a same-day appointment.
Complete questions 3 and 4.

STEP C: Bleeding

More than minimal bleeding is extremely rare after cryosurgery.
Confirm that the bleeding is not the patient's normal menstrual period.
If the bleeding soils more than one pad in 2 hours or is accompanied by heavy clots, the patient should be seen in the office immediately.
Continue to Question 4.

STEP D: Vaginal Odor

As frozen vaginal cells slough, the patient may notice a fleshy vaginal odor.

If the patient reports a foul or fishy odor or has a temperature greater than 100°F, schedule a same-day appointment to determine if she has an infection.

PATIENT EDUCATION

1. Cryosurgery is not done if the patient is pregnant or menstruating.
2. Advise the patient of the following:
   - Do not use tampons for at least 2 weeks.
   - Avoid intercourse for 2 weeks.
   - Watery discharge without odor is normal for 1–2 weeks.

Endometrial Ablation

KEY QUESTIONS

ASSESSMENT	ACTION
1. Are you considering an endometrial ablation?	**YES** Go to Step A. **NO** Go to Question 2.
2. Are you scheduled for an endometrial ablation?	**YES** Go to Step B. **NO** Continue to Question 3.
3. Have you had a recent endometrial ablation?	**YES** Go to Step C. **NO** No Action.

ACTIONS

STEP A: Overview of Endometrial Ablation

The lining of the uterus is known as the endometrium. Each month, the endometrium is shed during a woman's menstrual period. Some women, particularly those who are approaching menopause, may experience heavy, frequent, or lengthy menstrual periods. These types of menstrual periods can be managed with medications, but some women may not be able to take such medications or would like to control their menses by a procedure known as endometrial ablation.

Endometrial ablation uses sound waves, electrical, laser, or thermal (heat) energy to destroy a thin layer of the endometrium, resulting in either cessation of menstrual bleeding, much lighter menstrual flow, or spotting. Because endometrial ablation destroys a layer of the endometrium, it should not be done on women who would like to have more children. Although this procedure generally results in infertility, women who have had an ablation should use backup contraception until hormone and other tests indicate they are in menopause.

Endometrial ablation takes very little time and is usually done either in an outpatient surgicenter or an office. Patients typically receive mild sedation for the procedure, so they will need to be accompanied by someone who can drive them home. After the procedure, some women experience mild menstrual-like cramps for a day or two, a watery blood-tinged discharge, mild nausea, and increased urination for about 24 hours. Women typically return to their normal activities the day after the procedure.

Potential risks associated with ablation include blood loss, infection, fluid retention, uterine perforation, or reactions to any pain medications that are administered. The rate of such risks is extremely low.

STEP B: Preparing for an Endometrial Ablation

Before the ablation, the provider may order a complete blood cell count (CBC) to rule out anemia or infection. An ultrasound is usually ordered because the presence of a fibroid (benign growth in or on the uterus) or other uterine abnormality may help the gynecologist determine which type of ablation approach is best. If the provider suspects that the lining of the uterus is out of phase or wants to rule out a problem with the lining of the uterus, an EMB may be performed.

Ablation is usually avoided during menstruation. Ablation is usually a same-day surgery procedure and analgesia/anesthesia is required. Consequently, the patient should have no food or liquids for 10–12 hours prior to the ablation or per the protocol where the procedure will be performed.

No incisions are required for an ablation, and the patient can be expected to be discharged to home about 2 hours after the procedure is completed. Since patients receive sedation, they should be accompanied by someone who can drive them home. The majority of patients return to normal activities the day after the ablation.

STEP C: What to Expect Following an Endometrial Ablation

Common minor side effects associated with ablation include:

- mild, menstrual-like cramps for 1–2 days;
- increased urination for 24 hours after the procedure;
- a small amount of watery vaginal discharge. The discharge may be blood-tinged and this discharge can last for several weeks;
- nausea.

Douching, intercourse, or use of tampons is usually avoided for 2 weeks. Also, a method of contraception (such as condoms) is recommended.

If the patient reports heavy vaginal bleeding (more than a menstrual period) or shortness of breath, a provider should be contacted immediately. Women who complain of increased swelling, unusual vaginal odor, or fever should receive a same-day appointment.

Endometrial Biopsy (EMB)

KEY QUESTIONS

ASSESSMENT	ACTION
1. Is the patient scheduled for an office EMB?	**YES** Go to Step A.
	NO Proceed to Question 2.
2. Was the EMB ordered to evaluate postmenopausal bleeding?	**YES** Go to Step B.
	NO Continue to Question 3.
3. Was the EMB ordered to follow up an abnormal Pap smear?	**YES** Go to Step C.
	NO Go to Question 4.
4. Was the EMB ordered to evaluate abnormal uterine bleeding in a premenopausal woman?	**YES** Go to Step D.
	NO Go to Patient Education.

ACTIONS

STEP A: Provide General Information About the EMB Procedure

An EMB is a procedure in which a tissue sample is obtained from the uterine lining, or endometrium. EMBs are generally done to see if the lining of the uterus is growing in an organized way, is out of phase with what typically should be occurring, or is growing abnormally. The EMB is performed in the office and requires no anesthesia. If the provider has ordered any preprocedure medications (such as an NSAID or diazepam [Valium]), the patient should be instructed to take them ½ hour before the procedure. EMB cannot be performed during pregnancy.

The EMB sample is obtained by passing a thin straw-like device (called a pipelle) or a narrow instrument (called a curette) through the cervix and into the uterus. Gentle suction is applied to draw the tissue through the pipelle or curette. The client should be advised that she might experience a cramping sensation during the procedure. The tissue sample is sent to the laboratory for analysis. The procedure takes 5–10 minutes. Results may take 1–2 weeks.

After the EMB, the patient may experience cramping. She may note a small amount of bleeding or spotting. Heavy bleeding, purulent discharge, or fever should be reported to the health care provider.

STEP B: EMB for Postmenopausal Bleeding (Intact Uterus)

Postmenopausal bleeding is almost always considered abnormal and requires evaluation. Causes of bleeding in postmenopausal women include endometrial cancer, cervical cancer, endometrial polyps, and uterine fibroids.

STEP C: EMB for Abnormal Pap Smear

EMB is performed in addition to colposcopy when the Pap smear is reported to have abnormal glandular cells. Follow the protocol for colposcopy for additional information and instructions.

Pregnancy must be ruled out prior to performing the EMB.

STEP D: EMB for Abnormal Uterine Bleeding in a Premenopausal Woman

Abnormal uterine bleeding in premenopausal women, especially those in the perimenopausal period, is commonly due to an overgrowth of the uterine lining (endometrial hyperplasia) that is caused by hormonal imbalance and anovulation. Other causes include uterine fibroids, endometrial polyps, endometrial cancer, cervical cancer, and pregnancy.

A negative pregnancy test is required prior to the EMB if pregnancy is a possibility.

PATIENT EDUCATION

1. Some providers may advise the patient to take an NSAID (such as Advil, Motrin, or Aleve) ½–1 hour before the procedure to decrease the cramping sensation. Diazepam (Valium) or a similar tranquilizer may be prescribed for patients who are unusually nervous. Providers may ask the patient to have someone accompany them in the event they feel unsteady or unable to transport themselves after the procedure.
2. The results of the EMB are typically available within 1–2 weeks. The provider may either contact the patient over the telephone regarding the results of this test, or schedule a follow-up visit to discuss the results and any further tests or treatments that may be required.
3. Occasionally, an EMB is performed as part of an infertility evaluation. The instructions and procedure are the same in this situation.

Laparoscopy

ASSESSMENT

ACTION

1. Are you experiencing abdominal soreness?

YES Go to Step A.

NO Go to Question 2.

2. Are you experiencing neck or shoulder pain?

YES Go to Step B.

NO Go to Question 3.

3. Do you have an oral temperature greater than 100°F?

YES Go to Step C.

NO Go to Question 4.

4. Are you experiencing any bleeding?

YES Go to Step D.

NO Go to Question 5.

5. Is your incision clean, dry, and intact?

YES If the answer to the four previous questions is "no," the patient should have a follow-up appointment 4 to 6 weeks after laparoscopy.

NO Go to Step E.

ACTIONS

STEP A: Abdominal Soreness

Some abdominal soreness may occur after laparoscopy.

For soreness, the patient can take acetaminophen 650 mg every 4–6 hours or an analgesic prescribed by the provider who performed the laparoscopy.

If soreness persists or pain is reported as severe, schedule a same-day appointment for the patient.

If the soreness is accompanied by bleeding that is heavier than a normal menstrual period, see the patient immediately.

Be certain to check allergies if recommending pain medication as per your office or clinic protocol.

STEP B: Neck or Shoulder Pain

Neck or shoulder pain may occur as a result of the gas used to inflate the abdomen.

If neck or shoulder pain is accompanied by shortness of breath or faintness, the patient should contact the provider who performed the laparoscopy.

If there are no symptoms other than shoulder pain, the patient can take an analgesic prescribed at the time of laparoscopy or acetaminophen 650 mg every 4–6 hours, as directed by the manufacturer.

Be certain to check allergies if recommending pain medication as per your office or clinic protocol.

Application of a heating pad or heat pack to the neck and shoulder may help relieve soreness.

STEP C: Fever

A low-grade fever may be present. However, an oral temperature greater than 100°F may be a sign of infection.

If the patient's temperature is greater than 100°F, she should be scheduled for a same-day appointment.

STEP D: Bleeding

Minimal blood loss should occur after a laparoscopy.

Small amounts of oozing or bleeding may occur at the site of the incision. If there is more than slight bleeding or oozing, the patient should be scheduled for a same-day appointment. If bleeding is minimal, the incision site may be cleansed with hydrogen peroxide.

Vaginal bleeding should not exceed that of a normal menstrual period. Make sure that any vaginal bleeding is not the patient's normal menstrual period.

If vaginal bleeding is heavier than a period, have the patient perform a pad count. If more than one pad is saturated in a 2-hour period or there are clots larger than a quarter, the patient should be seen immediately.

STEP E: Incision

A normal incision should be clean, dry, and intact.

If the incision has a foul odor or the discharge is colored, have the patient take her temperature and refer to Step C.

The patient should receive a same-day appointment for evaluation of her incision.

PATIENT EDUCATION

Advise the patient that discomfort from gas reabsorption may be significant during the first 24–48 hours.

Lost Pessary

KEY QUESTIONS

ASSESSMENT	ACTION
1. Is the pessary in your vagina?	**YES** Go to Question 3.
	NO Go to Question 2.
2. Do you want to reinsert your pessary?	**YES** Go to Question 4.
	NO Instruct the patient to follow up with her care provider.
3. Is the pessary embedded in your vagina?	**YES** Go to Step B.
	NO Go to Question 4.
4. Do you suspect that you presently have a vaginal/pelvic infection?	**YES** Instruct the patient to follow up with her care provider.
	NO Go to Step A.

ACTION

STEP A: How to Reinsert a Pessary

Provide the patient with the following instructions regarding pessary insertion:
- Clean the pessary with mild soap and water before insertion.
- Wash your hands.
- Lubricate the pessary with a water-soluble lubricant and fold it in half before insertion. Spread the lips of your vagina, press down on the perineum, and push the pessary as far back in the vagina as possible. Insertion can be done while standing, sitting, or lying down.
- Fit the pessary as taught by your care provider.
- After the pessary is inserted, try different positions, such as standing, sitting, walking, and squatting, to determine if the pessary fits well without pain.

Follow up with your health care provider a few days after you have reinserted the pessary to have the fitting checked. It is possible the pessary fell out because it is too small. If you have symptoms that indicate a possible vaginal infection (vaginitis) or a pelvic infection, do **not** reinsert the pessary. Infections are contraindications to pessary placement.

STEP B: How to Manage an Embedded Pessary

A pessary can become embedded in the vaginal mucosa and may be difficult to remove. Instruct the patient to lubricate the vagina around the pessary with some estrogen cream. This may decrease vaginal inflammation, making it easier to remove
the pessary. This method may take several applications and a little bit of time.

Instruct the patient to find the rim of the pessary, gently pull down/up on it, gently
squeeze it to reduce its size, and slowly pull it from her vagina. If the patient cannot do this successfully, she should make an appointment with her care provider
for assistance with pessary removal.

PATIENT EDUCATION

A pessary cannot get lost in the body. It is either located in the vagina or has fallen out
of the body. If the patient cannot feel the pessary with her fingers anywhere in her
vagina, it most likely has fallen out. If the patient cannot find the pessary but does not
think it has fallen out, she may want to see her care provider for a speculum examination to see if the pessary can be located.

There are many types of pessaries, including the doughnut, Gehrung, Gellhorn,
Hodge's with knob, ring, Risser, Shaatz, Smith's, and tandem cube. Because of their
various shapes and styles, each is fitted slightly different. The patient should notify
her care provider if she does not remember what kind of pessary she has or can't remember the insertion/removal instructions, or cleaning instructions.

Pelvic Pain

ASSESSMENT	ACTION
1. Are you having pelvic pain?	**YES** Go to Question 2.
	NO No treatment necessary.
2. Are you having vaginal bleeding associated with the pain?	**YES** Go to Question 3.
	NO Go to Step A. Continue to Question 3.
3. Do you think you could be pregnant?	**YES** Go to Step A.
	NO Go to Question 4.
4. Are you having any of the following associated symptoms: fever, chills, nausea, vomiting, diarrhea, or abnormal vaginal discharge?	**YES** Go to Step B.
	NO Go to Question 5.
5. Have you had unprotected sex or possible exposure to a sexually transmitted disease?	**YES** Go to Step B.
	NO Go to Question 6.
6. Do you have any urinary symptoms, such as increased frequency, urgency, or blood in the urine? Is there any back pain associated with the symptoms?	**YES** Go to Step C.
	NO Go to Question 7.
7. Do you have a history of abdominal or pelvic surgeries?	**YES** Go to Step D.
	NO No further action.

ACTIONS

STEP A: Pelvic Pain, Vaginal Bleeding, and Pregnancy Possible

If the patient meets the criteria for serious, heavy bleeding, she should be seen ASAP. The patient should not drive herself. If there is any loss of consciousness or sensorimotor skills, the patient or her agent should call 911. If the bleeding is light, proceed as follows:

- Refer to protocol 1st Trimester Bleeding.
- Rule out the possibility of ectopic pregnancy before any other evaluation.
- Even if the patient thinks pregnancy is not possible, the possibility of ectopic pregnancy should be eliminated.

If pelvic pain is present, with or without bleeding, and pregnancy has been eliminated as a possibility, the timing of evaluation of the patient should be based on the severity of pain.

- If the patient reports severe pain, she should be seen within 1–3 hours or go to an ER or urgent care center.
- If the patient reports moderate pain, she should be seen within 24 hours. Advise her to call back or go to the ER if the pain worsens.
- If the patient reports mild pain, she should be seen within 48–96 hours. Advise the patient to call back or go to the ER if the pain worsens.

STEP B: Pelvic Pain, Possible Exposure to Sexually Transmitted Infection

If the patient's temperature is greater than 100.4° F, she should be seen that day for appropriate evaluation.

If the patient has a mild temperature elevation with or without the other symptoms mentioned, she should be seen within 24–48 hours.

Advise the patient to avoid sexual intercourse until she has undergone evaluation.

STEP C: Pelvic Pain With Blood in the Urine and/or Back Pain

Ask the patient if she has a fever. If her temperature is greater than 100.4° F, she should be seen that day for evaluation for a kidney infection.

Question the patient regarding any history of kidney stones. If she has such a history or her symptoms are consistent with spasmodic, moderate to severe pain, she should see her primary care provider or go to the ER or an urgent care center.

STEP D: Pelvic Pain, History of Abdominal Surgeries, Possible Adhesions

Question the patient regarding the timing and nature of her last surgery.

If the procedure was done within the last 2–10 days, refer the patient to her surgeon within 24 hours.

If the patient's temperature is greater than 100.4° F and she had surgery within the last 2 weeks, she should report her symptoms to her surgeon that day.

If the patient has a history of surgery (more than 4–6 weeks ago), she should discuss her symptoms with her surgeon to decide on the timing of an appointment. Depending on the type of surgery, some discomfort may be expected for as long as 6 months.

PATIENT EDUCATION

1. Pelvic pain can have a variety of causes, including a vaginal infection, an ectopic pregnancy, an ovarian cyst, adhesions from old surgeries, kidney stones, or constipation.
2. It is important to have this pain evaluated because of the following potential complications:
   - infertility,
   - ruptured ectopic pregnancy,
   - tubo-ovarian abscess,
   - pelvic adhesions, and
   - chronic pelvic pain.

Trapped Tampon

KEY QUESTIONS

ASSESSMENT

ACTION

1. Is the tampon in your vagina?

YES Go to Step A.

NO Go to Question 2.

2. Do you suspect that you have a vaginal/pelvic infection?

YES Go to Step B.

NO No further action.

ACTIONS

STEP A: How to Manage a Lost Tampon

A tampon can become lost in the vagina and may be difficult to remove. Instruct the patient to try lubricating her vagina around the tampon with some water-soluble lubricant. This may decrease vaginal inflammation and make it easier to remove the tampon. This method may take several applications and a little bit of time.

Once the patient finds the end of the tampon or the string, she should gently pull down/up on it, gently squeeze it to reduce its size, and slowly pull it from her vagina. If the patient cannot do this successfully, she should make a same-day appointment with her care provider for assistance with tampon removal.

STEP B: Suspected Infection

If the tampon has been in place for more than 24–48 hours, the patient should come to the office for additional evaluation.

Signs of potential infection include:

- fever,
- pelvic pain,
- fishy or foul odor, and
- unusual vaginal discharge.

If any of these signs are present, the patient should be scheduled for a same-day clinical evaluation.

Urinary Tract Infection Symptoms

ASSESSMENT

ACTION

1. Are you experiencing symptoms of burning while urinating, frequency of urination, or urgency to void?

YES Go to Question 2.

NO Not applicable.

2. Are you experiencing any back pain, nausea, or fever?

YES Go to Step A.

NO Go to Question 3.

3. Is the pain occurring as urine flows over the vulvar region?

YES Go to Step B.

NO Go to Step C.

ACTIONS

STEP A: Symptoms Accompanied by Back Pain, Nausea, or Fever

The patient may be at risk for a kidney infection.

Instruct the patient to come into the office or clinic ASAP to leave a urine sample for culture. (The patient should not collect the sample at home.)

The patient should have an opportunity to discuss symptoms with a provider when she leaves the clean-caught urine sample because a prescription for antibiotics may be given.

Encourage the patient to drink lots of fluids until she is seen for evaluation.

Instruct the patient to call if her symptoms worsen before her scheduled appointment. If necessary, she should go to the ER after office/clinic hours.

STEP B: Vulvar Burning With Urination

The patient may have lesions in the vulvar area. Her symptoms may not be urinary in origin, but the lesions are irritated by the presence of urine.

The patient should be seen within 24–48 hours for evaluation.

Instruct the patient to wash her hands thoroughly after urination.

Cold compresses or tepid baths may be soothing.

Instruct the patient not to apply creams or lotions to lesions until her condition has been diagnosed.

STEP C: Urinary Tract Infection Symptoms Not Complicated by Nausea, Back Pain, Fever, or Vulvar Burning

Instruct the patient to come in to leave a clean-caught urine sample for culture and sensitivity testing.

Encourage the patient to drink lots of fluids until she is seen for evaluation.

PATIENT EDUCATION

1. Patients often begin taking an antibiotic they previously have had prescribed. Instruct the patient to take no antibiotics; taking such drugs may taint the urine culture and delay proper treatment.
2. Patients may use over-the-counter Uristat as a bladder analgesic or another product your office or clinic recommends.

Vaginal Discharge With Pessary

ASSESSMENT

ACTION

1. Have you noticed a change in your vaginal
   discharge without any other symptoms?

   YES Go to Step A.

   NO Go to Question 2.

2. Do you have any of the following symptoms:
   vaginal itching, burning while urinating, frequency
   or urgency of urination, fever or chills, or low back/
   abdominal pain?

   YES Go to Step B.

   NO No further action.

ACTIONS

STEP A: Change in Discharge

If discharge is present, advise the patient as follows:

Remove your pessary.
Reinsert your pessary as directed:
  • Clean your pessary with mild soap and water before insertion.
  • Wash your hands.
  • Lubricate the pessary with a water-soluble lubricant and fold in half before insertion. Spread the lips of your vagina, press down on the perineum, and push the pessary as far back in the vagina as possible. Insertion can be done while standing, sitting, or lying down.
  • Fit your pessary as you were taught by your care provider.
  • After insertion, you should try different positions, such as standing, sitting, walking, and squatting, to determine if the pessary fits well without pain.
Instruct the patient to follow up with her care provider a few days after reinserting the pessary to have the fitting checked. It is possible that the pessary fell out because it is too small.

STEP B: What to Do if Having Symptoms

Instruct the patient to remove the pessary.
If the patient's temperature is greater than 100°F, schedule a same-day appointment for her.
If the patient has no fever and no bleeding, schedule an appointment for her within 3–5 days.

If the patient experiences burning on urination, instruct her to provide a urine sample for culture.

Instruct the patient to call back if her symptoms worsen before her scheduled appointment.

PATIENT EDUCATION

Vaginal discharge is the most common side effect of pessary wear.

Vulvovaginitis With Lesions

ASSESSMENT

ACTION

1. Is there a change in the odor, color, or amount of vaginal discharge?

YES Go to Question 2.

NO Go to Question 2.

2. Are you experiencing vaginal itching or burning?

YES Go to Question 3.

NO Go to Question 3.

3. Do you have any burning during or after urination?

YES Go to Question 4.

NO Go to Question 4.

4. Can you feel any bumps or lesions?

YES Go to Step A.

NO Not applicable.

5. Do you have a history of any vulvovaginal lesions?

YES Go to Step B.

NO Go to next question.

6. Are you concerned you may have been exposed to an STI?

YES Go to Step C.

NO Go to Step A.

ACTIONS

STEP A: Lesions Present

Although indications may be pointing to an STI, it is important patients are reminded there are benign lesions in the vaginal area, such as skin tags and sebaceous cysts. Emphasize that a diagnosis cannot be given over the telephone!

Schedule an appointment for the patient to come in within 24 hours.

Advise the patient to wash her hands thoroughly after urination.

Advise the patient to avoid sexual intercourse until she has been seen for evaluation.

STEP B: Recurrent Lesions

Patients may know they have a recurrence of herpes or genital warts. Patients may also have a recurring medical condition such as dysplastic mole, previously diagnosed melanoma, or vaginal intraepithelial neoplasia, which makes them think they have a return of the disorder.

If patient has a history of recurrent herpes, she may request suppressive therapy that has worked in the past.

If the patient thinks she has a recurrence of any lesion, she should be offered an appointment within 72 hours to confirm her suspicions.

If the patient has a history of serious lesions, she should be seen as soon as possible to relieve her anxiety.

Instruct the patient to avoid intercourse if she thinks she has a return of lesions that could be transmitted to others.

STEP C: Possible Exposure to a Sexually Transmitted Infection

The anxiety level will be high in these patients!

Ask the patient if she is experiencing pain associated with the lesion.

If the patient is experiencing pain, offer comfort measures as recommended by your providers.

Advise the patient to wash her hands after urination.

Advise the patient to avoid sexual intercourse until she has been seen for evaluation.

Make an appointment for the patient to be seen within 24 hours.

PATIENT EDUCATION

1. Patients with vulvovaginitis symptoms associated with lesions are always anxious and often distraught. Offer as much comfort as possible without giving false reassurances.
2. Patients may want to know what you think they "have." Be consistent in letting them know such conditions cannot be diagnosed over the telephone. Encourage her to avoid self-diagnosis over the internet.
3. For questions about specific diseases, see Common Questions Regarding Sexually Transmitted Diseases.
4. Patients need to be informed of when they should return for follow-up, for evaluation of reinfection.

Vulvovaginitis Without Lesions

KEY QUESTIONS

ASSESSMENT

ACTION

1. Is there a change in odor, color, or the amount of vaginal discharge?

YES Go to Question 2.
NO Go to Question 2.

2. Are you having vaginal itching?

YES Go to Question 3.
NO Go to Question 3.

3. Do you have any burning with urination?

YES Go to Step A.
NO Go to Question 4.

4. Are you concerned you could have been exposed to a sexually transmitted infection?

YES Go to Step B.
NO Go to Question 5.

5. Have you been douching frequently?

YES Go to Step C.
NO Go to Question 6.

6. Is there any possibility there is a foreign body in your vagina?

YES Go to Step D.
NO Go to Step E.

ACTION

STEP A: Vulvovaginitis Symptoms With Dysuria

This patient may have lesions present and should be seen within 24–48 hours.
Instruct the patient to wash her hands thoroughly after urination.
Advise the patient to avoid applying creams or lotions to the area until she has been seen for evaluation.
Instruct the patient in the use of comfort measures, such as cold compresses or tepid baths, that may be soothing.
Advise the patient to avoid sexual intercourse until she has been seen for evaluation.
Yeast infections also can mimic urinary tract infection symptoms. Explain to the patient that she may be asked to provide a clean-caught urine sample.

STEP B: Possible Exposure to a Sexually Transmitted Infection

The patient should be instructed to come in within 24 hours for a thorough evaluation.
Advise the patient that she may have to undergo cultures and blood tests.
Advise the patient to avoid sexual intercourse until she has been seen for evaluation.

STEP C: Frequent Douching

Inquire as to what the patient has used as a douche.

Educate the patient regarding disruption of the acid/base balance.

Recommend the patient stop douching.

If symptoms do not abate with cessation of douching, the patient should be seen within 72 hours.

STEP D: Possible Foreign Body

Instruct the patient to try to remove a trapped tampon or diaphragm in the bath or shower, where warm water may help with relaxation.

Advise the patient that discharge usually will cease once the article is removed. If odor or discharge persists beyond 24 hours, the patient should call back to schedule an appointment.

If the patient is uncomfortable trying to examine herself or fails to remove the article, instruct her to come into the office or clinic within 24 hours.

STEP E: Vulvovaginitis Symptoms, Etiology Unknown

Question the patient about recent antibiotic use or changes in toilet tissue, bubble baths, or laundry detergent.

Question the patient regarding the time of her last menstrual cycle.

Question the patient regarding frequency of this problem.

Instruct the patient in the comfort measures recommended by your providers.

Make an appointment for the patient to come in within 72 hours.

PATIENT EDUCATION

1. As mentioned, many patients self-diagnose these conditions and may request specific medication prescriptions based on past symptom resolution. Whether or not to treat over the telephone without seeing the patient will be at the discretion of your providers. Many offices or clinics have a policy to treat simple symptoms of yeast infections or bacterial vaginosis without seeing the patient, however, most providers will treat only once. If the patient experiences no improvement, she should be seen for evaluation.

2. Our goal is not to miss a more serious, possibly communicable infection. If a patient is fairly certain she has been exposed to an STI, encourage her to have her partner(s) tested and to refrain from intercourse until she has been seen for evaluation and treated.

3. Many providers may bring the patient back at an appropriate time interval, based on original diagnosis, to evaluate for reinfection or change in risky behavior.

CHAPTER 22

Systemic Hormonal Contraception Overview—Combined Oral Contraceptive Pills, NuvaRing, Ortho Evra, and Progesterone-Only Pills

With the development of new delivery systems for systemic hormonal contraceptives, specifically NuvaRing and Ortho Evra (the Patch), the emphasis in this section shifts to the similarities, and not the differences, between methods. Much of the advice that applies to combined oral contraceptive pills (COCPs) can be applied to these methods as well. The similarities are presented first, and problems unique to each method are highlighted at the end of the chapter. Other methods that work systemically to prevent ovulation (such as Depo-Provera and Implanon) are discussed in separate sections. For the purposes of this book, we will focus on OCPs, NuvaRing, and Ortho Evra.

Questions regarding the proper use of OCPs make up a large portion of telephone triage calls to OB/GYN offices and clinics. It is imperative that nurses in such triage roles be familiar with proper pill names and dosages. Many pills have similar names but come in varying dosages. Name confusion can lead to inappropriate prescribing and patient frustration. It should be a point of professional pride to know the names and available doses of the pills prescribed most often in your facility. Triage nurses should use every opportunity to reinforce the correct name when talking to patients because they often are confused about which pill they are taking.

All users of systemic hormonal contraceptives need to be aware of the potential warning signs of serious complications associated with their chosen method. Patients are initially instructed about what to look for but may forget over time. The acronym ACHES is used to remind patients (and providers) what warning signs need attention:

A. Abdominal pain (severe)
C. Chest pain (severe, cough, shortness of breath, or sharp pain on inspiration)
H. Headaches (severe, dizziness, weakness or numbness, especially if one sided)
E. Eye problems (vision loss or blurring)
S. Severe leg pain (calf or thigh)

The primary cause of most major systemic hormonal problems is the hormone component estrogen. Although some labeling information states otherwise, the conventional wisdom is that progesterone-only pills (POPs) do not carry the same risks.

Contraceptives in this category also provide many noncontraceptive benefits, including lighter and easier periods, less anemia, a beneficial effect on acne, less menstrual cramps, and, in some instances, decreased risk for endometrial and ovarian carcinoma. This is one good reason why systemic hormonal contraceptives are the most popular group of options among contraceptive methods.

BASIC TRIAGE ASSESSMENT FORM FOR SYSTEMIC HORMONAL CONTRACEPTIVES

1. When was your last menstrual period? _____ Was it normal?   Yes   No
2. Which method are you using? _____
3. What regimen (continuous or cyclic) are you using? _____
4. If taking oral contraceptives, are you using a combined product or a progesterone-only product? _____ Generic? _____
   Do you know the correct name? _____
   What time of day do you take your pill? _____ Have you missed any? _____
5. If using Ortho Evra, did you change your patch on the usual day? _____
   Any trouble with adherence? _____
6. If using NuvaRing, is the ring properly in place? _____
   How many days has it been in place? _____
7. Are you taking any other medication(s)? Drug name _____
   Dose _____ Duration of use _____
8. Are you taking any supplements? _____
9. Do you routinely use a backup method of contraception?   Yes   No
   If yes, what method do you use? _____

Abdominal Pain and Systemic Hormonal Contraceptives

KEY QUESTIONS

ASSESSMENT

ACTION

1. Is the pain severe in nature and did it start recently (in the past 24–48 hours)?

YES Go to Step A.

NO Go to Question 2.

2. Is the pain mild/moderate in nature, or has it been present longer than 24–48 hours?

YES Go to Step B.

NO Go to Question 3.

3. Is the abdominal pain recent and accompanied by nausea, vomiting, diarrhea, or fever?

YES Go to Step C.

NO Have patient describe symptoms.

ACTIONS

STEP A: Severe Pain

The patient may have an ectopic pregnancy, acute abdominal problem, or vascular condition; immediate referral to a primary care provider is indicated. The patient or her agent should call 911. The patient should not drive herself.

STEP B: Prolonged Pain

The patient still may have an acute abdominal problem and needs evaluation, but the disease process may be milder. Refer the patient within 24 hours.

STEP C: Nausea, Vomiting, Diarrhea, or Fever

The patient may have gastroenteritis. If she has no other complications, her condition may be managed at home (see Patient Education).

Referral of the patient to a physician or ER is appropriate when evolving appendicitis is possible; instruct the patient to call back if she experiences:

- increasing fever;
- pain localized in the right lower quadrant; or
- symptoms not resolving during a period of 12–24 hours.

Other disease conditions are present (cardiovascular, pregnancy, diabetes, cancer, HIV). Signs of significant dehydration are evident:

- The patient is unable to keep down any fluids (not even sips of water).
- The patient has not voided in the past 8 hours.
- The patient reports dizziness.

PATIENT EDUCATION

1. All patients need to be taught the serious warning signs associated with oral contraceptive use (see Oral Contraceptives Overview).
2. The patient with symptoms of gastroenteritis should be instructed to modify her diet for the next 24–48 hours.
   - avoid milk and milk products;
   - slowly rehydrate with sips of water (two sips of water every 5–10 minutes);
   - begin the BRAT (bananas, rice, applesauce, toast) diet after tolerating clear liquids;
   - remember that diarrhea often is the last symptom to resolve;
   - remember that diarrhea may persist for several days after nausea and vomiting subside.
3. The patient should be instructed to call back if:
   - her symptoms do not begin to resolve within 1–2 days;
   - her symptoms increase in intensity (more vomiting/nausea); or
   - she begins to run a fever.
4. If you suspect the GI complaints are only related to her contraception, refer to protocol on Gastrointestinal Complaints and Systemic Hormonal Contraceptives, page 367.

Acne and Systemic Hormonal Contraceptives

ASSESSMENT

ACTION

1. Have your skin care practices changed recently (using different soaps, new makeup, sunscreen, or moisturizers; or washing frequency)?

   YES Go to Step A.

   NO Go to Question 2.

2. Is there any change in facial or body hair associated with the skin changes?

   YES Go to Step B.

   NO Go to Question 3.

3. Do you have a single lesion that has become asymmetrical, has irregular borders, changed color, or has increased in size?

   YES Go to Step C.

   NO Go to Question 4.

4. Is this a red rash with papules/pustules over the central portion of the face and that is associated with facial flushing after hot/spicy foods are eaten or alcohol is consumed?

   YES Go to Step D.

   NO Go to Question 5.

5. Do you have scattered papules/pustules under the surface of your skin or directly on the skin, with or without additional whiteheads or blackheads?

   YES Go to Step E.

   NO Have patient describe symptoms.

ACTIONS

STEP A: Recent Skin Care Changes

This patient may have come into contact with an allergenic agent and could be experiencing dermatitis.

Instruct the patient to stop using the offending agent. If there is no improvement in 7 days, the patient should call back for an appointment.

For severe reaction, the patient should see her care provider within 24–48 hours.

STEP B: Change in Facial or Body Hair

This patient may be experiencing androgen excess, which may be caused by hormone use.

Have the patient discuss her symptoms with the prescribing provider.

STEP C: Skin Lesions

This lesion may indicate skin cancer or another skin problem. Refer the patient to her primary care provider or a dermatologist for an appointment within the next 7 days.

STEP D: Associated Symptoms

This may be rosacea, an acneform disorder in older adults characterized by vascular dilatation of the central face.

Rosacea is common in women older than 30 years.

Rosacea is more common in fair-complected women of northern European descent.

Rosacea is associated with a "rosy cheek" appearance.

Rosacea commonly requires topical antibiotic treatment.

Refer the patient to a dermatologist or her primary care provider for an appointment within the next 2–4 weeks.

STEP E: Papules or Pustules (Pimples)

This could be acne, a common skin condition, which may improve or worsen with hormonal use.

Follow the treatment suggestions in Patient Education.

If the patient experiences no improvement in 4–6 weeks of therapy, she should see her primary care provider.

PATIENT EDUCATION

1. Oral Contraceptives may be prescribed to improve acne.
   - It may take several months to see a significant improvement.
   - Many oral contraceptives, not just those products with FDA labeling that allows them to be marketed as such, are excellent for improving skin breakouts.
2. Patients should be instructed in proper skin care for mild-to-moderate acne.
   - Wash affected areas twice a day with a washcloth and noncreamy soap.
   - Consider using cleansers such as Cetaphil lotion or Benzoyl Peroxide Wash 10%.
   - Avoid picking at lesions.
   - Avoid oil-based cosmetics/face creams.
   - Avoid moisturizers, such as Vaseline, or baby oil.
   - For dryness, use Moisturelle or Nutraderm.

Amenorrhea and Systemic Hormonal Contraceptives

KEY QUESTIONS

ASSESSMENT	ACTION
1. Have you been taking systemic hormonal contraceptives containing both estrogen and progesterone (COCPs, NuvaRing, or Ortho Evra) for more than 3 months?	**YES** Go to Step A.
	NO Go to Question 2.
2. Did you start using systemic hormonal contraceptives containing both estrogen and progesterone during the past 3 months?	**YES** Go to Step B.
	NO Go to Question 3.
3. Are you taking progesterone-only pills (POPs)?	**YES** Go to Step C.
	NO Go to Question 4.
4. If you are taking oral contraceptives, have you missed any pills?	**YES** Go to Step D.
	NO Go to Step E.
5. If you are using Ortho Evra, were you late in changing your patch?	**YES** Go to Step D.
	NO Go to Step E.
6. If you are using NuvaRing, was the ring outside of your vagina for more than 3 hours or were you late restarting with the ring?	**YES** Go to Step D.
	NO Go to Step E.
7. Did you start any new medication recently (particularly those known to interfere with hormonal contraceptives, such as Dilantin, rifampin, and griseofulvin, or broad-spectrum antibiotics)?	**YES** Go to Step E.
	NO No further action.

ACTIONS

STEP A: Amenorrhea

Be sure to ask the patient if she is using her method continuously, as amenorrhea is the desired effect with continuous dosing. Amenorrhea may also occur in some women who use the method cyclically. Reassure the patient that the amenorrhea can be normal. (Continuous use of Ortho Evra is not recommended.)

If the patient has missed two cycles, have her perform a home pregnancy test. If the result is positive, instruct the patient to see an OB/GYN provider within the next 2–3 weeks. If the test result is negative, reassure the patient. If she is unsettled by this side effect, she may need to select an alternative form of contraception.

STEP B: Method Started Within the Past 3 Months

Determine whether the patient is using her method continuously and reassure her that amenorrhea is expected with that dosing schedule.

Menstrual patterns can be very erratic during the first 3 months of systemic hormonal contraceptive use. However, it is unusual for a woman to experience amenorrhea during this time with cyclic dosing. A major concern is pregnancy. If the result of a home pregnancy test is negative, review the information in Step A with the patient.

STEP C: Progesterone-Only Pills (POPs)

POPs typically cause irregular spotting/bleeding. However, after several months of POP therapy, it is not uncommon for periods to stop completely. This is a desired effect for some women.

Have the patient take a home pregnancy test and follow the instructions in Step A.

STEP D: Missed Pills, Delayed Patch Change, or "Misplaced" or Delayed Ring

Patients who have made errors in using their method need to rule out the possibility of pregnancy. If a patient has made an error within the last 5 days, review the need for emergency contraception.

Have her do a sensitive home pregnancy test and follow the suggestions in Step A.

STEP E: New Medication

Have the patient do a home pregnancy test. If the results are positive, have the patient notify her OB/GYN provider because a medication change may be in order.

If the results are negative and the medication is for long-term use, encourage the patient to discuss possible interactions with her contraceptive method with her OB/GYN provider.

PATIENT EDUCATION

1. All patients need to be educated about the expected side effects of their chosen method.
2. All patients need to know a backup method and use of emergency contraception in the event a method error occurs or other problems alter the efficacy of their method.

Breakthrough Bleeding/Spotting and Systemic Hormonal Contraceptives

KEY QUESTIONS

ASSESSMENT	ACTION
1. Are you taking POPs (mini-pills)?	**YES** Go to Step A. **NO** Go to Question 2.
2. Did you start using Ortho Evra or NuvaRing in the last 3 months?	**YES** Go to Step B. **NO** Go to Question 3.
3. Were you late starting your method, or did you have adherence issues with the patch or leave your ring out for more than 3 hours?	**YES** Go to Step C. **NO** Go to Question 4.
4. Did you start using combined oral contraceptives (containing both estrogen and progesterone) in the last 3 months?	**YES** Go to Step B and Continue to Question 5.
5. If you are taking combined oral contraceptives, have you missed any pills?	**YES** Go to Step C. **NO** Go to Question 6.
6. Are you sexually active with a male partner and not using a backup method of contraception?	**YES** Go to Step D. **NO** Go to Step E.

ACTIONS

STEP A: Spotting While Taking POPs

Spotting is a completely normal side effect of taking POPs and may continue for many months or even years. If this is undesirable to the patient, she should see her provider to discuss other contraceptive options. See Patient Education.

STEP B: Spotting or Breakthrough Bleeding in the First 3 Months of Systemic Hormonal Contraceptive Use

Spotting or breakthrough bleeding is common during the first few months of systemic hormonal contraceptive use, regardless of the delivery system used. Reassure the patient that this is common and she is better off continuing with the method for at least 4 months before considering another method. Investigate other potential causes for spotting or breakthrough bleeding by continuing to Question 6.

STEP C: Missed OCPs, Patch Adherence Problems, or Delayed Patch or Ring Use

Basically, any action that disrupts the dose of systemic hormonal contraceptives can be a cause of spotting and breakthrough bleeding. Disruptions of deliverance of hormones will vary with the chosen method.

Missed oral contraceptives pills are a common cause of unexpected bleeding during their use. See "Problems Unique to Combined Oral Contraceptives" and "Problems Unique to Progesterone-Only Oral Contraceptive Pills" for management options.

Problems with patch adherence or a delay in changing patches can cause breakthrough bleeding with Ortho Evra use. See "Problems Unique to Ortho Evra" for detailed information.

Failing to insert the NuvaRing on time or leaving it out for more than 3 hours within an appropriate cycle can commonly cause spotting or breakthrough bleeding with this method. Refer to "Problems Unique to NuvaRing" for management options.

STEP D: Sexually Active and Not Using a Backup Contraceptive Method

A patient who is not using a backup method, such as a condom, may be at risk for sexually transmitted infections (STIs). The risk of STI exposure should be determined. Ideally, the patient should come in for evaluation within 3–5 days or sooner if other acute symptoms coexist. The patient should abstain from intercourse until evaluated and should be encouraged to use condoms in the future.

STEP E: Other Possible Causes of Spotting and Breakthrough Bleeding

Most women adjust to a chosen method of systemic hormonal contraceptives within a few months. If unexplained bleeding occurs after several months of use, and the cause is not found by answering the questions above, other possible causes should be explored. Question her as to other medication use that may interfere with systemic hormones. If she is taking COCPs, gastrointestinal (GI) disruption may interfere.

A "one-time" episode of irregular bleeding may only warrant reassurance after investigation of the issues raised above. However, persistent problems require a physical evaluation within 1–2 weeks. The patient may be experiencing complications due to an ovarian cyst, cervical polyp, or even an undiagnosed pregnancy.

Her complaints should not be dismissed.

PATIENT EDUCATION

1. Patients using POPs need to know how common bleeding and spotting are until they become diligent with the method. Some patients, despite perfect use, still experience this annoying side effect.
2. All patients, regardless of method, need to know how to use a backup method, such as condoms. Those at particular risk for STIs need to be especially careful.
3. All patients using systemic hormonal contraceptives need to know they can become pregnant, even with perfect use.

Breakthrough Bleeding/Spotting and Continuous Dosing With Systemic Hormonal Contraceptives

KEY QUESTIONS

ASSESSMENT	ACTION
1. Are you taking monophasic oral contraceptives continuously?	**YES** Go to Step A.
	NO Go to Question 2.
2. Are you taking triphasic oral contraceptives continuously?	**YES** Go to Step B.
	NO Go to Question 3.
3. Are you using NuvaRing continuously?	**YES** Go to Step C.
	NO Go to Question 4.
4. Are you using Ortho Evra continuously?	**YES** Go to Step D.
	NO No further action.

ACTIONS

STEP A: Bleeding Problems With Monophasic Oral Contraceptives Used Continuously

First, determine whether the patient is taking combined monophasic oral contraceptives or progesterone-only oral contraceptives. Progesterone-only oral contraceptives are designed to *only* be taken continuously and are "less forgiving" if pills are missed or skipped; for example, missing 3 hours with a POP may be similar to missing a day with a COCP. Counsel the patient on proper use and have her continue to take them continuously.

If the patient has been taking her monophasic COCPs correctly and has not skipped any pills, find out how long she has been taking them continuously. Sometimes a bleeding pattern will develop over time that is unique to each woman; i.e., some women may be able to take COCPs continuously for only 6 weeks before they have a tendency to bleed, and some may be able to take them for 12 weeks or longer without a tendency to bleed. Help her determine whether a pattern is developing that will guide her in the future.

If she has been spotting for 7 consecutive days or bleeding heavily for 3 days, have her stop and have a withdrawal bleed. She should restart her pills continuously in 3–4 days. Under no circumstances should she extend the pill-free interval longer than 7 days, as this is likely to induce ovulation. Please refer to Patient Education.

STEP B: Bleeding Problems With Triphasic Oral Contraceptives Used Continuously

Triphasic oral contraceptives may be likely to cause spotting or breakthrough bleeding if taken continuously. The dosage varies as the color or shape of the active pills changes. The original intent of this dosing regimen was to "mimic a natural cycle" as hormone levels fluctuate in a "normal" cycle of ovulation and menstruation. If a patient is trying to take her triphasic pills continuously and experiences spotting for 7 consecutive days or heavy bleeding for 3 days, have her stop and have a withdrawal bleed. She should decide whether to continue using her triphasic preparation, in which case she may be better served by having a monthly cycle. Or she may consider a monophasic pill, which she may be able to use more successfully. In any situation, she should restart a method within 3–4 days. Under no circumstance should she extend the pill-free interval longer than 7 days, as this is likely to induce ovulation. Please refer to Patient Education.

STEP C: Bleeding Problems With NuvaRing Used Continuously

While each NuvaRing may be appropriate for 4 weeks of continuous use, some women may notice spotting as the end of that interval approaches. In such cases, the patient may be best advised to consistently plan on changing her ring before the end of the 4-week interval. If she experiences spotting for 7 consecutive days or heavy bleeding for 3 days, she should remove her ring and restart with a new ring in 3–4 days. Under no circumstances should she extend her ring-free interval longer than 7 days, as this is likely to induce ovulation. Please refer to Patient Education.

STEP D: Bleeding Problems With Ortho Evra Used Continuously

It is not recommended that this method be used continuously. Please see the Continuous Dose Systemic Hormonal Contraceptives protocol for the rationale.

PATIENT EDUCATION

1. Breakthrough bleeding and spotting are common problems with continuous use of systemic hormonal contraceptives, regardless of the delivery system used. All women who choose this method should be counseled at the time of method selection as to how to deal with the problem.
2. Most women will develop a pattern to their bleeding that may guide them in choosing an appropriate time for a withdrawal bleed.

3. Many experts advise women to *never* extend the method-free interval even as long as 7 days, as is common in a 21/7 regimen. The thought is that the longer a method is used in a continuous fashion, the greater the tendency to ovulate spontaneously given the opportunity.

4. A 3- to 4-day method-free interval is usually enough to cause a significant withdrawal bleed, and, as stated above, should never be extended beyond 7 days.

5. It can be helpful if patients retain any "day labeling" material provided with their method. This can be used to relabel packages when the method is restarted.

Breast Pain and Systemic Hormonal Contraceptives

KEY QUESTIONS

ASSESSMENT	ACTION
1. Is the breast pain bilateral?	**YES** Go to Step A.
	NO Go to Question 2.
2. Is the breast pain unilateral?	**YES** Go to Question 3.
	NO Go to Step B.
3. Is the pain isolated to one particular area of the breast?	**YES** Go to Step B.
	NO Go to Step B.
4. Did you recently start using systemic hormonal contraceptives (within the last 3 months)?	**YES** Go to Step C.
	NO Go to Question 5.
5. Are you concerned you could be pregnant?	**YES** Go to Step D.
	NO Go to Question 6.
6. Could this pain be chest wall or muscular pain (such as myocardial infarction, pulmonary embolus, costochondritis, or a pulled muscle)?	**YES** Go to Chest Pain and Oral Contraceptive Therapy protocol.
	NO No further action.

ACTIONS

STEP A: Bilateral Breast Pain

Both estrogen and progesterone have been implicated in breast pain associated with hormone use. This pain is usually bilateral.

Initiate the Basic Triage Assessment Form for Breast Complaints.

Question the patient about her consumption of caffeine and foods that contain the amino acid tyrosine (bananas, nuts, red wine, and yellow cheese).

Ask the patient if she has experienced a change in bra size.

Go to Step C.

STEP B: Unilateral Breast Pain

Unilateral breast pain is rarely caused by hormone use. Other causes need to be investigated, such as breast cysts, fibroadenoma, costochondritis, and breast cancer.

Ask the patient whether or not she has felt a lump.

Ask the patient where she is in her menstrual cycle.

If the patient is older than 35 years, have her come in within 24–48 hours for a physical evaluation. Prepare her that she may need a mammogram.

For younger patients, particularly those taking triphasic pills, the patient may wait for an examination until her hormone-free week. This should be the patient's choice.

STEP C: Recent Pill Start

Reassure the patient that hormones can cause breast tenderness during the first few months of use.

Recommend a good supportive bra.

Recommend the patient avoid activities that cause aggravation of symptoms (for instance, the patient should walk, rather than jog).

Recommend the patient initiate diet changes of decreased caffeine and tyrosine consumption.

If the symptoms are intolerable, refer the patient to a provider for other recommendations or a change in her method.

STEP D: Possible Pregnancy

All patients who are sexually active with male partners, even those who do not miss a pill, are at risk for pregnancy.

Ask the patient if she has missed any pills (see protocol Late or Missed Combined Oral Contraceptive Pills on page 379) or if she has been late changing her patch or inserting NuvaRing.

Question the patient as to the normalcy of last menstrual period or absence of withdrawal bleeding.

Encourage the patient to perform a highly sensitive urine pregnancy test or have the patient come in for a blood pregnancy test.

PATIENT EDUCATION

1. One of the keys to successful use of systemic hormonal contraception is understanding the expected problems and usual course of action. Educating the patient regarding the possible nature of her pain, particularly in the case of recent method initiation with bilateral pain, may help the patient tolerate the symptoms until her body adjusts to the pill's hormone dose.
2. Particular sensitivity is needed for patients with unilateral pain who may be at risk for breast problems of a more serious nature. Refer to the Breast Complaints Overview for some approaches in dealing with women with additional concerns.

3. Many women really do not understand that they **can** get pregnant while using their method correctly. All women need education regarding backup methods of contraception.
4. Because of the greater exposure to estrogen with Ortho Evra, the patient may want to try another method with lower estrogen exposure, such as NuvaRing.
5. Switching to a progesterone-only method may be an alternative.

Chest Pain and Systemic Hormonal Contraceptives

KEY QUESTIONS

ASSESSMENT	ACTION
1. Is the pain recent in onset (within 1 to 2 hours), described as "pressure" or "crushing" in nature, accompanied by shortness of breath, unrelieved by rest, or radiating into the left arm or jaw? (If the patient answers "yes" to any one of these questions, this is a positive response.)	**YES** Go to Step A. **NO** Go to Question 2.
2. Is the pain intermittent, associated with activity, relieved by rest, or described with any of the terms used in Question 1?	**YES** Go to Step B. **NO** Go to Question 3.
3. Is the pain localized to the chest/lung or sudden in onset or accompanied by severe shortness of breath or significant anxiety?	**YES** Go to Step C. **NO** Go to Question 4.
4. Has the chest pain evolved more gradually than that described above? Does the pain/discomfort increase with inspiration?	**YES** Go to Step D. **NO** Go to Question 5.
5. Can the patient point to a specific painful spot on the chest wall? Does it hurt when this area is palpated? Does the pain increase with specific movement?	**YES** Go to Step E. **NO** Go to Question 6.
6. Is the pain described as "indigestion" or "burning" in the chest, particularly after meals? Does the patient report increased gas or belching?	**YES** Go to Step F. **NO** Go to Question 7.
7. Is the pain localized to the breast? (Have all of the above complaints been ruled out?)	**YES** Go to the Breast Pain protocol. **NO** No further action.

ACTIONS

STEP A: Severe Pain

This may be a myocardial infarction (heart attack). Immediate evaluation is required. The patient or her agent should call 911.

Instruct the patient to take 325 mg aspirin while waiting for transport.

STEP B: Chest Pain With Activity

This may be angina (coronary artery disease). Urgent evaluation is required.

Instruct the patient to go to the ER for evaluation. She should call 911.

Instruct her to take 325 mg aspirin.

STEP C: Shortness of Breath/Anxiety

This may be a pulmonary embolus or severe asthma. Immediate evaluation is required. The patient or her agent should call 911.

STEP D: Gradual Chest Pain With Inspiration

This may be pulmonary in origin (pneumonia, emphysema, pleurisy).

Instruct the patient to call her primary care provider and schedule an appointment within the next 12–24 hours.

STEP E: Point-Specific Pain With Movement

This may be a chest wall problem (costochondritis, shingles). Evaluation within the next 3–5 days by a primary care provider is recommended.

Advise the patient to try anti-inflammatory drugs (ibuprofen or naproxen). She should use such agents only if no allergies or contraindications to these drugs are evident (for example, no history of gastrointestinal bleeding).

The patient can also apply ice packs or heat to the affected area.

If a rash develops along the painful chest wall area, the patient may have shingles.

Once the rash develops, the patient needs to be seen within 24 to 48 hours for possible antiviral therapy.

STEP F: Indigestion or Burning After Meals

This may be GERD (acid indigestion). Evaluation within the next 7–10 days by a primary care provider is recommended. Referral to the ER may be indicated if the patient has tried the following therapies without relief (she may have evolving myocardial infarction.)

Try Tums, Rolaids, Maalox, or Mylanta.

PATIENT EDUCATION

1. Severe chest pain is one of the early warning signs of serious complications of hormonal contraceptive use. All patients should be instructed in the warning signs designated by the letters ACHES. (See Systemic Hormonal Contraceptive Overview).
2. Be aware that the usual denial tactics associated with a heart attack can be manifested by women taking hormones. Counsel them as to the potential serious nature of severe chest pain while taking systemic hormonal contraceptives.
3. Women using Ortho Evra need to be informed of a slightly higher chance of blood clots with this method.

Continuous-Dose Systemic Hormonal Contraceptives

KEY QUESTIONS

ASSESSMENT	ACTION
1. Are you taking monophasic OCPs?	**YES** Go to Step A.
	NO Go to Question 2.
2. Are you taking triphasic OCPs?	**YES** Go to Step B.
	NO Go to Question 3.
3. Are you using NuvaRing?	**YES** Go to Step C.
	NO Go to Question 4.
4. Are you using Ortho Evra (the Patch)?	**YES** Go to Step D.
	NO No further action.

ACTIONS

STEP A: Taking Monophasic OCPs Continuously

Monophasic OCPs (same hormone dose daily) are very conducive to being taken on a continuous dosing basis. Any monophasic pill, despite what the package label indicates, may be used in this fashion. To do so, skip the placebo pills if using a 21/7 or a 24/4 regimen pack. Take only active pills continuously. This applies to POPs as well, as they are designed to be taken continuously. Continue to Patient Education.

STEP B: Taking Triphasic OCPs Continuously

In triphasic OCPs the hormone dose varies as the pills change color or shape. The original concept behind this dosing regimen was to mimic a "natural cycle" in which hormone doses normally vary throughout the process of ovulation and menstruation. Continuous dosing is not well suited for this type of pill because varying the dosage may cause a withdrawal bleed. However, this does not mean that some patients will not succeed in extending their cycle for a few days or a week, and some may do so for a longer period. If a patient wants to continue with the "continuous dosing," point out the mechanism of action with triphasic regimens and recommend they discuss a change of dose with their provider if problems develop.

STEP C: Using NuvaRing Continuously

NuvaRing is appropriate for continuous-dose use and may be more cost-effective for
some patients because one ring can be used for 4 weeks of contraception. In some
studies, NuvaRing was found to contain adequate hormone stores for up to 35 days.
However, the manufacturer does not recommend use for that long. Some patients
have noted a tendency to spot at the end of the fourth week. Patients may try changing rings at the fourth week, but the regimen may need to be individualized for each
patient. Continue to **Patient Education.**

STEP D: Using Ortho Evra (the Patch) Continuously

It is not recommended that this method be used continuously.

Ortho Evra creates a higher circulating blood level of estrogen (about 60% higher than
in women on the pill), which builds up over the course of its regular 3 weeks of use.
It is assumed that it will be even higher in weeks 4 and 5 if used continuously, thus
potentially increasing the risk of blood clots and stroke.*

PATIENT EDUCATION

1. Continuous dosing with systemic hormonal contraceptives is becoming increasingly
   popular. Some patients may choose to do this occasionally to avoid menstruation at
   inconvenient times, such as a wedding or vacation. Many women are electing to do
   this every month.
2. This regimen has to be individualized for each woman because some may be more
   tolerant than others of occasional breakthrough bleeding or spotting.
3. One hint is to advise patients to save the "day labeling" strips that go with pill
   packs. These can be used with other packs to help keep them on track.
4. Please refer to the protocol Breakthrough Bleeding/Spotting and Continuous Dosing
   with Systemic Hormonal Contraceptives on page 352 for related problems.

Personal communication, Dr. Robert A. Hatcher, July 1, 2008.

Depression and Systemic Hormonal Contraceptives

KEY QUESTIONS

ASSESSMENT	ACTION
1. Did the depressed mood begin gradually after you started taking hormonal contraceptives?	**YES** Go to Step A.
	NO Go to Step B.
2. Do you have a history of depression or bipolar disorder?	**YES** Go to Question 3.
	NO Go to Question 4.
3. If you have a currently prescribed antidepressant medication, are you taking it?	**YES** Go to Step C.
	NO Go to Step C.
4. Do you have no history of depression but recent onset of sadness, depressed mood, withdrawal, sleep disturbances (insomnia or daytime somnolence), change in appetite, loss of energy (fatigue)?	**YES** Go to Step A.
	NO Not applicable.
5. Do you feel like harming yourself or others? Do you have a suicide plan?	**YES** Go to Step D.
	NO Go to Step A.

ACTIONS

STEP A: Depression on Initiation of Systemic Hormonal Contraceptives

Depression may be a side effect of oral contraceptive use and can be severe for some people. This may be a new onset of depression, and whether or not it is related to hormone use, it requires thorough evaluation.

If the patient suspects hormones are the underlying cause, have her speak with her OB/GYN care provider within the next 12–24 hours.

The patient should consider evaluation with a mental health professional within 7–10 days.

The patient should be instructed in a backup method of birth control in case her symptoms cause her to stop taking systemic hormonal contraceptives.

STEP B: Pre-existing Depression

This patient may have pre-existing depression, which could be aggravated by hormone use.

Refer the patient to an OB/GYN care provider if the patient thinks hormones have aggravated her condition.

Refer the patient to a mental health professional within 7 to 10 days.

Continue to the next question regarding medication use patterns.

STEP C: Depression History and Medication Use

This patient needs follow-up care by her mental health provider or referral to a mental health professional if she is not receiving regular care.

Question the patient to determine if her contraception may be adversely influencing her moods. If so, consider consulting an OB/GYN care provider to discuss alternative type/delivery method of contraception.

If the patient has discontinued use of any prescribed medication for depression, bipolar disorder, or other mood disorder, encourage her to be in touch with the prescribing provider.

STEP D: Suicidal Thoughts or Actions

This patient may be suicidal and requires immediate referral for appropriate evaluation.

Try to keep the patient on the telephone if her symptoms are severe.

Have another health care provider or agent of the patient call 911 while you keep the patient on the line, if possible.

You should have suicide outreach hotline telephone numbers close at hand.

PATIENT EDUCATION

1. It is appropriate and necessary that patients with new systemic hormonal contraceptive initiation be screened for history of depression and educated at the time of oral contraceptive initiation about the possibility of their condition worsening with hormone use.
2. All patients should be instructed in a backup method in case they need to stop their chosen method for a medical reason.
3. You must be prepared for this type of call by having hotline or emergency referral telephone numbers close at hand. Although serious calls indicative of suicidal thoughts may be rare, they certainly are not the time to be searching for telephone numbers for appropriate referral and help.

Eye and Visual Changes and Systemic Hormonal Contraceptives

KEY QUESTIONS

ASSESSMENT	ACTION
1. Have you had a sudden loss (central or peripheral blindness) or significant change (blurring, double vision) in your vision?	**YES** Go to Step A. **NO** Go to Question 2.
2. Do you have eye pain?	**YES** Go to Question 3. **NO** Go to Question 4.
3. Is the pain unilateral and intense and did it begin suddenly?	**YES** Go to Step B. **NO** Go to Question 4.
4. Is the eye red but painless and your vision unaffected?	**YES** Go to Step C. **NO** Go to Question 5.
5. Is your vision changing gradually and affecting normal activities, such as reading, sewing, or driving?	**YES** Go to Step D. **NO** No further action.

ACTIONS

STEP A: Sudden Loss of Vision

This patient may be experiencing a transient ischemic attack (stroke); may have acute angle glaucoma or retinal detachment; or may be experiencing a new onset of ocular migraine. The patient needs to be seen immediately; refer her to the ER or have her call 911.

STEP B: Eye Pain

This patient may have iritis, cluster headache, or an unusual ocular migraine presentation. This needs to be evaluated by the patient's primary care provider or in an ER within the next 2–4 hours.

STEP C: Eye Redness

This could be a spontaneous hemorrhage, conjunctivitis, or scleritis. This should be evaluated by the patient's primary care provider within the next 12–24 hours.

STEP D: Gradual Change of Vision

This patient may have changing central vision and need corrective lenses or an increase in her current eyewear prescription. The patient needs to see her eye care provider within the next week.

Gastrointestinal Complaints: Nausea/Vomiting and Systemic Hormonal Contraceptives

KEY QUESTIONS

ASSESSMENT	ACTION
1. Did you start using systemic hormonal contraceptives in the last 1–2 months?	**YES** Go to Question 2.
	NO Go to Question 2.
2. Are you sexually active with a male partner and not using backup contraception?	**YES** Go to Step A.
	NO Go to Question 3.
3. Have you missed any pills, delayed your patch or ring, or taken any medications known to interfere with your method?	**YES** Go to Step A.
	NO Go to Question 4.
4. Is the nausea/vomiting related to taking your pill, changing your patch, or starting a new ring?	**YES** Go to Step B.
	NO Go to Question 5.
5. Is the nausea/vomiting intermittent, associated with certain foods (fatty, greasy, or spicy), and accompanied by pain (right upper quad or shoulder)?	**YES** Go to Step C.
	NO Go to Question 6.
6. Did this nausea/vomiting start within the past 24 hours and is it accompanied by diarrhea and mild/moderate abdominal pain?	**YES** Go to Step D.
	NO No further action.

ACTIONS

STEP A: At Risk for Pregnancy

Patients who are not using backup contraception, missing pills, delaying ring or patch initiation, or taking medications known to interfere with their method may be at risk for pregnancy. They should be counseled to eliminate early pregnancy as a possible explanation for their GI symptoms before investigating other causes.

STEP B: Nausea or Vomiting Related to Method Initiation

GI symptoms that present when a method is initiated may be related to hormone use, particularly estrogen dose. If a patient is taking COCPs, she can try taking them at a different time of the day. Switching to a lower dose may help. Since there is only one patch and one ring, switching dosages is not an option. The ring provides the lowest dose of estrogen of all methods; therefore, this may be an option if she experiences problems with the patch. However, if she has problems with nausea when using the ring, systemic hormonal contraceptives may not be a pleasant option for her.

For those who experience such symptoms only after a method-free interval, continuous dosing may help.

STEP C: Symptoms Associated With Eating

This may be gastroesophageal reflux disease (GERD), acid reflux, or gallbladder disease. She should switch to a bland diet and contact her primary care provider (PCP) for evaluation.

STEP D: Nausea/Vomiting Accompanied by Mild to Moderate Abdominal Pain and/or Diarrhea

This patient may have gastroenteritis. If she has no other complications, her condition may be managed at home (see Patient Education).

Refer the patient to a physician or ER when evolving appendicitis is possible. She should seek help if she experiences:
- increasing fever;
- pain localized in the right lower quadrant; or
- symptoms that do not resolve in the next 12–24 hours.

She should contact her PCP or the nearest ER if she has an ongoing medical condition that may be made worse by debilitating GI symptoms.

She should contact her PCP or nearest ER if signs of dehydration occur, such as an inability to keep fluids down for 24 hours, no voiding in 8 hours, or dizziness.

PATIENT EDUCATION

1. If the patient has acute GI symptoms that can be managed at home, have her modify her diet in the following manner for the next 24–48 hours:
   - Avoid milk and milk products.
   - Slowly rehydrate with sips of water every 5–10 minutes. Ice chips may help.
   - Begin BRAT diet (bananas, rice, applesauce, and toast) only after tolerating clear liquids.
   - Diarrhea is often the last symptom to go.
   - Diarrhea may persist for several days after nausea and vomiting have subsided.

2. She should see her PCP if:
   - symptoms do not resolve in 1–2 days;
   - symptoms increase in intensity;
   - fever develops; or
   - she has other concerns.

Hair Growth or Loss and Systemic Hormonal Contraceptives

KEY QUESTIONS

ASSESSMENT	ACTION
1. Did the hair change begin 1–3 months after you started using systemic hormonal contraceptive?	**YES** Go to Step A.
	NO Go to Question 2.
2. Is hair loss a problem?	**YES** Go to Step B.
	NO Go to Question 3.
3. Is hair excess a problem?	**YES** Go to Step C.
	NO No further action.

ACTIONS

STEP A: Hair Change Associated With Hormone Use

Hair loss or increase may be a consequence of hormonal imbalance. Have the patient contact her OB/GYN care provider to determine if she should change her method.

STEP B: Hair Loss

This could be thyroid disease, an infection, a skin condition, or an androgen imbalance causing male pattern baldness. Refer the patient to her primary care or OB/GYN care provider.

Women are at higher risk for thyroid disorders. Screening is appropriate when women present with complaints consistent with thyroid disease.

Certain infections, such as scabies or other conditions, may result in hair loss.

STEP C: Excess Hair

The patient may have androgen excess (adrenal gland dysfunction, Cushing disease, or an androgen-secreting tumor.) Refer the patient to her primary care provider.

Headaches and Systemic Hormonal Contraceptives

KEY QUESTIONS

ASSESSMENT   **ACTION**

1. Did the headache begin within the last 1–2 hours, and is it the worst headache you have ever had in your life?

   YES Go to Step A.
   NO Go to Question 2.

2. Is the headache accompanied by visual changes?

   YES Go to Step B.
   NO Go to Question 3.

3. Is the headache accompanied by any numbness, tingling, loss of bowel or bladder control, or seizure?

   YES Go to Step A.
   NO Go to Question 4.

4. Is the headache accompanied by neck stiffness?

   YES Go to Step C.
   NO Go to Question 5.

5. Do you have upper respiratory tract infection symptoms (such as congestion, fever, or cough)?

   YES Go to Step D.
   NO Go to Question 6.

6. Do you have a predictable monthly headache, such as when you begin placebo pills with COCPs or remove your patch or ring before a withdrawal bleed?

   YES Go to Step E.
   NO Go to Question 7.

7. Have you had more frequent, debilitating headaches since you started using a form of hormonal contraception?

   YES Go to Step F.
   NO No further action.

ACTIONS

STEP A: Severe Headache (Worst She's Ever Had)

This may be an aneurysm or an evolving cerebrovascular accident. Have her or her agent call 911.

STEP B: Visual Changes

The patient may have a cluster headache or an unusual ocular migraine presentation. The patient needs to be evaluated by her PCP within the next 2–4 hours unless she has a diagnosis of recurring cluster or ocular migraines. In that case, she may have a plan, including prescribed medication for this problem. These patients are usually not good candidates for systemic hormonal contraceptives and should have a medical evaluation before continuing with this method.

STEP C: Neck Stiffness

This patient may have spinal meningitis. She should contact her PCP and will most likely need to be seen in the ER for immediate evaluation.

STEP D: Congestion, Fever, and Cough

This patient may have a sinus headache. She may try a usual pain reliever for this condition if such agents are not contraindicated by allergies or other medical conditions. If symptoms persist or worsen, she should make an appointment to see her PCP within 2–4 days to be evaluated for a sinus infection.

STEP E: Cyclic Headaches Related to Systemic Hormonal Contraceptive Use

Cyclic headaches at the time of withdrawal bleed (placebo week of pills, "free" week with patch or ring) are often due to estrogen withdrawal. Possible options for this patient include continuous use of a hormonal method, switching to a progesterone-only method, or, with approval from her PCP, supplementing the withdrawal period with a low dose of estrogen. Pill users can accomplish this by switching to a product related to Mircette or by using a hormonal patch usually used in menopause, such as Climara. Because this would be an "off label" use of such a patch, she would have to discuss this with her GYN care provider.

STEP F: More Frequent Debilitating Headaches with Systemic Hormonal Contraceptive Use

This patient may not be a good candidate for her current method. If she is using COCPs, she may try a different dose. Unfortunately, we only have one patch and one ring, so her options for switching either of those methods involves a change in delivery system. Trying a progesterone-only method may help. Since NuvaRing delivers the lowest dose of estrogen, she may want to try that method if she is not happy with progesterone-only options.

PATIENT EDUCATION

1. Headaches are common in women. There are several good books about the subject, such as *What Women Need to Know: From Headaches to Heart Disease and Everything in Between* (Colman and Legato; Chicago: Olmstead Press, 2000).

2. Patients who are headache sufferers should be apprised of comfort measures for headaches. Cold compresses, a quiet environment, meditation, and acupuncture are alternatives that do not involve medications and may bring relief.
3. Patients should know that the diagnosis of "migraine" involves a medical evaluation. Many patients who say they have this condition have not been properly diagnosed. If you suspect this is the case, encourage her to get proper evaluation and treatment.

Leg Cramps/Pain and Systemic Hormonal Contraceptives

KEY QUESTIONS

ASSESSMENT

ACTION

1. Do you have unilateral pain, localized pain in one calf, or unilateral leg swelling?

YES Go to Step A.

NO Go to Question 3.

2. If you are having unilateral leg problems, have you been immobile recently (recent surgery or sitting for prolonged periods in a car or airplane)?

YES Go to Step A.

NO Go to Question 3.

3. Is the pain bilateral, worse when reclining at night, or keeping you from sleeping?

YES Go to Step B.

NO Go to Question 4.

4. Does this feel like a charley horse (sharp leg cramp that commonly awakens people during sleep)? Is it related to a recent increase in activity?

YES Go to Step C.

NO No further action.

ACTIONS

STEP A: Exclude Possible Deep Vein Thrombosis

This patient may have a deep vein thrombosis (DVT). Refer her immediately to her primary care provider (within 12–24 hours).
Proceed to Question 2.

STEP B: Problem Occurs at Bedtime

This may be restless leg syndrome. Refer the patient to her primary care provider within the next 1–2 weeks.

STEP C: Charley Horse

This may be muscle fatigue or cramping. Offer some management suggestions.
If it is a charley horse, try the following:
- gentle stretching;
- massage; and
- hot packs.

If it is muscle strain/fatigue, the patient should try taking anti-inflammatory agents, if they are not contraindicated by such factors as ulcers, stomach problems, or the patient taking anticoagulant agents.

If the pain is persistent or symptoms worsen, the patient should see her primary care provider within the next 1–2 weeks.

PATIENT EDUCATION

1. Severe leg pain is one of the early warning signs of hormonal contraceptive use.
2. All women should be familiar with the warning signs described in the Systemic Hormonal Contraceptive Overview on page 342.
3. Women using Ortho Evra should be informed of a slightly higher incidence of blood clots with this method.
4. Chronic "charley horse" pain may indicate a calcium/phosphorus imbalance.

Libido Decrease and Systemic Hormonal Contraceptives

ASSESSMENT

ACTION

1. Did this change in libido begin concurrently with hormone use?

YES Go to Step A.
NO Go to Question 2.

2. Is this decrease in libido associated with a depressed mood?

YES Go to Step B.
NO Go to Question 3.

3. Is this change in libido associated with painful intercourse?

YES Go to Step C.
NO No further action.

ACTIONS

STEP A: Libido Decrease With Oral Contraceptive Use

The patient should consult her OB/GYN care provider. She may need a change of contraceptive method (sex hormone-binding globulins may be affected by hormones, resulting in changes in libido).

STEP B: Associated Depression

Libido changes (particularly decreased libido) often are associated with relationship problems. They also can be associated with cumulative life stressors. Offer referral to a psychiatric/mental health provider or to a primary care provider to discuss these issues.
Possible causes:
- depression;
- marital/relationship discord; or
- significant emotional stress (ill child, elderly parents, financial stressors).

STEP C: Decreased Libido and Painful Intercourse

Dyspareunia is a common complaint among women. It is commonly caused by vaginal infection, vaginal lesions, or more complex pelvic floor complications (such as vulvar vestibulitis). It may also be caused by decreased estrogen, common with some hormonal contraceptives.

If this is a chronic problem, refer the patient to her OB/GYN care provider within the next 2–4 weeks.

If this is an acute problem, refer the patient to her OB/GYN care provider within the next 2–4 days.

She may try using a lubricant with intercourse.

Problems Unique to Combined Oral Contraceptive Pills (COCPs)

A major category of problems unique to COCPs involves simply taking the pill orally! Many women choose to take "the pill" because the act of swallowing (or chewing) is *not* a passive act. They like to be aware, on a daily basis, of the fact that they are providing themselves with contraception. Women who already take daily medication may not mind taking another oral medication. Some women who desire the benefits and excellent efficacy of systemic methods may not be comfortable with the patch or the ring.

Problems involving the ingestion of pills cover a range from simply forgetting to take the pills to nausea/vomiting and, therefore, possibly not digesting the pill. The following protocol unique to COCPs involves missing a pill, for whatever reason. Missing pills can be a source of side effects such as breakthrough bleeding, and if enough are missed or they are missed at an inopportune time, pregnancy may result. Please refer to the protocol on Gastrointestinal Complaints and Systemic Hormonal Contraceptives for nausea/vomiting concerns.

Late or Missed Combined Oral Contraceptive Pills

ASSESSMENT	ACTION
1. Are you taking 21-day combined pills?	**YES** Go to Question 3.
	NO Go to Question 2.
2. Are you taking 28-day combined pills? (Remind the patient that missing any of the placebo pills does not place a woman at increased risk for pregnancy.)	**YES** Go to Question 3.
	NO N/A.
3. Have you missed pills in weeks 1 or 2 (pills 1–7 or 8–14)?	**YES** Go to Step A.
	NO Go to Question 4.
4. Did you miss a pill during week 3 of the pill pack (pills 16–21)?	**YES** Go to Step B.
	NO Go to Question 5.
5. Did you miss any of the placebo pills (pills 22–28)?	**YES** Go to Step C.
	NO No further action.

ACTIONS

STEP A: Missed Pills in Week 1 or 2

If the patient is less than 24 hours late in taking the pill, she should:
- take the missed pill immediately;
- return to the daily pill schedule, taking the next pill at the regularly scheduled time; and
- use a backup method or abstain from intercourse for the next 7 days.

If the patient is 24 hours late in taking the pill, she should:
- take both the missed pill and today's pill at the same time (she may experience some nausea); and
- use a backup method or avoid intercourse for the next 7 days.

If the patient is more than 24 hours late in taking the pill, she should:
- take the last missed pill immediately;
- take the next scheduled pill at the regularly scheduled time;
- throw out the other missed pills;
- take the rest of the pills on schedule; and
- use a backup method or avoid intercourse for the next 7 days.

STEP B: Completely Missed Pills During Week 3

The patient should finish all hormone pills in the pack.

If the patient uses 21-day pills, she should not take a week off between pill packs.

If the patient uses 28-day pills, she should not take the placebo pills.

As soon as the patient has completed the hormone pills in her current pack, she should begin taking a new pack of pills.

The patient should not necessarily expect a period until she finishes the second pack of pills.

If the patient did not take the pills as scheduled and had unprotected intercourse within the last 72 hours, she should consider emergency contraception (see the protocol Emergency Contraception With Oral Contraceptive Pills).

STEP C: Missing Any of the Seven Placebo Pills

The patient should throw out any missed pills.

She should take one pill per day until the pack is finished (making certain not to extend the placebo period more than 7 days).

Additional protection is not needed unless there has been more than a 7-day interval without hormone pills.

The patient should start the next pill pack at the regularly scheduled time.

PATIENT EDUCATION

1. It is important for patients to understand that extending the pill-free week, either by missing pills at the end or beginning of a pack, creates the greatest opportunity for spontaneous ovulation and unintended pregnancy.
2. Certain medications may interfere with pill effectiveness. Missing pills while taking medications that may interfere with OCP therapy may increase the risk of unintended pregnancy. (See Hatcher et al. *Contraceptive Technology* (18th ed.), New York: Ardent Media, 2004. p. 436.)
3. All users of oral contraceptives need instruction in a back-up method, not just for protection from STIs. Even a married, monogamous woman needs to know what to do if she is on vacation without her OCPs!
4. These instructions apply to the newer regimens with 24/4 pill packs (4 placebo pills).
5. Patients missing any pills in Week 1 should be offered emergency contraception (see Protocol Emergency Contraception with Plan B or Combined Oral Contraceptives). The same applies to missing 5 pills in ANY week of the pack.

Problems Unique to NuvaRing

NuvaRing is a design that allows for once-a-month vaginal insertion for systemic contraception. Its acceptance as a reliable and easy-to-use systemic contraceptive method is growing. However, the very design that makes it unique may make it unacceptable to women who are squeamish about touching their vagina, or who do not feel comfortable about leaving something in place in their vagina for an extended period.

The vagina is a remarkable receptacle for medication. Because it has exceptional blood flow and an absence of glands and fat cells, less medication may be used to accomplish the same effect achieved by transdermal (Ortho Evra) or oral (combined or progesterone-only oral contraceptives) administration. This may minimize some troubling side effects of other routes of administration, notably nausea/vomiting and breast pain. The NuvaRing may be a good choice for women who are unduly susceptible to side effects when using other methods.

However, the vagina also poses some unique problems. Changes in vaginal discharge may be reported. Particularly troublesome may be the case of a "lost" NuvaRing. Insertion and removal problems are also unique to this method. The following protocols focus on "lost" rings and insertion and removal issues.

"Lost" NuvaRing

KEY QUESTIONS

ASSESSMENT

1. Was your NuvaRing in place 3 hours ago?

ACTION

YES Go to Step A.
NO Go to Step B.

ACTIONS

STEP A: NuvaRing Out for Less Than 3 Hours

If the ring has been out for less than 3 hours, it can be rinsed with tepid water and reinserted. No interruption in contraception will occur.

If the ring has been out but is truly lost, inserting a new ring before 3 hours will allow the patient to continue on her same ring cycle.

STEP B: Nuva Ring Out More Than 3 Hours

If this happens in week 1 or 2, contraceptive effectiveness may be reduced. Insert the ring as soon as possible and use a backup method of contraception until the ring has been used for 7 consecutive days.

If the ring is out of the vagina for more than 3 consecutive hours in week 3, choose one of the following options:

1. Insert a new ring immediately and begin a new cycle. The patient may not menstruate at her usual time and may have spotting or breakthrough bleeding. Use a backup method for 7 continuous days.
2. Do not reinsert the ring or use a new ring. Stop and have a period. Reinsert the ring within 7 days. Use a backup method for 7 continuous days.

PATIENT EDUCATION

1. Some patients may choose to remove the NuvaRing during intercourse. They need to be educated to keep track of the time the NuvaRing is outside of the vagina.
2. It is unusual for a NuvaRing to be truly lost, but women with prolapse, cystocele, or rectocele may be more likely to expel the device.

Insertion/Removal Problems With NuvaRing

KEY QUESTIONS

ASSESSMENT	ACTION
1. Are you having trouble inserting the NuvaRing?	**YES** Go to Step A.
	NO Go to Next Question.
2. Are you having trouble removing the NuvaRing?	**YES** Go to Step B.
	NO No further action.

ACTIONS

STEP A: Trouble Inserting the NuvaRing

Proper positioning before attempting insertion may be helpful. Try putting one leg up on a small stool, lying on your back with your knees bent and slightly apart, or perch on the edge of a chair or toilet. Squeeze the ring between your thumb and forefinger. Gently insert the ring into the vagina. You may need to push it until you cannot feel any pressure at the introitus (vaginal opening). If you can feel the ring, just gently push it further into your vagina. It is not important for the ring to be in any one place to be effective. The vaginal muscles will hold the ring in place.

An alternate method is to use a tampon as an applicator. Remove the tampon from its applicator and insert the ring halfway into the applicator. Insert as you would a tampon. Dispose of the applicator appropriately.

STEP B: Trouble Removing the NuvaRing

Hook your forefinger (index finger) under the closest rim and gently pull down and out. An alternate method is to use the index finger and middle finger to grasp the ring and gently pull down and out.

Attempting to remove the ring in a warm bath or during a shower may facilitate muscle relaxation.

PATIENT EDUCATION

1. Comfort with this method is key in learning to insert the ring and remove it easily. Encourage the patient to practice if she is concerned. She can practice as long as the ring does not remain out of the vagina for more than 3 hours.
2. If possible, have her pick up extra samples at your office. She can use them for practice as well.

Problems Unique to Ortho Evra (the Patch)

Ortho Evra users are exposed to about 60% more estrogen than users of typical 35-microgram OCPs. Generally, estrogen is responsible for the more serious risks of systemic hormonal contraceptives, notably blood clots. Studies have not been consistent, but one study found the risk of blood clotting events to be double that of traditional COCPs.

Many of the more minor problems of the patch have to do with problems with the adhesive. A small percentage of women will be sensitive to the adhesive and therefore may be unable to use this method. Some just complain that the patch looks like "a dirty band-aid" at the end of a week of use, but tolerate this appearance if they are not experiencing skin irritation. Some complain that the patch does not adhere well enough to give them confidence in its use. The protocol that follows addresses problems with the patch adhesive.

Despite these considerations, Ortho Evra remains a popular contraceptive choice. Many women find that the convenience of the patch outweighs the potential for risk. However, all patch users should be informed of the increased estrogen exposure and advised to "stay tuned" for updates on this issue.

Adhesive Issues With Ortho Evra

KEY QUESTIONS

ASSESSMENT	ACTION
1. Does the patch seem loose, lift off your skin, or fail to stick?	**YES** Go to Question 2.
	NO No further action.
2. Did this happen in the last 24 hours?	**YES** Go to Step A.
	NO Go to Question 3.
3. Did this happen longer than 24 hours ago, or are you uncertain when it happened?	**YES** Go to Question 4.
	NO No further action.
4. Did you have unprotected intercourse during this time?	**YES** Go to Step B.
	NO Go to Step C.

ACTIONS

STEP A: Less Than 24 Hours Since Patch Has Had Trouble Adhering

Try to reapply your patch or apply a new patch immediately.
You will not need a backup method or need to change your "patch change day."

STEP B: Unprotected Intercourse and More Than 24 Hours After or Uncertain When Patch Started to Have Trouble Adhering

Offer patient emergency contraception (refer to Emergency Contraception Overview and protocols for Management Options on page 227).
Continue to Step C for patients choosing to continue with Ortho Evra.

STEP C: More than 24 Hours After or Uncertain When Patch Started to Have Trouble Adhering

Start a new 4-week patch cycle immediately.
You will have a new Day 1 for your cycle and a new patch change day.
You will need to use a backup method of contraception for the next 7 days.

PATIENT EDUCATION

1. This is a good opportunity to determine how satisfied the patient is with the method and to review proper use.
2. If the patient thinks her skin is irritated by the patch, she should consider another method.
3. Under no circumstances should a patient use any other adhesive to try to get the patch to adhere to her skin.

Problems Unique to Progesterone-Only Oral Contraceptive Pills (POPs)

Progesterone-only OCPs, also known as POPs or mini-pills, are unlike COCPs because they only contain the hormone progesterone. They are an excellent form of birth control for women who cannot use estrogen. This includes nursing women as well as those who have medical indications that preclude the use of estrogen. Problems unique to this method center on the need to be very diligent in taking the POPs.

The demands of taking POPs make patients who take them more prone to spotting, particularly if the POP is not taken about the same time every day. Some women report bothersome spotting even when they take the pills regularly. The effectiveness of POPs may also be decreased if these pills are taken late. For example, being 3 hours late taking POPs is similar to missing an entire day of a COCP. Consequently, all patients using POPs need to be instructed in a backup method of contraception (such as condoms). Additionally, women who miss even one dose of their POPs should be aware of how to use and obtain emergency contraception.

POPs are designed to be taken continuously. Unlike the use of continuous COCPs, where one might advise a patient to briefly stop the method to have a withdrawal bleed, POPs *must* be taken continuously to remain effective. When taken properly, this can lead to amenorrhea, a desired state for some women. Certainly patients need to be aware that amenorrhea is a possibility when they take the product as directed.

Problems unique to this method can be summed up in this phrase: timing is everything!

Dosing Schedule and Progesterone-Only Contraceptives

KEY QUESTIONS

ASSESSMENT

1. Are you taking POPs (mini-pills)?

2. POPs are designed to be taken continuously at the same time each day. Is this how you are taking them?

ACTION

YES Go to Question 2.
NO No further action.

YES No further action.
NO Go to Step A.

ACTIONS

STEP A: Improper Dosing Schedule With POPs

As stated in the overview on POPs, timing of dosing is most important with this method. Patients need to be instructed that being 3 hours late is similar to missing a day of COCPs. Reviewing the protocol on Continuous Dose Systemic Hormonal Contraceptives on page 361 may be helpful. Remind patients that amenorrhea is an expected and often desired side effect of this method.

Quick Start Method and Systemic Hormonal Contraceptives

KEY QUESTIONS

ASSESSMENT	ACTION
1. Do you suspect you are pregnant?	**YES** Go to Step A.
	NO Go to Question 2.
2. Do you want to start your systemic hormonal contraceptive method as soon as possible?	**YES** Go to Step B.
	NO Go to Step C.

ACTIONS

STEP A: Suspected Pregnancy

If the patient suspects she may be pregnant, she should use a backup method until she gets her period or determines her pregnancy status. In this case a "Day 1 start" or "Sunday start" is a better choice.

STEP B: Starting Systemic Hormonal Contraception With the Quick Start Method

Advise the patient that she may start her systemic hormonal contraceptive any time in her cycle. She should use a backup method for 7 days. See Patient Education.

STEP C: Starting Systemic Hormonal Contraceptive Methods with the Day-1-Start or Sunday-Start Method

The Day-1-start regimen refers to beginning the systemic hormonal method on the first day of menstruation. In the case of combined systemic hormonal contraceptive pills or Ortho Evra, no backup method is necessary. If this method is used with NuvaRing, a backup method should be used for 7 days. It is recommended that the NuvaRing be started between days 1–5 of the menstrual cycle.

The Sunday-start regimen refers to beginning the systemic method chosen on the first Sunday after menstruation starts. Some women prefer a Sunday start because they usually will not menstruate on a weekend. This is not necessarily true with the new 24/4 regimens of oral contraceptives.

With all methods, it is recommended that a backup method be used for 7 days.

PATIENT EDUCATION

1. The Quick Start method has been used with all forms of systemic hormonal contraceptives. Studies have shown high patient acceptance and breakthrough bleeding rates similar to those of more conventional starting regimens.
2. Patient compliance may be enhanced because of the immediate start. It may be particularly helpful when device demonstration is part of the educational process, such as in NuvaRing insertion.
3. Let the patient know her menstrual period may be delayed until the method-free interval.

Weight Gain and Systemic Hormonal Contraceptives

KEY QUESTIONS

ASSESSMENT	ACTION
1. Did you recently (within the past 3 months) start a systemic hormonal contraception?	**YES** Go to Question 2.
	NO Go to Question 2.
2. Is this weight gain associated with foot, ankle, or leg swelling or shortness of breath?	**YES** Go to Step A.
	NO Go to Question 3.
3. Have you gained more than 5 pounds in the past 7–10 days?	**YES** Go to Step B.
	NO Go to Question 4.
4. Do you think you might be pregnant?	**YES** Go to Step C.
	NO Go to Question 5.
5. If pregnancy has been excluded, and your weight has increased slowly, has your activity level decreased or your nutritional habits changed significantly (Are you eating more processed/convenience foods? Do you have more life stressors, such as an altered living situation [divorcing, homeless]?)	**YES** Go to Step D.
	NO Go to Question 6.
6. Has your weight increased slowly during the past 3–6 months?	**YES** Go to Step E.
	NO No further action.

ACTIONS

STEP A: Foot, Ankle, or Leg Swelling or Shortness of Breath

This may be a significant adverse effect of hormonal contraception. This patient may have a thromboembolic disorder (DVT or pulmonary embolus) This patient needs to be evaluated by her provider within the next 2–4 hours. If she has shortness of breath, she needs to be seen immediately (may need to call 911).

STEP B: Rapid Weight Gain Not Accompanied by Other Symptoms

This may be an adverse hormonal effect and should be evaluated by the OB/GYN care provider or the primary care provider within the next 1 to 2 days.

If additional symptoms develop, the patient may need to be seen sooner.

STEP C: Potential Pregnancy

Pregnancy should always be considered in women of reproductive age. A pregnancy test is indicated.

Inquire as to whether the patient has other symptoms of pregnancy, such as breast tenderness, fatigue, or missed or abnormal menses.

STEP D: Changes in Diet or Activity

Decreases in activity or changes in nutritional intake may result in an increase in body weight. Advise the patient to monitor her activities and caloric intake. The patient may need to consult a dietitian or seek stress management counseling.

STEP E:

If the patient's activity levels and caloric intake are stable and she continues to gain weight, recommend she seek an evaluation by her primary care provider. This may be an early sign of an underactive thyroid.

PATIENT EDUCATION

Occasionally, women experience bloating for the first hormonal contraceptive cycles. After you have ruled out other causes for the weight gain, reassure the patient that the gain is normal and usually subsides with time. If the weight gain is a significant problem, suggest she talk with her provider and consider changing the type or route of hormonal contraception. The patient also may elect to discontinue hormonal contraception because of this side effect and select another method of contraception.

PART IV

OTHER WOMEN'S HEALTH PROTOCOLS

CHAPTER 23

Overview of Other Women's Health Issues

Many women see their OB/GYN health care provider as their *only* health care provider. It is true that some health insurance carriers may allow women to choose an OB/GYN as a primary care provider. However, most providers in women's health do not feel qualified to provide general health services, and many do not want to provide these services. In any case, it is important that those who work in women's health have a basic understanding of some of the problems that, in general, are major health issues for women.

The inclusion of all health issues is beyond the scope of this book. We have chosen those which we feel are common concerns women may express at the time of their annual well-woman exam or during the course of another related telephone call. They are:

• cholesterol Screening;
• depression;
• domestic Violence;
• hypertension;
• smoking Cessation.

Depression

ASSESSMENT

ACTION

1. Are you experiencing crying spells, insomnia, sadness, fatigue, anxiety, headache, poor concentration, or confusion?

   YES Go to Question 2.

   NO Go to Question 2.

2. Are you experiencing feelings that you want to harm yourself or someone else?

   YES Go to Step A.

   NO Go to Question 3.

3. Do you have a history of depression or any other factors that may make you prone to depression?

   YES Go to Step B.

   NO Review Steps A and B.

ACTIONS

STEP A: Refer to Mental Health Counselor

If the patient is experiencing uncontrolled mood swings, thoughts about harming herself or others, feeling out of control, or becoming withdrawn, do the following:

- Make a same-day appointment with a mental health care provider and ensure that the patient is accompanied to the appointment by a friend, family member, or social services personnel.
- Do not leave a high-risk patient alone.

STEP B: Treatment for Depression

Risk Factors for Depression

- History of depression or mental illness
- Physical or sexual abuse, including domestic violence
- Family history of mental illness
- Increased situational or life factors that are stressful
- Financial burdens
- Recent death or loss of a family member or close friend

Symptoms of Depression

- Depressed mood (as reported by the patient or observed by others)
- Decreased interest in all or most activities most of the time
- More than 5% weight loss or weight gain in the past month
- Difficulty sleeping or difficulty getting out of bed
- Fatigue or low energy or hyperenergia
- Recurrent thoughts of death or suicide
- Feelings of low self-worth or excessive guilt
- Difficulty thinking or concentrating

If the patient is not experiencing severe depression with thoughts of suicide or harming someone, do the following:

- Refer her for mental health counseling (either to a counselor she has seen before or to a new counselor).
- Have her discuss her feelings with her partner, friends, and family.
- Recommend she look to the community, friends, and family for support.
- Recommend she get out and do something for herself every day.
- Advise her to do some physical activity that she enjoys (walking, gardening, bicycling).
- Suggest she try to put some balance in her life with family, work, exercise, and rest.

PATIENT EDUCATION

Research indicates that approximately 20% of all women will experience depression at some point in their lives. Unfortunately, only about one-fourth of these women will receive adequate and appropriate therapy. This protocol is designed to identify severe depression in women, which requires immediate attention, and ensure that women are given the opportunity to receive much needed mental health care services.

Domestic Violence

ASSESSMENT	ACTION
1. Is anyone currently threatening to hurt you or has actually hurt you?	**YES** Go to Step A.
	NO Go to Question 2.
2. Has anyone ever physically harmed you or forced you to have sex?	**YES** Go to Step B.
	NO Go to Question 3.
3. Are you ever afraid of either your partner or anyone else?	**YES** Go to Step B.
	NO Go to Question 4.
4. Do you have a safety plan?	**YES** No further action.
	NO Go to Step C.

ACTIONS

STEP A: Immediate Concern for Harm

Approximately 5 million women will be victims of violence every year, with 1.7 million experiencing a severe injury. About 30% of all women who are murdered in the United States are murdered by an intimate partner. Domestic violence often escalates during pregnancy.

If there is an immediate concern for the patient, see if she can escape to a neighbor's home to avoid additional injury. If this is not possible, call 911 for immediate police or ambulance assistance. The safety of the patient and any children or adults in the area should be the paramount concern at this point.

Document, as carefully as possible, any statements made by the patient. These may become important evidence in any subsequent legal action.

STEP B: Abuse History

Validate the patient's concerns and acknowledge the abuse.

Make sure the patient has a safety plan (see Step C).

Refer the patient to local or national abuse support services (see Appendix A for resources).

Make sure that ongoing support is provided for the patient.

Be aware that violence can be cyclical in nature, with the abuser often being quite remorseful after the abuse, followed by a pattern of escalating violence.

Document all interactions.

STEP C: Safety Plan

Because domestic abuse tends to be recurrent in nature, it is important the patient and her abuser receive counseling. Unfortunately, for many reasons, not all women will be ready to leave an abusive relationship. For those women, it is important that a safety plan is in place. This makes it easier for the patient to leave in the event additional abuse occurs or seems likely.

Safety Plan

The patient should pack a safety bag in advance and leave it with a neighbor who she thinks she can trust.

In the bag the patient should have:

- extra clothes for the patient and her children and a few toys for the children;
- extra cash, checks, or credit cards;
- birth certificates for the patient and her children;
- Social Security cards for the patient and her children;
- driver's license or photo identification;
- medications used regularly and health insurance or Medicare/Medicaid cards;
- deed or lease to the house or apartment;
- pay stub(s); and
- any court orders or other legal papers.

The patient should hide a set of car and house keys outside the house in the event that she has to leave quickly.

Provide the patient with the name and telephone number of a local women's shelter in case she finds she has no safe place to go.

Hyperlipidemia (Elevated Cholesterol)

ASSESSMENT

ACTION

1. Do you have concerns and questions about cholesterol screening and cholesterol levels?

YES Go to Step A.

NO Go to Step A.

2. Do you have any risks for heart disease, such as smoking, hypertension, diabetes, older age ($\geq$ 55), low HDL (<40) and have a first-degree male relative with CHD (such as a heart attack) before age 55 years and first-degree female relatives with CHD before age 65 years?

YES Go to Step B.

NO Go to Step A.

ACTIONS

STEP A: Provide General Information about Appropriate Screening

Generally, screening for lipid disorders is initially performed on adults beginning at age 20 and then every 5 years. A fasting lipid profile or non-fasting total cholesterol and HDL cholesterol is obtained for males >age 35 and females >age 45. Screening may occur earlier if you have any of the significant risk factors for heart disease.

It is best to have a blood test called a "lipoprotein profile" to find out your cholesterol numbers. This blood test is done after a 9- to 12-hour fast and gives information about your:

- total cholesterol;
- lDL (bad) cholesterol—the main source of cholesterol buildup and blockage in the arteries;
- hDL (good) cholesterol—helps keep cholesterol from building up in the arteries;
- triglycerides—another form of fat in your blood.

Encourage the patient to consider the testing if the time interval is appropriate. Continue on the Question 2.

STEP B: Refer Patient to Source of Care for Evaluation

If the patient has risk factors, particularly if she does not have a source of regular preventative care, encourage her to have lipid testing.

Even if the lab work is performed in your OB/GYN office, abnormalities in lab values are best managed by the patient's primary care provider (PCP) as other referrals may be needed. She may need assistance in finding a PCP. Let her know you can forward the results to the appropriate person.

Practitioners may use a coronary heart disease risk assessment scale to determine specific goals for your cholesterol levels.

In general the goals for cholesterol levels are:

Total cholesterol (mg/dl)

<200 Desirable
200–239 Borderline high
≥240 High

LDL cholesterol (mg/dl)

<100 Optimal
100–129 Near or above optimal
130–159 Borderline high
160–189 High
≥190 Very high

HDL cholesterol (mg/dl)

<40 Low (undesirable)
≥60 High (desirable)

Triglycerides (mg/dl)

<150 Normal
150–199 Borderline high
200–499 High
≥500 Very high

PATIENT EDUCATION

1. According to the American Heart Association, cardiovascular disease is the leading cause of death among American women.
2. Cholesterol is a "fat" (lipid) like substance that has been found in cells and other parts of the body. Cholesterol has been further divided into the good (HDL) and bad (LDL) components.
3. While it is an essential component of the body, elevations in LDL cholesterol have been associated with coronary heart disease.
4. High levels of HDL actually can help prevent a person from developing heart disease.
5. It is important to stress to patients that lowering LDL cholesterol can significantly reduce their risk of heart disease.
6. Treatment for hyperlipidemia or elevated cholesterol includes lifestyle modification and medication. Patients can be advised to initiate elements of a healthy lifestyle such as weight loss, healthy diet, and regular aerobic physical activity.

Hypertension (Elevated Blood Pressure)

KEY QUESTIONS

ASSESSMENT

ACTION

1. What is your blood pressure?

Continue on to Question 2.

Systolic	Diastolic	ACTION
<120	<80	Go to Step A
120–139	80–89	Go to Step A
140–159	90–99	Go to Step B
≥160	≥100	Go to Step B
>180	>110	Go to Step C

2. Along with an elevated blood pressure, are you also experiencing symptoms such as, headache, blurred vision or visual changes, epistaxis, or severe anxiety?

YES Go to Step C.

NO Go to Step that Correlates with BP.

ACTIONS

STEP A: Provide Reassurance and Education

Reported blood pressure:

- <120–<80 (Normal): inform patient that this is normal and that they should have blood pressure rechecked within two years.
- 120–139/80–89 (Prehypertensive): inform patient to have their blood pressure rechecked within 1 year.

STEP B: Refer Patient to Source of Care for Follow-Up Evaluation

Reported blood pressure:

- 140–159/90–99 (Stage 1): inform patient to follow up for confirmation and evaluation by their primary care provider within 2 months.
- ≥160 or ≥100 (Stage 2): inform patient to follow up for care within 1 month.

STEP C: Refer for Immediate Evaluation and Treatment

If patient reports that blood pressure reading is >180/110, then they should be referred for immediate evaluation and treatment to their primary care provider or if necessary, the closest emergency department.

If patient is experiencing an elevated blood pressure with a headache, blurred vision, epistaxis or severe anxiety, they should be referred to the nearest emergency department or urgent care center for further evaluation.

PATIENT EDUCATION

1. According to the *Seventh Report of the Joint National Committee on Prevention, Detection, Evaluation, and Treatment of High Blood Pressure*, approximately 7.1 million deaths annually may be attributed to high blood pressure.
2. The incidence of hypertension increases more rapidly in women (aged 50 and older) than in men, with over 75% of women aged 75 or older diagnosed with hypertension.
3. It is important to stress to patients that small decreases in blood pressure can significantly reduce their risk of stroke, heart disease and risk of death.
4. Patients should also be instructed on the importance of accurate blood pressure monitoring. Blood pressure measurements need to be obtained by adequately trained personnel with the proper equipment.
5. Treatment for hypertension includes lifestyle modification and medication. Patients can be advised to initiate elements of a healthy lifestyle such as: weight loss, healthy diet, regular aerobic physical activity, limited intake of alcohol & sodium, and elimination of tobacco use.
6. Blood pressure standards may vary for patients with certain health conditions, such as diabetes.

Smoking Cessation

ASSESSMENT   **ACTION**

1. Have you ever considered trying a smoking
   cessation program?
                                                          YES Go to Step B.

                                                          NO Go to Step A.

ACTIONS

STEP A: General Education and Referral

Inform patient that there are many resources available for women who desire to stop
   smoking. Because smoking cessation involves both a psychological and physical
   component, many programs include both pharmacological and counseling/behav-
   ioral treatment options.

Pharmacotherapy:

The medical options include: medications that replace nicotine and medications that
   theoretically suppress the desire for nicotine.
Nicotine Replacement Therapies:

There are five types of nicotine replacement therapies that have been approved by the
   Food and Drug Agency. These are nicotine patches, nicotine gum, nicotine inhalers,
   nicotine nasal spray, and nicotine lozenges. These nicotine replacement therapies
   replace the nicotine that individuals receive when they smoke, therefore minimizing the physical withdrawal symptoms that could occur with sudden cessation of
   nicotine (such as, dizziness, depression, feelings of frustration, impatience and
   anger, anxiety, irritability, sleep disturbances, trouble concentrating, restlessness,
   and headaches).
Other Medications:

Bupropion (Zyban) and varenicline (Chantix) are two other medications that may be
   prescribed to aid individuals in a smoking cessation program. Zyban is a prescription antidepressant in an extended-release form that reduces symptoms of nicotine
   withdrawal. Chantix is a prescription medicine that has been found to decrease some
   individual's desire for tobacco by interfering with nicotine receptors in the brain.
Counseling/Behavioral Therapies:

Inform patient that many individuals who wish to stop smoking benefit from involve-
   ment in a smoking cessation program. According to the American Heart Association,

smoking cessation programs are designed to help smokers recognize and cope with problems that come up during quitting and to provide support and encouragement in long-term smoking cessation. Intense programs with either one-on-one or group counseling appear to be more effective at enabling individuals to successfully stop smoking.

Refer patients to their primary care providers for a more complete discussion and implementation of a treatment plan.

STEP B: Encouragement

Inform patient that there are resources available if they are ever interested in help with smoking cessation. You should know the sources in your area.

PATIENT EDUCATION

1. Smoking cessation has immediate and long-term health benefits for women. According to the American Cancer Society, quitting smoking decreases the risk of lung cancers, heart attack, stroke and chronic lung disease. Specifically, women who quit smoking prior to or early in their pregnancy can reduce the risk of low birth-weight babies. These benefits are significantly greater than any small increase in weight that may be associated with smoking cessation.

2. The American Cancer Society offers free smoking cessation literature and programs to aid individuals with tobacco cessation. In fact, this organization offers a program entitled Quitline® that links callers with trained counselors. Smokers can get help finding a Quitline® phone counseling program in their area by calling the American Cancer Society at 1-800-ACS-2345 (1-800-227-2345).

Selected Important Community Resources

Type of Resource	Information Resources	Address and/or Website	Telephone Number	Comment
Adolescent genecology	Association of Reproductive Health Professionals	www.arhp.org 2401 Pennsylvania Ave, NW Washington, DC 20037-1718	202-466-3825	Research, education and practice information on reproductive health issues.
	AWARE (Adolescent Wellness through Access to Resources to Education)	www.awarefoundation. org		Provides information to teens, parents and health care providers on adolescent wellness, sexuality and reproductive health.
	North American Society of Pediatric and Adolescent Gynecology	www.naspag.org 1209 Montgomery Hwy Birmingham, AL 35216	Phone: 205-978-5011 FAX: 205-978-5005	Conducts education programs in pediatric and adolescent gynecology. Contains clinical resources and educational materials.
	The Society for Adolescent Medicine	www.adolescenthealth. org 1916 Cooper Oaks Circle Blue Springs, MO 64015	816-224-8010	Multidisciplinary organization dedicated to improving health and well-being for all adolescents.

(continued)

Type of Resource	Information Resources	Address and/or Website	Telephone Number	Comment
Adoption Agencies	Adoption.com	www.adoption.com		Information on unplanned pregnancy, parent profiles, adoptive parents, research and reunion.
	Adopting.com	www.adopting.com		Contains an index of adoption resources, sites available on the Internet.
	Birthright International	www.birthright.org		Provides pregnancy and adoption services.
Bed rest/ preterm labor support	Sidelines	www.sidelines.org P.O. Box 1808 Laguna Beach, CA 92652	888-447-4754	Provides online resources, articles and scheduled chats for those on bed rest.
	Bed rest Book Buddies	health.groups.yahoo. com/ bedrestbookbuddies		Online community for women on bed rest.
Breast Cancer Support	American Cancer Society— Reach for recovery	www.cancer.org/ docroot/ESN/content/ ESN_3_1x_Reach_to_ Recovery_5.asp	1-800-ACS-2345	Face-to-face or telephone support for women and men with a personal concern about breast cancer.
	Y-ME National Breast Cancer Organization	www.y-me.org	1-800-0221-2141 (English) 1-800-986-9505 (Spanish)	Hotline with interpreters in 150 languages available. Contains message boards and telephone support for cancer patients and families.
Breast-feeding Support	La Leche	www.llli.org		Support services for breastfeeding women
	Lactation Education Resources	www.leron-line.org	1-703-691-2069	How to become a certified lactation consultant; lactation information.

(continued)

Type of Resource	Information Resources	Address and/or Website	Telephone Number	Comment
	Medela	medelabreastfeedingus.com		Breastfeeding information from breast pump company. Times and solutions for pumping.
Childbirth Education	ASPO/Lamaze International	www.lamaze.org	1-800-368-4404	Provides directory of Lamaze instructors, how to become certified as an instructor, and information on Lamaze. Includes Spanish language version of site.
	Bradley Method	www.Bradleybirth.com	1-800-4-A-BIRTH	Information on becoming an instructor, classes and the Bradley method.
	International Childbirth Education (ICEA)	www.icea.org	1-952-854-8660	Directory of instructors, how to become certified and philosophy of CEA.
Contraceptive information	U.S. National Library of Medicine— National Institute of Health	www.nlm.nih.gov/medlineplus/birthcontrol.html		Selected online resources and links to additional web sites.
	CDC	www.cdc.gov/reproductivehealth/unintendedpregnancy/contraception.html		Latest News, Research, Organizations, Journal Articles and Clinical Trials.
Domestic abuse resources	Safe Horizon Domestic Violence	safehorizon.org	1-800-621-HOPE (4673)	24-hour domestic violence hotline; Resources for creating a safety plan.
	US National Library of Medicine— National Institute of Health	www.nlm.nih.gov/medlineplus/medlineplus/birthcontrol.html		Free computer-based literature searches.

(continued)

Type of Resource	Information Resources	Address and/or Website	Telephone Number	Comment
Emergency Contraception	Office of Population Research, Princeton University	ec.princeton.edu not-2-late.com		Explains emergency contraception, options, EC providers.
	The National Women's Health Information Center—U.S. Department of Health & Human Services	http://www.4woman. gov/FAQ/econtracep. htm		Provides valuable information on contraception.
Grief Support	Compassionate Friends	www.compassionate friends.org P.O. Box 3696 Oak Brook, IL 60522	1-877-969-0010	Grief Support after death of a child or loss of a pregnancy.
Infertility Information	Shady Grove Fertility Center	www.shadygrove fertility.com	1-888-IVF-0500	Explains common infertility workup, treatments, options.
Natural family planning resources	Billings Ovulation Method	www.billings-centre. ab.ca		Information in 22 languages on the Billings Method of Natural Family Planning.
	Couple to Couple League International/ USA	ccli.org PO Box 111194 Cincinnati, OH 45211	513-471-2000	Contains information on a variety of natural family options.
	Georgetown University— Institute for Reproductive Health	www.irh.org/nfp.htm		Good source for safety of medications in pregnancy.
Pregnancy/ Information Termination	Planned Parenthood of America	www.planned parenthood.org	800-230-PLAN	Information on local centers, reproduction information.
	Pregnancy Termination clinics online	www.clinicasdeaborto. com		Listing of Pregnancy Termination clinics by state, nation and category. Spanish language version available.

(continued)

APPENDIX A *(continued)*

Type of Resource	Information Resources	Address and/or Website	Telephone Number	Comment
Preterm labor	March of Dimes	www.marchofdimes.com/prematurity 1275 Mamaroneck Avenue White Plains, NY 10605	888-MODIMES	Website in both English and Spanish contain information on preterm labor
Rape crisis/ SANE	Rape, Abuse & Incest National Network	www.rainn.org		Info on rape, incest, and being a sexual assault nurse examiner.
	Sexual Assault Nurse Examiner Programs	www.sane-sart.com		Programs, conferences, data and links.
	US Department of Justice— Office of Justice Programs— Office for Victims of Crimes	www.ojp.usdoj.gov/ovc/publications/bulletins/sane_4_2001/welcome.html		Department of Justice bulletin on SANE programs.

Index

Note: Page numbers followed by *f* indicate figures; those followed by *t* indicate tables; and those followed by *b* indicate boxed material.

Dramamine, 167*t*
Dull headaches
  first trimester, 77
  second trimester, 104
  third trimester, 140
Dyspareunia, 294

E
Ectopic pregnancy, 70
Elevated blood pressure. *See*
  Hypertension
EMB. *See* Endometrial biopsy
Embryonic stem cells, 43
Emergency contraception. *See*
  Contraception, emergency
Emergency contraception in-
  formation resources, 407
Emetrol, 168*t*
Emotional patient, 21
Endometrial ablation,
  321–322
Endometrial biopsy (EMB), 324
Enpresse, 229*t*
Entex PSE (guaifenesin/
  pseudoephedrine), 168*t*
Epithelial cell abnormalities,
  304
Erythromycin, 168*t*
Estrogen tablet(s), missed, 295
Excess hair, hormone therapy,
  286
Exercise after birth, 177
Exposure to, 38*t*–40*t*
Eye and visual changes,
  hormone therapy
  eye pain, 282
  gradual change in vision,
    282
  red eye, 283
  severe symptoms, 282
Eye and visual changes,
  systemic hormonal
  contraception
  eye pain, 365
  eye redness, 366
  gradual change of vision, 366
  sudden loss of vision, 365
Eye changes, gradual
  hormone therapy, 282
  second trimester, 121
  systemic hormonal
    contraception, 366
  third trimester, 165

Eye pain
  hormone therapy, 282
  second trimester, 120–121
  systemic hormonal
    contraception, 365
  third trimester, 164
Eye redness, 283, 366

F
Facial and upper extremity
  swelling, 113, 157
Facial or body hair, change
  in, 346
Facial redness, 271
Fainting. *See* Dizziness/
  fainting
Fatigue, 75, 101–102
Fearful patient, 26
Feeding, bottle. *See* Bottle-
  feeding, neonatal
Feeding, breast. *See*
  Breastfeeding, neonatal
Fetal movement, decreased,
  99–100, 137–138
Fever
  cryosurgery, 319
  first trimester, 79
  headache, 372
  hormone therapy, 268–269
  laparoscopy, 326
  neonatal, 191, 193
  systemic hormonal contra-
    ception, 343–344
Fibroadenoma, 217*t*
Fifth disease (parvovirus
  B19), 38*t*
First menses, 199
First trimester, patient
  education
  abdominal pain, 66
  ambivalence/depression, 68
  bleeding, 70
  constipation, 72
  depression, 68
  dizziness/fainting, 74
  nausea/vomiting, 79
  vaginal discharge, 84
First trimester of pregnancy
  abdominal pain, 65–66
  ambivalence, 67–68
  bleeding, 69–70
  constipation, 71
  depression, 67–68

dizziness/fainting, 73–74
  fatigue, 75
  headache, 76–77
  nausea, 78–79
  urinary complaints, 80–81
  vaginal discharge, 82–84
  vomiting, 78–79
Fish, food safety and, 44–45
Flagyl (Metronidazole), 170*t*
Flu, 109, 146
Follicle stimulating hormone,
  recombinant (Follistim,
  Gonal-F), 54*t*
Follistim (follicle stimulating
  hormone [recombinant]),
  54*t*
Food intolerance, first
  trimester, 79
Food safety (in pregnancy),
  44–46
Food/fluid difficulties, first
  trimester, 78
Foot swelling, 297, 391
Forms, sample
  abnormal bleeding, 197
  amenorrhea, 209
  barrier contraceptives, 212
  bleeding, abnormal, 197
  breast complaints, 217
  communicable diseases,
    exposure to, 37
  contraception, emergency,
    226
  contraceptives, Implanon
    implantable, 234
  contraceptives, injectable,
    240
  contraceptives, intrauterine,
    254
  environmental and
    household chemicals,
    exposure to, 37
  hormone therapy, 266–267
  infertility, 37
  postpartum period, 175
  pregnancy assessment, 53
  systemic hormonal contra-
    ception, 342
  telephone triage, 2*f*
Frequent urination
  first trimester, 80
  second trimester, 115
  third trimester, 159–160
Fussy baby/colic, 194–195

breast pain, 221
perimenopausal patient not using hormonal contraception, 211
Hot flashes/sweats, 289–290
HPV. *See* Human Papilloma Virus
Human chorionic gonadotropin (Ovidrel, Pregnyl, Profasi, Novarel), 56*t*, 60
Human menopausal gonadotropin (Pergonal, Repronex, Humegon Menopur), 56*t*
Human Papilloma Virus (HPV), 316*t*
Humegon Menopur (human menopausal gonadotropins, purified urinary gonadotropins), 56*t*
Hyperlinks, 29
Hyperlipidemia
appropriate screening for, 398
HDL cholesterol, 399
LDL cholesterol, 399
lipid testing, 398
patient education, 399
risk factors, 398
total cholesterol, 399
triglycerides, 399
Hypertension (elevated blood pressure), 139, 400–401
Hysterectomy
abnormal bleeding/spotting, 207, 272, 274
hot flashes/sweats, 289
missed or late pills or patch, hormone therapy, 295

I

Implanon, 210, 233–234
In term delivery, 154
Inability to formulate a plan, 24
Incision, laparoscopy, 325–326
Incision care, postpartum, 186
incision draining blood, 187
incision increasing redness, 187
incision increasing tenderness, 187

incision looks dirty to patient, 187
incision separated, 187
incision warm to touch, 187
infection, care of, 186
Indigestion, second trimester. *See also* Nausea/vomiting
with additional symptoms, 105
history of, 106
onset pregnancy related, 105
patient education, 106
Indigestion, third trimester. *See also* Nausea/vomiting
with additional symptoms, 141
history of, 142
onset pregnancy related, 141
patient education, 142
Indigestion or burning after meals, 359
Infertility
chicken pox, 38*t*
cleaning agents, 41
communicable diseases, exposure to, 38*t*–40*t*
cord blood banking, 42–43
embryonic stem cells, 43
fifth disease, 38*t*
German measles, 39*t*
measles, 39*t*
parvovirus B19, 38*t*
rubella, 39*t*
rubeola, 39*t*
toxoplasma gondii, 40*t*
toxoplasmosis, 40*t*
triage assessment forms, 37
Varicella, 38*t*
work-up for women with 28-to-30-day cycles, 51–53
Infertility, medications
clomiphene citrate, 54*t*
follicle stimulating hormone, recombinant, 54*t*
gonadotropin releasing hormone analogs, 55*t*
gonadotropin releasing hormone antagonist, 55*t*
human chorionic gonadotropin, 56*t*, 60

human menopausal gonadotropin, 56*t*
purified urinary gonadotropins, 56*t*
steroids, 57*t*
Infertility, sample assessment forms
communicable diseases, 37
environmental and household chemicals, 37
pregnancy, 53
Information resources
adoption, 405
breast feeding, 405
childbirth education, 406
contraceptive, 406
domestic abuse, 406
grief support, 406
natural family planning, 406–407
preterm labor, 407
rape crisis/SANE, 408
Intense pressure, 151
Intercourse. *See* Sexual intercourse
International Childbirth Education Association (CEA), 406
Internet. *See* Online information retrieval
Intrauterine contraceptives, patient education
abdominal pain, 256
amenorrhea, 258
bleeding irregularities, 261
lost string, 264
Inverted nipples, 143, 180–181
IUD. *See* Contraceptives, intrauterine

J

Jaundiced skin, neonatal, 191, 193
JCAHO. *See* Joint Commission on Accreditation of Health Care Organizations
Joint Commission on Accreditation of Health Care Organizations (JCAHO), 4
Jolessa, 229*t*